Injury & Trauma Sourcebook

Learning Disabilities Sourcebook, 2nd Edition

Leukemia Sourcebook

Liver Disorders Sourcebook

Lung Disorders Sourcebook

Medical Tests Sourcebook, 2nd Edition

Men's Health Concerns Sourcebook, 2nd Edition

Mental Health Disorders Sourcebook, 3rd Edition

Mental Retardation Sourcebook

Movement Disorders Sourcebook

Muscular Dystrophy Sourcebook

Obesity Sourcebook

Osteoporosis Sourcebook

Pain Sourcebook, 2nd Edition

Pediatric Cancer Sourcebook

Physical & Mental Issues in Aging Sourcebook

Podiatry Sourcebook, 2nd Edition

Pregnancy & Birth Sourcebook, 2nd Edition

Prostate Cancer Sourcebook

Prostate & Urological Disorders Sourcebook

Rehabilitation Sourcebook

Respiratory Diseases & Disorders Sourcebook

Sexually Transmitted Diseases Sourcebook, 3rd Edition

Sleep Disorders Sourcebook, 2nd Edition

Smoking Concerns Sourcebook

Sports Injuries Sourcebook, 3rd Edition

Stress-Related Disorders Sourcebook

Stroke Sourcebook

Substance Abuse Sourcebook

Surgery Sourcebook

Thyroid Disorders Sourcebook

Transplantation Sourcebook

Traveler's Health Sourcebook

Urinary Tract & Kidney Diseases & Disorders Sourcebook, 2nd Edition

Vegetarian Sou[...]

Women's Heal[...]
2nd Edition

Workplace Health & Safety Sourcebook

Worldwide Health Sourcebook

Teen Health Series

Abuse & Violence Information for Teens

Alcohol Information for Teens

Allergy Information for Teens

Asthma Information for Teens

Body Information for Teens

Cancer Information for Teens

Complementary & Alternative Medicine Information for Teens

Diabetes Information for Teens

Diet Information for Teens, 2nd Edition

Drug Information for Teens, 2nd Edition

Eating Disorders Information for Teens

Fitness Information for Teens

Learning Disabilities Information for Teens

Mental Health Information for Teens, 2nd Edition

Pegnancy Information for Teens

Sexual Health Information for Teens

Skin Health Information for Teens

Sports Injuries Information for Teens

Suicide Information for Teens

Tobacco Information for Teens

Adult Health
Concerns
SOURCEBOOK

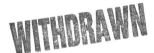

Health Reference Series

First Edition

Adult Health Concerns
SOURCEBOOK

Basic Consumer Health Information about Medical and Mental Concerns of Adults, Including Facts about Choosing Healthcare Providers, Navigating Insurance Options, Maintaining Wellness, Preventing Cancer, Heart Disease, Stroke, Diabetes, and Osteoporosis, and Understanding Aging-Related Health Concerns, Including Menopause, Cognitive Changes, and Changes in the Coronary and Vascular Systems

Along with Tips on Caring for Aging Parents and Dealing with Health-Related Work and Travel Issues, a Glossary, and a Directory of Resources for Additional Help and Information

Edited by
Sandra J. Judd

Omnigraphics WITHDRAWN

P.O. Box 31-1640, Detroit, MI 48231-1640

Bibliographic Note

Because this page cannot legibly accommodate all the copyright notices, the Bibliographic Note portion of the Preface constitutes an extension of the copyright notice.

Edited by Sandra J. Judd

Health Reference Series

Karen Bellenir, *Managing Editor*
David A. Cooke, M.D., *Medical Consultant*
Elizabeth Collins, *Research and Permissions Coordinator*
Cherry Stockdale, *Permissions Assistant*
EdIndex, Services for Publishers, *Indexers*

* * *

Omnigraphics, Inc.

Matthew P. Barbour, *Senior Vice President*
Kay Gill, *Vice President—Directories*
Kevin M. Hayes, *Operations Manager*

* * *

Peter E. Ruffner, *Publisher*

Copyright © 2008 Omnigraphics, Inc.

ISBN 978-0-7808-0999-4

Library of Congress Cataloging-in-Publication Data

Adult health concerns sourcebook / edited by Sandra J. Judd. -- 1st ed.
   p. cm. -- (Health reference series)
   "Basic consumer health information about medical and mental concerns of adults, including facts about choosing healthcare providers, navigating insurance options, maintaining wellness, preventing cancer, heart disease, stroke, diabetes, and osteoporosis, and understanding aging-related health concerns, including menopause, cognitive changes, and changes in the coronary and vascular systems; along with tips on caring for aging parents and dealing with health-related work and travel issues, a glossary, and a directory of resources for additional help and information."
   Includes bibliographical references and index.
   ISBN 978-0-7808-0999-4 (hardcover : alk. paper) 1. Medicine, Popular--Handbooks, manuals, etc. 2. Self-care, Health--Handbooks, manuals, etc. 3. Health--Handbooks, manuals, etc. I. Judd, Sandra J.
   RC82.A38 2008
   616--dc22

                                                        2007043690

Table of Contents

Visit www.healthreferenceseries.com to view *A Contents Guide to the Health Reference Series*, a listing of more than 13,000 topics and the volumes in which they are covered.

Part II: Maintaining Your Health

Part III: Disease Prevention: What Adults Should Know

Part VII: Other Concerns That Impact Adult Health

Part VIII: Additional Help and Information

Preface

About This Book

Adults make decisions every day about what to eat, whether to exercise, whether to drink or smoke, or whether to see a doctor or have a screening test. These types of decisions all play an important role in overall health. According to the Centers for Disease Control and Prevention, 12 percent of all adults report a limitation in normal activities due to chronic health conditions. Statistics also reveal that 66 percent of adults twenty years of age and older are overweight, only 30 percent engage in regular exercise, and 21 percent currently smoke.

Adult Health Concerns Sourcebook provides information for adults who need to make health-related choices. It discusses how to choose healthcare providers and understand insurance options. It talks about the importance of maintaining a healthy weight, breaking free of such risky behaviors as smoking and drug use, and preventing cancer, heart disease, diabetes, kidney and liver disease, and osteoporosis. It describes recommended screening tests and self-examinations, adult vaccinations, and other aging-related health concerns, including menopause, prostate problems, cognitive changes, and changes in the bones and joints, coronary and vascular systems, and hair and skin. Tips on caring for aging parents are also included, along with information on work- and travel-related health concerns. A glossary of related terms and a directory of additional resources provide additional help and information.

How to Use This Book

This book is divided into parts and chapters. Parts focus on broad areas of interest. Chapters are devoted to single topics within a part.

Part I: Making Routine and Emergency Decisions about Health Care provides information about choosing a doctor or hospital, getting a second opinion, and recognizing a medical emergency. It offers tips to guide readers through the often-confusing process of choosing health insurance and making a health insurance claim or disputing a denial. It also discusses patients' health privacy rights and describes the most commonly used medications.

Part II: Maintaining Your Health describes recommended preventative healthcare measures and adult vaccinations. It offers suggestions for following a healthy diet, keeping physically active, maintaining a healthy weight, and managing stress. It provides information about how to reduce behaviors that can put health at risk, including smoking, using alcohol or drugs, indoor tanning, and aggressive driving.

Part III: Disease Prevention: What Adults Should Know offers suggestions for preventing the most common diseases and disorders affecting adults as they age. These include high blood pressure, coronary heart disease, high cholesterol, diabetes, cancer, stroke, and osteoporosis. Suggestions for preventing liver disease and hepatitis and preserving oral health are also included.

Part IV: Screening for Common Diseases and Disorders describes the screening tests and self-examinations most commonly recommended for adults. It details each testing procedure and explains when and how often the tests should be performed. It provides step-by-step procedures for the most common self-examination practices, explains what to look for, and offers suggestions for what to do if something unusual is found.

Part V: Understanding How the Aging Process Affects Wellness discusses how the aging process affects the body and offers tips on how to manage the most common age-related physical and mental challenges. Cognitive and mental health issues related to aging are described, as well as changes likely to affect the senses, coronary and vascular systems, bones and joints, and prostate. Age-related changes in sleep patterns and sexuality are also described.

Part VI: Menopause describes the changes that occur with menopause and offers tips for managing the more bothersome symptoms. It discusses the pros and cons of hormone therapy and other symptom management techniques, including complementary and alternative therapies. It also describes medical problems that often accompany menopause, including depression and insomnia. In addition, a section on male menopause is included.

Part VII: Other Concerns That Impact Adult Health provides insight into the life experiences that often impact adult health. It discusses common work-related concerns, including ergonomics, carpal tunnel syndrome, noise-induced hearing loss, and job stress, and it offers suggestions for minimizing these issues. It also offers tips for managing health concerns related to travel, including vaccination requirements, cruise safety, jet lag, and traveler's diarrhea. The part concludes with a discussion of common concerns related to caring for aging parents, including managing caregiver stress and making choices about housing options for elders.

Part VIII: Additional Resources for Help and Information provides a glossary of terms related to adult health concerns and a directory of organizations able to provide additional help and support.

Bibliographic Note

This volume contains documents and excerpts from publications issued by the following U.S. government agencies: Administration on Aging; Agency for Healthcare Research and Quality (AHRQ); Centers for Disease Control and Prevention (CDC); Department of Health and Human Safety (HHS); National Cancer Institute (NCI); National Center for Complementary and Alternative Medicine (NCCAM); National Heart, Lung, and Blood Institute (NHLBI); National Institute of Allergy and Infectious Diseases (NIAID); National Institute of Arthritis and Musculoskeletal and Skin Diseases (NIAMS); National Institute of Diabetes and Digestive and Kidney Diseases (NIDDK); National Institute of Neurological Disorders and Stroke (NINDS); National Institute on Aging (NIA); National Institute on Alcohol Abuse and Alcoholism (NIAAA); National Institute on Deafness and Other Communication Disorders (NIDCD); National Institutes of Health (NIH); National Kidney Disease Education Program (NKDEP); National Women's Health Information Center (NWHIC); NIH Senior Health; President's Council on Physical Fitness and Sports; U.S. Department of Agriculture; and the U.S. Food and Drug Administration (FDA).

In addition, this volume contains copyrighted documents from the following organizations and individuals: A.D.A.M., Inc.; American Academy of Family Physicians; American College of Emergency Physicians; American Council on Exercise; American Federation for Aging Research; American Geriatrics Society Foundation for Health in Aging; American Heart Association; American Institute for Cancer Research; American Lung Association; American Osteopathic Association; American Society for Dermatologic Surgery; American Urological Association; Bereaved Families of Ontario - York Region; Better Health Channel, Victoria, Australia; Cleveland Clinic; College of American Pathologists; Family Caregiver Alliance; Geriatric Mental Health Foundation; Hepatitis Foundation International; Hormone Foundation; Immunization Action Coalition; International Society of Hair Restoration Surgery; Iowa State University Extension Service; Michigan Office of Financial and Insurance Services; National Jewish Medical and Research Center; National Osteoporosis Foundation; National Sleep Foundation; Nemours Foundation; Norman Endocrine Surgery Clinic; North Dakota Insurance Department; Portland Community College - Office for Students with Disabilities; Public Health - Seattle and King County; Skin Cancer Foundation; University of Connecticut Health Center - Pat and Jim Calhoun Cardiology Center; University of Florida Cooperative Extension - Institute of Food and Agriculture Sciences; University of Michigan Depression Center; and the University of Rochester/Strong Health.

Full citation information is provided on the first page of each chapter. Every effort has been made to secure all necessary rights to reprint the copyrighted material. If any omissions have been made, please contact Omnigraphics to make corrections for future editions.

Acknowledgements

Thanks go to the many organizations, agencies, and individuals who have contributed materials for this *Sourcebook* and to medical consultant Dr. David Cooke and document engineer Bruce Bellenir. Special thanks go to managing editor Karen Bellenir and permissions coordinator Liz Collins for their help and support.

About the Health Reference Series

The *Health Reference Series* is designed to provide basic medical information for patients, families, caregivers, and the general public. Each volume takes a particular topic and provides comprehensive coverage. This is especially important for people who may be dealing with a newly diagnosed disease or a chronic disorder in themselves or in a family member. People looking for preventive guidance, information about disease warning signs, medical statistics, and risk factors for health problems will also find answers to their questions in the *Health Reference Series*. The *Series*, however, is not intended to serve as a tool for diagnosing illness, in prescribing treatments, or as a substitute for the physician/patient relationship. All people concerned about medical symptoms or the possibility of disease are encouraged to seek professional care from an appropriate healthcare provider.

A Note about Spelling and Style

Health Reference Series editors use *Stedman's Medical Dictionary* as an authority for questions related to the spelling of medical terms and the *Chicago Manual of Style* for questions related to grammatical structures, punctuation, and other editorial concerns. Consistent adherence is not always possible, however, because the individual volumes within the *Series* include many documents from a wide variety of different producers and copyright holders, and the editor's primary goal is to present material from each source as accurately as is possible following the terms specified by each document's producer. This sometimes means that information in different chapters or sections may follow other guidelines and alternate spelling authorities. For example, occasionally a copyright holder may require that eponymous terms be shown in possessive forms (Crohn's disease *vs.* Crohn disease) or that British spelling norms be retained (leukaemia *vs.* leukemia).

Locating Information within the Health Reference Series

The *Health Reference Series* contains a wealth of information about a wide variety of medical topics. Ensuring easy access to all the fact sheets, research reports, in-depth discussions, and other material contained within the individual books of the series remains one of our highest priorities. As the *Series* continues to grow in size and scope, however, locating the precise information needed by a reader may become more challenging.

A Contents Guide to the Health Reference Series was developed to direct readers to the specific volumes that address their concerns. It presents an extensive list of diseases, treatments, and other topics of general interest compiled from the Tables of Contents and major index headings. To access *A Contents Guide to the Health Reference Series*, visit www.healthreferenceseries.com.

Medical Consultant

Medical consultation services are provided to the *Health Reference Series* editors by David A. Cooke, M.D. Dr. Cooke is a graduate of Brandeis University, and he received his M.D. degree from the University of Michigan. He completed residency training at the University of Wisconsin Hospital and Clinics. He is board-certified in Internal Medicine. Dr. Cooke currently works as part of the University of Michigan Health System and practices in Ann Arbor, MI. In his free time, he enjoys writing, science fiction, and spending time with his family.

Our Advisory Board

We would like to thank the following board members for providing guidance to the development of this series:

Dr. Lynda Baker, Associate Professor of Library and Information Science, Wayne State University, Detroit, MI

Nancy Bulgarelli, William Beaumont Hospital Library, Royal Oak, MI

Karen Imarisio, Bloomfield Township Public Library, Bloomfield Township, MI

Karen Morgan, Mardigian Library, University of Michigan-Dearborn, Dearborn, MI

Rosemary Orlando, St. Clair Shores Public Library, St. Clair Shores, MI

Health Reference Series *Update Policy*

The inaugural book in the *Health Reference Series* was the first edition of *Cancer Sourcebook* published in 1989. Since then, the *Series* has been enthusiastically received by librarians and in the medical community. In order to maintain the standard of providing high-quality health information for the layperson the editorial staff at Omnigraphics felt it was necessary to implement a policy of updating volumes when warranted.

Medical researchers have been making tremendous strides, and it is the purpose of the *Health Reference Series* to stay current with the most recent advances. Each decision to update a volume is made on an individual basis. Some of the considerations include how much new information is available and the feedback we receive from people who use the books. If there is a topic you would like to see added to the update list, or an area of medical concern you feel has not been adequately addressed, please write to:

Editor
Health Reference Series
Omnigraphics, Inc.
P.O. Box 31-1640
Detroit, MI 48231
E-mail: editorial@omnigraphics.com

Part One

Making Routine
and Emergency Decisions
about Health Care

Chapter 1

Finding Quality Health Care

Chapter Contents

Section 1.1

Choosing a Doctor

Reprinted from "Choosing a Doctor," National Institute on Aging, November 2006.

Mrs. Wiley had a big surprise the other day when she called her doctor's office to make an appointment. The receptionist told her that Dr. Horowitz was retiring at the end of the year. After all this time—after the doctor had treated her for strep throat, bladder infections, and that nasty broken wrist; after he had helped her through menopause—she felt like she was losing a trusted friend. Mrs. Wiley worried that she wouldn't be able to find a new doctor she would like.

There are many reasons why you might be looking for a new doctor. You may have moved to another city, or your doctor could be retiring. Whatever the reason, the following ideas can help you find a doctor who is right for you.

What Type of Doctor?

For your primary care doctor, you might want a general or family practitioner, an internist, or a geriatrician.

General practitioners provide health care for a wide range of medical problems. They do not focus on any one area of medicine.

Family practitioners are similar to general practitioners, with extra training on health care for all family members, regardless of age.

Internists are doctors for adults. Some internists take additional training to become specialists. For example, cardiologists are internists who specialize in diseases of the heart.

Geriatricians specialize in the care of older adults. A geriatrician is trained in family practice or internal medicine, but has additional training in caring for older people.

Finding a New Doctor

Once you have a sense of what kind of doctor you need, ask people you know about doctors they use and like. Friends, coworkers, and other health professionals may be helpful. You can make it easier for them to tell you about the doctors they like by asking questions such as, "What do you like about your doctor?"

A doctor whose name comes up often might be a good one to try. It may help to have several names to choose from in case the doctor you select is not taking new patients or does not take part in your health insurance plan. If you need more help finding names of doctors, contact a local hospital or medical center, medical society, physician referral service, or nearby medical schools.

If you belong to a managed care plan, you can get a list of doctors from the plan's membership services office. Your choices will be limited to the doctors who are part of the plan.

What Does Medicare Cover?

Most people age sixty-five and older are eligible for Medicare hospital insurance (Part A). They also can enroll in Medicare medical insurance (Part B) for a monthly fee. Medicare medical insurance helps pay for visits to the doctor. It also covers many other medical services and supplies not covered by Medicare's Part A.

Medicare prescription drug coverage (Part D) is a voluntary Medicare program that helps pay for both brand name and generic prescription drugs at participating area pharmacies. Everyone with Medicare can get this coverage. There is a monthly fee and a deductible cost. Patients must select among the drug plans available in their area.

There are many different Medicare plans. Their benefits, costs, and rules vary. Be sure to compare each plan and consider the type of insurance that is best for you. For information about Medicare benefits, call the Social Security Administration office listed in your phone book.

When Your Doctor Stops Seeing Patients

Often when a doctor leaves a medical practice, he or she can arrange for you to see another doctor who will have access to all your medical records. You should go for an office visit with the new doctor before deciding if you want him or her to be your physician.

What Should You Look for in a Doctor?

Of course you want a doctor who is well trained and capable. But, in addition, a doctor who takes the time to know you well may be able to help you prevent some health problems and manage problems that do come up. Once you have chosen two or three doctors, call their offices. The office staff can give you information about the doctor's education and training. You can say, "Before I make an appointment, I have some questions about the office and the practice. Can I speak to an office manager or a nurse?" This person can tell you about office policies, standard insurance the office takes, whether or not they file the insurance claims for you, payment methods, and the hospitals where the doctor sends patients. When choosing a new doctor you may want to know about all of the following:

- **Board certification:** Board-certified doctors have extra training after medical school to become specialists in a field of medicine such as family practice, internal medicine, or geriatrics.

- **Communication:** Because communication is important to good health care, you want a doctor who will listen carefully to your concerns, answer your questions, and explain things clearly and fully.

- **Type of health insurance:** Does the doctor accept your health insurance? What about Medicare?

- **Location of the doctor's office:** Will it be easy for you to get there? Is there parking?

- **Lab work:** Will I need to go to another location for blood tests or are lab tests done in the doctor's office?

- **Group practice:** If this is a group practice, who are the other doctors and what are their specialties?

- **Coverage:** Who sees patients for the doctor if he or she is out of town or not available?

How Do You Make a Good Choice?

Find out as much as you can about the doctor and the practice. Here are more questions you may want to ask the office staff:

- Does the doctor see many older patients?

- Does the doctor see patients who have many health problems?

- Does the doctor refer patients to other doctors for special problems?

- Does the doctor treat many patients with the same chronic health problem that I have (for example, diabetes)?

6

The First Appointment

After choosing a doctor, make your first medical appointment. Before going to the doctor's office, write down any questions you may have. It's a good idea to bring a list of your medicines. Include both prescription and over-the-counter drugs, even vitamins, supplements, and eye drops. The nurse is often the first person you'll talk to in the office. The nurse usually takes your blood pressure and asks about your medications. If you're having a problem with a medicine, the nurse will explain how to take it.

During your first visit, the doctor will probably take a medical history and ask questions about your health and the medical history of people in your family. The doctor will examine you. If you go to a new doctor, be sure to bring your past medical records or have them sent. Your former doctor may charge you for this service. Make a list of any drug allergies or serious drug reactions you've had. During this visit, take time to ask any questions you may still have about the doctor and the practice.

For instance, you may want to ask the doctor the following questions:

- Will you give me written instructions about my care?

- May I bring a family member (spouse, daughter, or son) to my office visits?

- Are you willing to talk with my family about my condition?

- Will you maintain my privacy if I ask you not to discuss my condition with anyone else?

After the meeting, ask yourself if you felt comfortable and confident with this doctor. Were you at ease asking questions? Did the doctor clearly answer your questions? If you are not sure, schedule a visit with one of the other doctors on your list.

Once you have found a doctor you like, your job is not finished. A good doctor-patient relationship is a partnership. Both you and your doctor need to work together to solve your medical problems and maintain your good health. Finding a doctor that suits your needs is an important first step. Good communication with the doctor and the office staff is key.

Section 1.2

How to Talk with Your Doctor

Reprinted from "Next Steps After Your Diagnosis: Finding Information and Support," Agency for Healthcare Research and Quality, Publication No. 05-0049, July 2005. http://www.ahrq.gov/consumer/diaginfo.htm

Your Doctor Is Your Partner in Health Care

You probably have many questions about your disease or condition. The first person to ask is your doctor.

It is fine to seek more information from other sources; in fact, it is important to do so. But consider your doctor your partner in health care—someone who can discuss your situation with you, explain your options, and help you make decisions that are right for you.

It is not always easy to feel comfortable around doctors but research has shown that good communication with your doctor can actually be good for your health. It can help you to feel more satisfied with the care you receive and have better outcomes (end results), such as reduced pain and better recovery from symptoms.

Being an active member of your health care team also helps to reduce your chances of medical mistakes, and it helps you get high-quality care.

Of course, good communication is a two-way street. Following are some ways to help make the most of the time you spend with your doctor.

Prepare for Your Visit

- Think about what you want to get out of your appointment. Write down all your questions and concerns.

- Prepare and bring to your doctor visit a list of all the medicines you take.

- Consider bringing along a trusted relative or friend. This person can help ask questions, take notes, and help you remember and understand everything once you leave the doctor's office.

Give Information to Your Doctor

- Do not wait to be asked.

- Tell your doctor everything he or she needs to know about your health—even the things that might make you feel embarrassed or uncomfortable.

- Tell your doctor how you are feeling—both physically and emotionally.

- Tell your doctor if you are feeling depressed or overwhelmed.

Get Information from Your Doctor

- Ask questions about anything that concerns you. Keep asking until you understand the answers. If you do not, your doctor may think you understand everything that is said.

- Ask your doctor to draw pictures if that will help you understand something.

- Take notes.

- Tape record your doctor visit, if that will be helpful to you. But first ask your doctor if this is okay.

- Ask your doctor to recommend resources such as websites, booklets, or tapes with more information about your disease or condition.

Do Not Hesitate to Seek a Second Opinion

A second opinion is when another doctor examines your medical records and gives his or her views about your condition and how it should be treated.

You might want a second opinion in order to:

- Be clear about what you have;

- Know all of your treatment choices;

- Have another doctor look at your choices with you.

It is not pushy or rude to want a second opinion. Most doctors will understand that you need more information before making important decisions about your health.

Check to see whether your health plan covers a second opinion. In some cases, health plans require second opinions.

Here are some ways to find a doctor for a second opinion:

- Ask your doctor. Request someone who does not work in the same office, because doctors who work together tend to share similar views.

- Contact your health plan or your local hospital, medical society, or medical school.

Get Information about Next Steps

- Get the results of any tests or procedures. Discuss the meaning of these results with your doctor.

- Make sure you understand what will happen if you need surgery.

- Talk with your doctor about which hospital is best for your health care needs.

Finally, if you are not satisfied with your doctor, you can do two things:

1. Talk with your doctor and try to work things out.

2. Switch doctors, if you are able to.

It is very important to feel confident about your care.

Ten Important Questions to Ask Your Doctor after a Diagnosis

These ten basic questions can help you understand your disease or condition, how it might be treated, and what you need to know and do before making treatment decisions.

1. What is the technical name of my disease or condition, and what does it mean in plain English?

2. What is my prognosis (outlook for the future)?

3. How soon do I need to make a decision about treatment?

4. Will I need any additional tests, and if so what kind and when?

5. What are my treatment options?

6. What are the pros and cons of my treatment options?

7. Is there a clinical trial (research study) that is right for me?

8. Now that I have this diagnosis, what changes will I need to make in my daily life?

9. What organizations do you recommend for support and information?

10. What resources (booklets, websites, audiotapes, videos, DVDs, etc.) do you recommend for further information?

Section 1.3

How to Get a Second Opinion

Reprinted from "Tools to Help You Build a Healthier Life! How to Get a Second Opinion," National Women's Health Information Center, October 2006.

Even though doctors may get similar medical training, they can have their own opinions and thoughts about how to practice medicine. They can have different ideas about how to diagnose and treat conditions or diseases. Some doctors take a more conservative, or traditional, approach to treating their patients. Other doctors are more aggressive and use the newest tests and therapies. It seems like we learn about new advances in medicine almost every day.

Many doctors specialize in one area of medicine, such as cardiology or obstetrics or psychiatry. Not every doctor can be skilled in using all the latest technology. Getting a second opinion from a different doctor might give you a fresh perspective and new information. It could provide you with new options for treating your condition. Then you can make more informed choices. If you get similar opinions from two doctors, you can also talk with a third doctor.

Tips: What to Do

Ask your doctor for a recommendation. Ask for the name of another doctor or specialist, so you can get a second opinion. Don't worry about hurting your doctor's feelings. Most doctors welcome a second opinion, especially when surgery or long-term treatment is involved.

Ask someone you trust for a recommendation. If you don't feel comfortable asking your doctor for a referral, then call another doctor you trust. You can also call university teaching hospitals and medical societies in your area for the names of doctors. Some of this information is also available on the internet.

Check with your health insurance provider. Call your insurance company before you get a second opinion. Ask if they will pay for this office visit. Many health insurance providers do. Ask if there are any special procedures you or your primary care doctor need to follow.

Ask to have medical records sent to the second doctor. Ask your primary care doctor to send your medical records to the new doctor. You need to give written permission to your current doctor to send any records or test results to a new doctor. You can also ask for a copy of your own medical records for your files. Your new doctor can then examine these records before your office visit.

Learn as much as you can. Ask your doctor for information you can read. Go to a local library. Search the internet. Find a teaching hospital or university that has medical libraries open to the public. The information you find can be hard to understand, or just confusing. Make a list of your questions, and bring it with you when you see your new doctor.

Do not rely on the internet or a telephone conversation. When you get a second opinion, you need to be seen by a doctor. That doctor will perform a physical examination and perhaps other tests. The doctor will also thoroughly review your medical records, ask you questions, and address your concerns.

Section 1.4

How to Choose a Hospital

Reprinted from "Your Guide to Choosing Quality Health Care," Agency for Healthcare Research and Quality, U.S. Department of Health and Human Services, AHRQ Publication No. 99-0012, July 2001. Reviewed by David A. Cooke, M.D., May 2007.

How can you choose the best quality hospital for the care you need? It is important to consider quality, because research shows that some hospitals simply do a better job than others. For example, we know that hospitals that do a greater number of the same surgeries have better outcomes for their patients.

Quick Check for Quality

Look for a hospital that:

- Is accredited by the Joint Commission on Accreditation of Healthcare Organizations;

- Is rated highly by state, consumer, or other groups;

- Is one where your doctor has privileges, if that is important to you;

- Is covered by your health plan;

- Has experience with your condition;

- Has had success with your condition;

- Checks and works to improve its own quality of care.

Questions to Ask When Choosing a Hospital

The following questions can help you make the best choices.
You may not have a choice of hospitals right now because of your health plan or doctor, but keep these questions in mind for when you might make a change.

Does the hospital meet national quality standards?

Hospitals can choose to be surveyed by the Joint Commission on Accreditation of Healthcare Organizations (JCAHO) to make sure they meet certain quality standards. The standards address the quality of staff and equipment, and—most recently—the hospital's success in treating and curing patients. If a hospital meets those standards, it becomes accredited (gets a "seal of approval"). Reviews are done at least every three years. Most hospitals participate in this program.

The JCAHO prepares a performance report on each hospital that it surveys. The report lists the following information:

- Accreditation status (six levels, from the lowest, "Not Accredited," to the highest, "Accredited with Commendation")

- Date of the survey

- Evaluation of the key areas reviewed during the survey

- Results of any follow-up activity

- Areas needing improvement

- Comparison with national results

You can order JCAHO's performance reports free of charge by calling 630-792-5800. Or, check the JCAHO's website at http://www.jcaho.org for a hospital's performance report or for its accreditation status.

How does the hospital compare with others in my area?

One important way to learn about hospital quality is to look at hospital report cards developed by states and consumer groups. A recent study about such reports found that besides helping consumers make informed choices, they also encourage hospitals to improve their quality of care. This is a very good reason to look for and use consumer information about hospitals. Here are some ways to find such information:

- Some States—for example, Pennsylvania, California, and Ohio—have laws that require hospitals to report data on the quality of their care. The information is then given to the public so consumers can compare hospitals.

- Some groups gather information on how well hospitals perform and how satisfied their patients are. An example is the Cleveland Health Quality Choice Program, which is made up of businesses, doctors, and hospitals.

- Consumer groups publish guides to hospitals and other healthcare choices in various cities. Find out what kind of information is available where you live by calling your state department of health, healthcare council, or hospital association. Also, ask your doctor what he or she thinks about the hospital.

Does my doctor have privileges at the hospital (is permitted to admit patients)?

If not, you would need to be under the care of another doctor while at the hospital.

Does my health plan cover care at the hospital?

If not, do you have another way to pay for your care?

If going to a certain hospital is important to you, keep that in mind when choosing a doctor or health plan. In general, you will go to the hospital where your doctor has "privileges."

Does the hospital have experience with my condition?

For example, "general" hospitals handle a wide range of routine conditions, such as hernias and pneumonia. "Specialty" hospitals have a lot of experience with certain conditions (such as cancer) or certain groups (such as children). You may be able to choose General Hospital "X" for gallbladder surgery, Specialty Hospital "Y" if you need care for a heart condition, and Specialty Hospital "Z" for your children.

You also may want to find out if the hospital has a special team of health professionals that works with people with your condition or treatment.

Has the hospital had success with my condition?

Research shows that hospitals that do many of the same types of procedures tend to have better success with them. In other words, "practice makes perfect." Ask your doctor or the hospital if there is information available on the following topics:

- How often the procedure is done there

- How often the doctor does the procedure
- Patient outcomes (how well the patients do)

Also, some health departments and others publish reports on "outcomes studies" about certain procedures. These studies show, for example, how well patients do after having heart bypass surgery. Such studies can help you compare which hospitals and surgeons have had the most success with a procedure.

How well does the hospital check and improve on its own quality of care?

More and more hospitals are trying to improve the quality of their care. One way to do this is to keep track of patient outcomes for certain procedures. Another way is to keep track of patient injuries and infections that occur in the hospital. By finding out what works and what doesn't, the hospital can improve the way it treats patients.

Ask the hospital quality management (or assurance) department how it monitors and improves the hospital's quality of care. Also, ask for any patient satisfaction surveys the hospital has done. These will tell you how other patients have rated the quality of their care.

Chapter 2

How to Recognize a Medical Emergency

Chapter Contents

Section 2.1

Symptoms of Serious Health Conditions

Reprinted from "Tools to Help You Build a Healthier Life! Pay Attention: Symptoms of Serious Health Conditions," National Women's Health Information Center, October, 2006.

Following are some symptoms that could be signs of serious health conditions, which should be checked by a doctor or which should be checked by a doctor or nurse. It is important to note that you might feel symptoms in one part of your body that could actually mean a problem in another part. Even if the symptoms don't seem related, they could be. Keep track of your symptoms. If you have any of these symptoms, make an appointment to see your doctor. Listen to what your body is telling you, and be sure to describe every symptom in detail to your provider.

Signs of a Heart Attack

Some symptoms of a heart attack can happen a month or so before the heart attack. Before a heart attack, people may have had one or more of these symptoms:

- Unusual tiredness
- Trouble sleeping
- Problems breathing
- Indigestion
- Anxiety

During a heart attack, people may have one or more of these symptoms:

- Pain or discomfort in the center of the chest
- Pain or discomfort in other areas of the upper body, including the arms, back, neck, jaw, or stomach
- Other symptoms, such as shortness of breath, breaking out in a cold sweat, nausea, or light-headedness

If you have any of these symptoms, go to an emergency room right away or call 911.

Signs of a Stroke

Signs of a stroke happen suddenly and are different from signs of a heart attack:

- Sudden or developing problems with speaking or understanding
- Sudden or developing problems with sight
- Sudden or developing problems with balance, coordination, walking, and dizziness
- Sudden numbness or weakness in the face, arms, or legs
- Sudden severe headache with no known cause

If you have any of these symptoms, go to an emergency room right away or call 911.

Symptoms of Reproductive Health Problems in Women

- Bleeding or spotting between periods
- Itching, burning, or irritation (including bumps, blisters, or sores) of the vagina or genital area
- Pain or discomfort during sex
- Severe or painful bleeding with periods
- Moderate to severe pelvic pain
- Unusual (for you) vaginal discharge of any type or color or with strong odor

Symptoms of Breast Problems in Women

- Nipple discharge
- Unusual breast tenderness or pain
- Breast or nipple skin changes: ridges, dimpling, pitting, swelling, redness, or scaling
- Lump or thickening in or near breast or in underarm area, or tenderness

Symptoms of Lung Problems

- Coughing up blood
- Persistent cough that gets worse over time
- Repeated bouts of bronchitis or pneumonia
- Shortness of breath
- Wheezing

Symptoms of Stomach or Digestive Problems

- Bleeding from the rectum
- Blood or mucus in the stool (including diarrhea) or black stools
- Change in bowel habits or not being able to control bowels
- Constipation, diarrhea, or both
- Heartburn or acid reflux (feels like burning in throat or mouth)
- Pain or feeling of fullness in stomach
- Unusual abdominal swelling, bloating, or general discomfort
- Vomiting blood

Symptoms of Bladder Problems

- Difficult or painful urination
- Frequent urination or loss of bladder control
- Blood in urine
- Feeling the urge to urinate when bladder is empty

Symptoms of Skin Problems

- Changes in the skin, such as changes in existing moles or new growths
- Moles that are no longer round or have irregular borders
- Moles that change colors or change in size (usually get bigger)
- Frequent flushing (a sudden feeling of heat)
- Jaundice (when the skin and whites of the eyes turn yellow)
- Painful, crusting, scaling, or oozing sores that don't heal
- Sensitivity to sun

Symptoms of Muscle or Joint Problems

- Muscle pains and body aches that are persistent, or that come and go often
- Numbness, tingling (pins and needles sensation), or discomfort in hands, feet, or limbs
- Pain, stiffness, swelling, or redness in or around joints

Symptoms of Emotional Problems

- Anxiety and constant worry
- Depression: feeling empty, sad all the time, or worthless
- Extreme fatigue, even when rested
- Extreme tension that can't be explained
- Flashbacks and nightmares about traumatic events
- No interest in getting out of bed or doing regular activities, including eating or sex
- Thoughts about suicide and death
- Seeing or hearing things that aren't there (hallucinations)
- Seeing things differently from what they are (delusions)
- For women, "baby blues" that haven't gone away two weeks after giving birth and seem to get worse over time
- For women, thoughts about harming yourself or your baby after giving birth

Note: These symptoms can have a physical cause and are usually treatable.

Symptoms of Headache Problems

- Headaches between the eyes
- Headaches that come on suddenly
- Headaches that last longer than a couple of days
- Seeing flashing lights or zigzag lines and temporary vision loss before a headache starts

- Spreading pain in face that starts in one eye

- Severe pain on one or both sides of head with upset stomach, nausea, or vision problems

Symptoms of Eating or Weight Problems

- Extreme thirst or hunger

- Losing weight without trying

- Desire to binge on food excessively

- Desire to vomit on purpose

- Desire to starve (not eat at all)

Section 2.2

When Should I Go to the Emergency Department?

More than 300,000 Americans on average are treated in our nation's emergency departments every day, according to the latest government statistics, and patients are treated for a wide variety of medical conditions.

How do you decide when a medical condition rises to the level of a medical "emergency"? The American College of Emergency Physicians (ACEP) offers a list of warning signs that indicate a medical emergency, which are also available with addition health and safety information on the organization's website:

- Difficulty breathing, shortness of breath

- Chest or upper abdominal pain or pressure

- Fainting, sudden dizziness, weakness

- Changes in vision

- Confusion or changes in mental status

- Any sudden or severe pain

- Uncontrolled bleeding

- Severe or persistent vomiting or diarrhea

- Coughing or vomiting blood

- Suicidal feelings

- Difficulty speaking

- Shortness of breath

- Unusual abdominal pain

Children have unique medical problems and may display different symptoms than adults. Symptoms that are serious for a child may not be as serious for an adult. Children may also be unable to communicate their condition, which means an adult will have to interpret the behavior. Always get immediate medical attention if you think your child is having a medical emergency.

"If you or a loved one think you need emergency care, come to the emergency department and have a doctor examine you," said Dr. Frederick Blum, president of ACEP. "If you think the medical condition is life-threatening or the person's condition will worsen on the way to the hospital, then you need to call 9-1-1 and have your local emergency medical services provider come to you."

Emergency departments see patients based on the severity of their illnesses or injuries, not on a first-come, first serve basis. With that in mind, ACEP offers the following tips to patients when they come to an emergency department in order to get the best possible care as quickly as possible:

- **Bring a list of medications and allergies:** What's the name of the medication you are taking? How often do you take it and for how long? A list of allergies is important, especially if there are many of them. Be sure to include medications, foods, insects, or any other product that may cause an allergic reaction. Bring a medical history form with you.

- **Know your immunizations:** This will likely be a long list for children; mainly tetanus, flu, and Hepatitis B for adults.

- **Remain calm:** Obviously it is difficult to remain composed if you've been badly injured, but a calm attitude can help increase communication with the doctors and nurses who are caring for you.

"Communication is important when you arrive at an emergency department," said Dr. Blum. "I want to know as much about the patient as I can, as quickly as I can, so the proper treatment can begin. There can be long waits in the emergency department as doctors and nurse tend to those with the most severe conditions, but by all means tell us if you are in pain or there is any change in your condition while you're at the hospital."

Section 2.3

What to Do in Case of a Heart Attack, Stroke, or Cardiac Arrest

"Heart Attack, Stroke and Cardiac Arrest Warning Signs," reproduced with permission from www.americanheart.org. © 2007, American Heart Association.

Dial 9-1-1 Fast

Heart attack and stroke are life-and-death emergencies—every second counts. If you see or have any of the listed symptoms, immediately call 9-1-1. Not all these signs occur in every heart attack or stroke. Sometimes they go away and return. If some occur, get help fast! Today heart attack and stroke victims can benefit from new medications and treatments unavailable to patients in years past. For example, clot-busting drugs can stop some heart attacks and strokes in progress, reducing disability and saving lives. But to be effective, these drugs must be given relatively quickly after heart attack or stroke symptoms first appear. So again, don't delay—get help right away!

Statistics

Coronary heart disease is America's No. 1 killer. Stroke is No. 3 and a leading cause of serious disability. That's why it's so important to reduce your risk factors, know the warning signs, and know how to respond quickly and properly if warning signs occur.

Heart Attack Warning Signs

Some heart attacks are sudden and intense—the "movie heart attack," where no one doubts what's happening. But most heart attacks start slowly, with mild pain or discomfort. Often people affected aren't sure what's wrong and wait too long before getting help. Here are signs that can mean a heart attack is happening:

- **Chest discomfort:** Most heart attacks involve discomfort in the center of the chest that lasts more than a few minutes, or that goes away and comes back. It can feel like uncomfortable pressure, squeezing, fullness, or pain.

- **Discomfort in other areas of the upper body:** Symptoms can include pain or discomfort in one or both arms, the back, neck, jaw, or stomach.

- **Shortness of breath:** May occur with or without chest discomfort.

- **Other signs:** These may include breaking out in a cold sweat, nausea, or lightheadedness

As with men, women's most common heart attack symptom is chest pain or discomfort. But women are somewhat more likely than men to experience some of the other common symptoms, particularly shortness of breath, nausea/vomiting, and back or jaw pain.

If you or someone you're with has chest discomfort, especially with one or more of the other signs, don't wait longer than a few minutes (no more than five) before calling for help. Call 9-1-1. Get to a hospital right away.

Calling 9-1-1 is almost always the fastest way to get lifesaving treatment. Emergency medical services staff can begin treatment when they arrive—up to an hour sooner than if someone gets to the hospital by car. The staff are also trained to revive someone whose heart has stopped. Patients with chest pain who arrive by ambulance usually receive faster treatment at the hospital, too.

25

If you can't access the emergency medical services (EMS), have someone drive you to the hospital right away. If you're the one having symptoms, don't drive yourself, unless you have absolutely no other option.

Stroke Warning Signs

The American Stroke Association says these are the warning signs of stroke:

- Sudden numbness or weakness of the face, arm, or leg, especially on one side of the body
- Sudden confusion, trouble speaking or understanding
- Sudden trouble seeing in one or both eyes
- Sudden trouble walking, dizziness, loss of balance or coordination
- Sudden, severe headache with no known cause

If you or someone with you has one or more of these signs, don't delay! Immediately call 9-1-1 or the emergency medical services (EMS) number so an ambulance (ideally with advanced life support) can be sent for you. Also, check the time so you'll know when the first symptoms appeared. It's very important to take immediate action. If given within three hours of the start of symptoms, a clot-busting drug can reduce long-term disability for the most common type of stroke.

Cardiac Arrest

Cardiac arrest strikes immediately and without warning. Here are the signs:

- Sudden loss of responsiveness (no response to tapping on shoulders).
- No normal breathing (the victim does not take a normal breath when you tilt the head up and check for at least five seconds).

If these signs of cardiac arrest are present, tell someone to call 9-1-1 and get an automated external defibrillator (AED), if one is available, and you begin cardiopulmonary resuscitation (CPR) immediately.

If you are alone with an adult who has these signs of cardiac arrest, call 9-1-1 and get an AED (if one is available) before you begin CPR.

Use an AED as soon as it arrives.

Chapter 3

Commonly Used Medications

Chapter Contents

Section 3.1

Taking Medicines: Common Questions

Excerpted from "Taking Medicines: Frequently Asked Questions," National Institutes of Health (NIH) Senior Health, March 21, 2007.

What is the difference between prescription drugs and over-the-counter drugs?

There are two types of medications: drugs your doctor prescribes for you, called prescription drugs, and those you can get without a doctor's prescription, called over-the-counter drugs. It is important to realize that over-the-counter products include many different substances such as vitamins and minerals, herbal and dietary supplements, laxatives, cold medicines, and antacids.

After you swallow a pill or capsule, what happens to the drug inside the body?

When you swallow a pill or a capsule, it moves through the digestive tract to the liver, the place where the body processes chemicals. The drug then enters the bloodstream, where it can interact with many body organs.

How does the body get rid of medicines?

After a medicine has done its job in the body, the drug is broken down through a process called metabolism, which occurs mostly in the liver. Once inactive, a drug enters the excretion stage and exits the body in the urine or feces.

What is an active ingredient?

An active ingredient is the chemical substance in a medicine that works with your body to bring relief of your symptoms. Many drugs, such as over-the-counter pain relievers, contain one or more of four different active pain relief ingredients.

Does aging affect how the body processes medicines?

Yes. As the body ages, its ability to absorb and process foods and drugs changes. As people age, metabolism changes, so that older people often process drugs less extensively than they once did. Older people often need smaller doses of medicine per pound of body weight.

Do medicines work the same in all people?

No. Many factors, including exercise habits, diet, general state of health, and heredity can influence how a person responds to medications.

How do genes affect how people respond to drugs?

Genes determine the make-up of all the body's proteins, and as drugs travel through the body they interact with proteins. So, small variations in your genetic make-up can produce proteins that act differently with drugs. This can affect how you respond—or don't respond—to a medicine.

How can I remember when to take all my medications?

Keep a checklist of all the prescription and over-the-counter medications you take. For each medicine, mark the amount you take, the time of day you take it, and whether it should be taken with food. Store two copies of the list: one on the refrigerator door or where your medications are stored, and one in your wallet or purse.

Should I inform my doctor or pharmacist about all the different medications I am taking?

Yes. You should always be sure to tell your doctor or pharmacist about any and all medications that you take every day or even once in a while. Unwanted effects can occur when a drug interacts, or interferes with, another drug or with certain foods. These chemical interactions change the way your body handles one or both medicines.

If I have questions about my medicine after I leave the doctor's office, what should I do?

Call your doctor's office and see if the doctor or a nurse can answer your questions. Your pharmacist is another good source of information about taking medicines.

Why do some medications need to be taken with meals?

Taking some medicines with food can help the drug be absorbed by the body, although certain foods actually slow down absorption. Foods can also sometimes prevent stomach upset, a common side effect that can occur when a drug irritates the stomach's lining. Taking medicine with a full glass of water can reduce the chance of getting an upset stomach because the water helps the medicine dissolve faster.

Should all medicines be taken with food?

No. It is very important that you read the labels on all medications, both prescription and over-the-counter drugs. Food can interact with some medicines, affecting their action. These types of medicines should be taken with a full glass of water—not milk or juice—to help prevent them from becoming lodged in your throat or esophagus.

What are drug interactions?

Drug interactions occur when a medicine interacts chemically with another drug or with certain foods. These interactions change the way your body handles one or both medicines, which can change the effectiveness of either or both drugs.

What are side effects?

Side effects are unwanted or unexpected symptoms or feelings that occur when you take medicine. Side effects can be relatively minor, such as a headache or a dry mouth. They can also be life threatening, such as severe bleeding or irreversible damage to the liver or kidneys.

Stomach upset, including diarrhea or constipation, is a side effect common. Often, this side effect can be lessened by taking certain drugs with meals. However, check with your doctor, nurse, or pharmacist first because food can increase the absorption of certain medications.

What are some ways to avoid side effects?

- Always inform your doctor or pharmacist about all medicines you are already taking, including herbal products and over-the-counter medications.

- Tell your doctor, nurse, or pharmacist about past problems you have had with medicines, such as rashes, indigestion, dizziness, or not feeling hungry.

Here are some tips to help avoid side effects:

- Ask whether the drug may interact with any foods or other over-the-counter drugs or supplements you are taking.

- Read the prescription label on the container carefully and follow directions. Make sure you understand when to take the medicine and how much to take each time.

- If you experience side effects, write them down so you can report them to your doctor accurately.

- Call your doctor right away if you have any problems with your medicines or if you are worried that the medicine might be doing more harm than good. He or she may be able to change your medicine to another one that will work just as well.

- Don't mix alcohol and medicine unless your doctor or pharmacist says it's okay. Some medicines may not work well or may make you sick if taken with alcohol.

What is the "grapefruit juice effect?"

Taking certain medications with a glass of grapefruit juice can lead to higher levels of medicine in the blood, which can cause health problems. Scientists originally discovered the "grapefruit juice effect" by luck, after giving volunteers grapefruit juice to mask the taste of a medicine.

Researchers now know that grapefruit juice blunts the effects of an enzyme that processes several types of drugs, including many of those commonly used to treat heart conditions.

If I feel better, can I stop taking my medication?

No. Don't stop taking a prescription drug unless your doctor says it's okay—even if you are feeling better. Also, never share prescription drugs with another person.

What's the best place to store my medications?

Be sure to ask your doctor or pharmacist or read a medication's label to determine how it should be stored. Some medications must be stored in the refrigerator. Contrary to what you may think, your bathroom medicine cabinet is not a good place to store most medications due to the moist, warm conditions that can cause drugs to break down more quickly. Keep medicines in their original containers, and never put more than one kind of medicine in the same container.

How can doctors be sure new drugs work as they should?

The Food and Drug Administration, or FDA, is the federal agency responsible for making sure that foods and cosmetics are safe, and that drugs and medical devices are safe and effective. The FDA requires that new drugs be tested in clinical trials before they are put on the market.

What are clinical trials and who conducts them?

A clinical trial is a research study with people to find out if a new drug or treatment is both safe and effective. Clinical trials may be sponsored by pharmaceutical companies, federal agencies like the National Institutes of Health, foundations, individuals, and voluntary groups. Trials can take place in a variety of locations, such as hospitals, universities, doctors' offices, or community clinics.

Are there risks involved in participating in clinical trials?

Enrolling in a clinical trial offers benefits and risks. Patients who participate in a clinical trial may get therapies not yet available to most patients. Clinical trials do pose risks, however. Scientists who wish to test drugs in people must follow strict rules that are designed to protect patient volunteers. Special groups called institutional review boards, or IRBs, evaluate all proposed research with humans to determine the potential risks and expected benefits.

Are researchers working on medicines for diseases of aging?

Yes. Currently, hundreds of new medicines are in development for diseases of aging. Among these are potential new drugs for heart disease, stroke, cancer, Alzheimer disease, diabetes, and osteoporosis.

What is pharmacogenetics research?

Many scientists around the country are conducting research to understand how genes affect the way people respond to medicines. This type of research is called pharmacogenetics.

What are some exciting new therapies on the horizon?

Many novel treatments are in the drug discovery pipeline. Among these are a new medicine for chronic pain that came from a poison found in cone snails and self-tying stitches made from new body-friendly plastics.

Section 3.2

Pain Medicines

Pain Treatments: Nonprescription

What are OTC pain medicines?

Over-the-counter (OTC) medicines are those that are available without a prescription from a doctor. Some examples of OTC pain relievers are acetaminophen and nonsteroidal anti-inflammatory drugs (NSAIDs). Acetaminophen products include Tylenol®. NSAIDs include aspirin, ibuprofen (Motrin®), ketoprofen (Orudis® KT), and naproxen sodium (Aleve®). Some products contain both aspirin and acetaminophen (Extra Strength Excedrin®).

Both acetaminophen and NSAIDs reduce fever and relieve pain caused by muscle aches and stiffness, but only NSAIDs can also reduce inflammation (swelling and irritation). Acetaminophen and NSAIDs also work differently. NSAIDs relieve pain by reducing the production of prostaglandins, which are hormone-like substances that cause pain and inflammation. Acetaminophen works on the parts of the brain that receive the "pain messages."

What are topical pain relievers?

OTC pain treatments also include topical pain relievers. These products include creams, lotions, or sprays that are applied to the skin in order to relieve pain from sore muscles and arthritis. Some examples of topical pain relievers include the brands Aspercreme® and Ben-Gay®. Some topical treatments contain a medicine like aspirin, but there is no evidence that putting aspirin on the skin is effective. Other topical medicines "mask" the feelings of pain by making the skin feel warm or cold. (An example of this is capsaicin, which comes from the extracts of chili peppers.) Some topical treatments block the "pain message" from reaching the brain. In general these medicines are safe, even for long-term use.

Pain Treatments: Prescription

What are corticosteroids?

Corticosteroids are cortisone-like medicines that are used to provide relief for inflamed areas of the body. These medicines help to ease swelling, redness, itching, and allergic reactions. Often, corticosteroids are used for conditions such as allergies, asthma, and arthritis. Corticosteroids are similar to the natural corticosteroid hormones that are produced by the cortex (outer part) of the adrenal glands. Some corticosteroids are available over the counter, such as lower-strength hydrocortisone creams (Cortaid®, Cortizone®).

Other common types of corticosteroids require prescriptions. These include the following: prednisone; prednisolone; methylprednisolone; and dexamethasone.

Prescription corticosteroids are strong medicines and might have serious side effects. Side effects might include weight gain, diabetes, upset stomach, headache, mood changes, and trouble sleeping. These medicines might also make it harder for the body to fight off infections. Efforts are underway to develop safer corticosteroids.

What are opioids?

Opioids are narcotic pain medicines that contain natural, synthetic, or semi-synthetic derivatives of morphine. Opioids are often used for acute pain, such as short-term pain after surgery. Some examples of opioids include the following: morphine; fentanyl; oxycodone; and codeine.

Opioids are effective for severe pain and do not cause bleeding in the stomach or other parts of the body. It is rare for people to become addicted to opioids if the drugs are used for acute pain (such as after surgery). However, there is always a risk of dependence. Some side effects of opioids include drowsiness, nausea, constipation, and itching. The drugs can also interfere with breathing when given in large doses to patients that are not accustomed to the drugs' effects.

What are antidepressants?

Antidepressants are drugs that can treat pain or emotional conditions by adjusting levels of neurotransmitters (natural chemicals) in the brain. These medicines can increase the availability of the body's signals for well-being and relaxation, enabling pain control for people with chronic pain conditions that do not completely respond to the usual treatments.

Chronic pain conditions treated by low-dose antidepressants include some types of headaches (like migraines) and menstrual pain. Some antidepressant medicines include the following:

- **Selective serotonin reuptake inhibitors (SSRIs):** citalopram (Celexa®), fluoxetine (Prozac®), paroxetine (Paxil®), and sertraline (Zoloft®)

- **Tricyclic antidepressants:** amitriptyline (Elavil®), desipramine (Norpramin®), doxepin (Sinequan®), imipramine (Tofranil®), and nortriptyline (Pamelor®)

Antidepressants usually are prescribed for a few months. These drugs, especially tricyclics and SSRIs, depend on having a steady dose of the medicine build up in the body over a period of time. In general, antidepressants have fewer long-term side effects than frequent, ongoing use of other pain medicines.

The most common side effects of antidepressants include blurry vision, constipation, difficulty urinating, dry mouth, fatigue, nausea, and headache. Generally, SSRIs have fewer side effects than tricyclic antidepressants.

Other Pain Treatments

Another means of topical pain relief comes in the form of a lidocaine patch (Lidoderm®), which is a prescription medicine.

If your pain is not relieved by the usual treatments, your doctor might refer you to a pain management specialist. Doctors who specialize in pain management might try other treatments such as certain types of physical therapy or other types of medicine. They might also recommend a transcutaneous electrical nerve stimulator (TENS) unit, a device that uses patches placed on the skin to send signals that stop pain.

Section 3.3

Use Caution with Pain Relievers

Excerpted from *FDA Consumer* magazine, January–February 2003 issue, revised September 2005.

Taking too much acetaminophen can lead to serious liver damage. The drug is sold under brand names such as Tylenol and Datril®, but it is also available in many cough and cold products and sleep aids, and is an ingredient in many prescription pain relievers. The Food and Drug Administration warns consumers that all over-the-counter pain relievers should be taken with care to avoid serious problems that can occur with misuse.

Acetaminophen can cause liver injury through the production of a toxic metabolite. The body eliminates acetaminophen by changing it into substances (metabolites) that the body can easily eliminate in the stool or urine. Under certain circumstances, particularly when more acetaminophen is ingested than is recommended on the label, more of the harmful metabolite is produced than the body can easily eliminate. This harmful metabolite can seriously damage the liver.

To avoid accidental overdosing, it's very important not to take more than the recommended dose on the label. Also, you should not take acetaminophen for more days than recommended, or take more than one drug product that contains acetaminophen at the same time. Consumers should be aware that taking more than the recommended dose will not provide more relief.

If you're taking a prescription pain medicine, check with your doctor first before taking over-the-counter (OTC) acetaminophen. You also need to check the labels of other OTC drug products for the ingredient. In some cases of accidental acetaminophen overdose, it appears that consumers used two or more acetaminophen-containing products at the same time.

Some individuals appear to be more susceptible to acetaminophen-induced liver toxicity than others. People who use alcohol regularly may be at increased risk for toxicity, particularly if they use more than the recommended dose. Parents should be cautious when giving acetaminophen to children.

Consumers should also know that there is a potential for gastrointestinal bleeding associated with the use of aspirin and other nonsteroidal anti-inflammatory drugs (NSAIDs) such as ibuprofen and naproxen. Aspirin is sold under brand names such as Bayer® and St. Joseph's®. Ibuprofen is sold under names such as Advil® and Motrin®. Naproxen is sold under the name Aleve®. There are generic versions available for all of these products, as well.

The risk for bleeding is low for those who take these products intermittently. For those who take the products on a daily or regular basis, the risk is increased, particularly for those over sixty-five years of age or those who take corticosteroids (such as prednisone).

In addition, consumers should ask healthcare providers about NSAID use if they have kidney disease or are taking diuretics (fluid pills).

Always read labels carefully, be sure you are getting the proper dose, and check with your healthcare provider to be sure that you can use these drugs safely.

Section 3.4

Know the Facts about Taking Aspirin to Reduce Your Risk of Heart Attack and Stroke

Reprinted from "Aspirin for Reducing Your Risk of Heart Attack and Stroke: Know the Facts," Center for Drug Evaluation and Research, U.S. Food and Drug Administration, August 17, 2005.

You can walk into any pharmacy, grocery, or convenience store and buy aspirin without a prescription. The drug facts label on medication products will help you choose aspirin for relieving headache, pain, swelling, or fever. But what about using aspirin for a different use, time period, or in a manner that is not listed on the label? For example, using aspirin to lower the risk of heart attack and clot-related strokes. In these cases, the labeling information is not there to help you with how to choose and how to use the medicine safely. Since you don't have the labeling directions to help you, you need the medical knowledge of your doctor, nurse practitioner, or other health professional.

You can increase the chance of getting the good effects and decrease the chance of getting the bad effects of any medicine by choosing and using it wisely. When it comes to using aspirin to lower the risk of heart attack and stroke, choosing and using wisely means knowing the facts and working with your health professional.

Daily Use of Aspirin Is Not Right for Everyone

Aspirin has been shown to be helpful when used daily to lower the risk of heart attack, clot-related strokes, and other blood flow problems. Many medical professionals prescribe aspirin for these uses. There may be a benefit to daily aspirin use for you if you have some kind of heart or blood vessel disease, or if you have evidence of poor blood flow to the brain. However, the risks of long-term aspirin use may be greater than the benefits if there are no signs of or risk factors for heart or blood vessel disease.

Every prescription and over-the-counter medicine has benefits and risks—even such a common and familiar medicine as aspirin. Aspirin use can result in serious side effects, such as stomach bleeding, bleeding in the brain, kidney failure, and some kinds of strokes. No medicine is completely safe. By carefully reviewing many different factors, your health professional can help you make the best choice for you.

When you don't have the labeling directions to guide you, you need the medical knowledge of your doctor, nurse practitioner, or other health professional.

Daily Aspirin Can Be Safest When Prescribed by a Medical Health Professional

Before deciding if daily aspirin use is right for you, your health professional will need to consider the following things:

- Your medical history and the history of your family members
- Your use of other medicines, both prescription and over-the-counter
- Your use of other products, such as dietary supplements, including vitamins and herbals
- Your allergies or sensitivities, and anything that affects your ability to use the medicine
- What you have to gain, or the benefits, from the use of the medicine

- Other options and their risks and benefits

- What side effects you may experience

- What dose, and what directions for use are best for you

- How to know when the medicine is working or not working for this use

Make sure to tell your health professional all the medicines (prescription and over-the-counter) and dietary supplements, including vitamins and herbals, that you use—even if only occasionally.

Aspirin Is a Drug

If you are at risk for heart attack or stroke your doctor may prescribe aspirin to increase blood flow to the heart and brain. But any drug—including aspirin—can have harmful side effects, especially when mixed with other products. In fact, the chance of side effects increases with each new product you use.

New products include prescription and other over-the-counter medicines, dietary supplement, (including vitamins and herbals), and sometimes foods and beverages. For instance, people who already use a prescribed medication to thin the blood should not use aspirin unless recommended by a health professional. There are also dietary supplements known to thin the blood. Using aspirin with alcohol or with another product that also contains aspirin, such as a cough-sinus drug, can increase the chance of side effects.

Your health professional will consider your current state of health. Some medical conditions, such as pregnancy, uncontrolled high blood pressure, bleeding disorders, asthma, peptic (stomach) ulcers, and liver and kidney disease, could make aspirin a bad choice for you.

Make sure that all your health professionals are aware that you are using aspirin to reduce your risk of heart attack and clot-related strokes.

Safe Use Depends on Following Your Doctor's Directions

There are no directions on the label for using aspirin to reduce the risk of heart attack or clot-related stroke. You may rely on your health professional to provide the correct information on dose and directions for use. Using aspirin correctly gives you the best chance of getting the greatest benefits with the fewest unwanted side effects. Discuss with your health professional the different forms of aspirin products that might be best suited for you.

Aspirin has been shown to lower the risk of heart attack and stroke, but not all over-the-counter pain and fever reducers do that. Even though the directions on the aspirin label do not apply to this use of aspirin, you still need to read the label to confirm that the product you buy and use contains aspirin at the correct dose. Check the drug facts label for "active ingredients: aspirin" or "acetylsalicylic acid" at the dose that your health professional has prescribed.

Remember, if you are using aspirin every day for weeks, months, or years to prevent a heart attack or stroke, or for any use not listed on the label without the guidance from your health professional, you could be doing your body more harm than good.

Section 3.5

Over-the-Counter Antacids and Acid Reducers for Heartburn and Acid Reflux

Reprinted with permission from "Antacids and Acid Reducers: OTC Relief for Heartburn and Acid Reflux," Updated December 2006, http://familydoctor.org/online/famdocen/home/otc-center/otc-medicines/854.html. © 2006 American Academy of Family Physicians. All rights reserved.

What types of OTC products treat heartburn?

Over-the-counter (OTC) products are medicines you can buy without a doctor's prescription. Many OTC products are advertised to relieve heartburn or acid reflux. These include antacids, bismuth subsalicylate, H_2 blockers, proton pump inhibitors, and combination medicines. Combination medicines may include two or more drugs.

How do antacids and acid reducers work?

Antacids neutralize the acid in your stomach. They can provide fast, short-term relief. Many OTC drugs combine different antacids.

H$_2$ blockers reduce the amount of acid your stomach makes. While they don't relieve symptoms right away, H$_2$ blockers relieve symptoms for a longer period of time than antacids.

Some products combine antacids and an H$_2$ blocker. One example combines famotidine, calcium carbonate, and magnesium hydroxide (brand name: Pepcid® Complete). These combination medicines can relieve symptoms right away and the relief can last for many hours.

Bismuth subsalicylate works by balancing the way fluid moves through your bowels. It also binds toxins (poisons) from bacteria so

Table 3.1. Common Antacids and Acid Reducers

Category	Generic Name	Brand Name(s)
Antacids	Aluminum hydroxide and magnesium carbonate	Gaviscon®
	Calcium carbonate	Maalox® Regular Strength Antacid, Tums® Regular Antacid, Pepcid® Complete Chewable Tablets
	Calcium carbonate and magnesium hydroxide (milk of magnesia)	Mylanta® Gelcaps, Rolaids® Antacid Tablets
	Magnesium hydroxide (milk of magnesia)	Ex-Lax® Milk of Magnesia Stimulant Free Liquid Laxative/ Antacid, Phillips'® Chewable Tablets Antacid-Laxative Stimulant Free
	Sodium bicarbonate and citric acid	Alka-Seltzer® Heartburn Relief
Bismuth Subsalicylate	Bismuth subsalicylate	Kaopectate®, Pepto-Bismol®, Maalox® Maximum Strength Total Stomach Relief
H$_2$ Blockers	Cimetidine	Tagamet® HB 200
	Famotidine	Pepcid® AC
	Ranitidine	Zantac® 75
Proton Pump Inhibitor	Omeprazole	Prilosec® OTC

that they are not harmful and helps kill germs. It's also used as an antiemetic (medicine to treat nausea and vomiting) and as an antidiarrheal (medicine to treat diarrhea).

Proton pump inhibitors stop your body's production of acid. This type of drug requires one to four days to work. Only people who have heartburn often—at least two days a week—should use this drug.

To find out which product is right for you, talk to your doctor.

What problems can OTC antacids and acid reducers help?

These medicines can help relieve heartburn or dyspepsia (pain or an uncomfortable feeling in the upper middle part of your stomach). Heartburn is also called acid reflux disease or gastroesophageal reflux disease (GERD). OTC antacids and acid reducers may also be used as part of a plan to treat ulcers. For treating ulcers, these medicines may be used together or combined with antibiotics (drugs that kill bacteria) prescribed by your doctor.

If you aren't getting enough calcium from your diet, your doctor might suggest that you take additional calcium to help treat or prevent osteoporosis. Antacids that contain calcium carbonate can be used with vitamin D to supplement the calcium in your diet.

What are some common side effects of heartburn medicines?

Antacids and acid reducers usually cause only minor side effects that go away on their own. These may include headaches, nausea, constipation, or diarrhea. Bismuth subsalicylate can cause your tongue or stool to turn dark. This is a short-term side effect.

If side effects make it hard for you to take medicine for heartburn, talk to your family doctor. He or she may suggest a different drug or have ideas about how to make the side effects less of a problem.

Who shouldn't take OTC antacids and acid reducers?

Don't take these drugs if you have an allergy to any of the ingredients. Phenylalanine is an example of an ingredient in some antacids that can cause a problem for certain people. If you have a condition called phenylketonuria, you shouldn't take a medicine that contains phenylalanine.

Don't take bismuth subsalicylate if you've ever had an allergy to aspirin or any other product that contains salicylates. Also don't give bismuth subsalicylate to children who may have the flu or chickenpox because they will have a higher risk of Reye syndrome.

Other ingredient-related warnings concern your diet while you're taking an antacid or acid reducer. For example, unless your doctor tells you it's okay, don't use products that contain sodium bicarbonate or aluminum hydroxide and magnesium carbonate if you're on a low-salt diet. Don't take magnesium hydroxide if you're following a magnesium-restricted diet.

If you have kidney disease, you shouldn't use products containing calcium carbonate or aluminum hydroxide and magnesium carbonate without your doctor's recommendation

Can OTC antacids or acid reducers cause problems with any other medicines I take?

If certain drugs are taken at the same time, they can react with each other and change the way your body processes them. This is called a drug interaction. When this happens, the risk of side effects increases.

Don't use more than one antacid or acid reducer at a time. Don't mix acid reducers and antacids without first talking to your doctor.

If you take any prescription drugs and you're thinking about taking an antacid, H_2 blocker, or proton pump inhibitor, talk to your doctor first. These drugs can cause problems with other medicines you take.

The following drugs may be of special concern for people who are taking H_2 blockers or proton pump inhibitors:

- Theophylline: oral asthma drug
- Warfarin (brand name: Coumadin®): blood-thinning drug
- Phenytoin (brand name: Dilantin®): seizure drug
- Prescription medicine for fungal or yeast problems
- Diazepam: anxiety drug
- Digoxin: heart drug

Bismuth subsalicylate may affect some drugs so that they don't work as well. It also may cause side effects if combined with other drugs. If you take any of the following drugs, talk to your doctor before taking bismuth subsalicylate:

- Blood-thinning drugs
- Drugs to treat gout
- Drugs to treat arthritis
- Drugs for diabetes

Also, check with your doctor or pharmacist before taking bismuth subsalicylate if you take pain relievers, cold products, or some prescription drugs. These medicines may contain aspirin, which is a salicylate, or they may contain some other type of salicylate. Because bismuth subsalicylate contains salicylate, you may take more salicylate than you intend if you take more than one of these products.

Should I call my doctor for any other reasons?

Before taking an antacid or acid reducer, talk to your doctor if you have any of the following symptoms:

- Trouble or pain when you swallow

- Bloody vomit

- Bloody or black stools

- Ongoing stomach pain

- Lightheaded, dizzy, or sweaty feeling

- Chest pain, shoulder pain, or pain that spreads to your arms, neck, or shoulders with shortness of breath

- Weight loss for no reason

- Nausea or vomiting

- Wheezing (you'll hear a squeaky or musical sound in your chest)

- Heartburn that has lasted more than three months

You should stop using antacids or acid reducers and call your doctor if any of the following are true:

- Your stomach pain doesn't get better when you use the medicine, or it gets worse.

- You need to take the medicine for more than fourteen days.

- You're taking Omeprazole (brand name: Prilosec®) and feel like you need to take more than one course in four months.

Don't try to treat yourself if you have any of these symptoms. They may be signs that you have an ulcer or a more serious problem that needs to be checked by your doctor.

What should I look for on the drug label?

When choosing an OTC antacid or acid reducer, check the drug label for possible side effects or interactions with other drugs you're taking. This information will appear in the "warnings" section of the label.

Be sure to check that you're not taking two medicines that contain the same ingredient. You'll find this information in the "active ingredient" section.

Always read and follow the directions on the label. Be sure you understand what the label says before taking the medicine. If you have any questions, ask your family doctor or pharmacist.

Section 3.6

Antihistamines: Understanding Your Options

Reprinted with permission from "Antihistamines: Understanding Your Options," Updated 10/2006, http://familydoctor.org/online/famdocen/home/otc-center/otcmedicines/857.html. © 2006 American Academy of Family Physicians. All Rights Reserved.

What types of over-the-counter (OTC) antihistamines are available?

OTC drugs are medicines you can buy without a doctor's prescription. Two types of OTC antihistamines are available: first-generation and the newer second-generation antihistamines.

First-Generation OTC Antihistamines. These include the following:

- Brompheniramine (brand names: Dimetapp® Cold & Allergy Elixir, Robitussin® Allergy & Cough Liquid)

- Chlorpheniramine (one brand name: Singlet®)

- Dimenhydrinate (one brand name: Dramamine® Original)

- Diphenhydramine (some brand names: Benadryl® Allergy, Nytol®, Sominex®)

- Doxylamine (two brand names: Vicks NyQuil®, Alka-Seltzer Plus® Night-Time Cold Medicine)

Second-Generation OTC Antihistamines. These include the following:

- Loratadine (some brand names: Alavert®, Claritin®)

Note: Both types of antihistamines often are mixed with other drugs, such as pain relievers or decongestants. Many of the brand names above are for these combination medicines, which are meant to treat many symptoms at once.

How do antihistamines work?

Histamines are substances that try to attach to the cells in your body and irritate them. Histamines can cause itching, sneezing, a runny nose, and watery eyes. Antihistamines prevent histamines from attaching to your cells and causing symptoms.

Antihistamines also work in the part of the brain that controls nausea and vomiting. This is why they can help prevent motion sickness.

What symptoms can OTC antihistamines treat?

Antihistamines can help prevent and treat the symptoms of allergies, colds, and the flu (influenza). These symptoms include sneezing, itchy and watery eyes, and a runny nose. Antihistamines can also relieve itchiness caused by insect bites and stings, poison ivy, and poison oak.

Some antihistamines are used to prevent motion sickness. Because one of the most common side effects of antihistamines is feeling sleepy, they are sometimes used to help people who have insomnia.

Will an OTC antihistamine work as well as a prescription one?

In general, OTC antihistamines work as well as prescription medicines.

What are some common side effects of OTC antihistamines?

Side effects from antihistamines aren't common for healthy adults. However, side effects can be a concern for older adults or people who have health problems.

First-generation antihistamines can make you feel very sleepy. This can affect your ability to drive or operate machines. It can also make it hard for you to think clearly. Antihistamines can cause your mouth and eyes to feel dry. Second-generation antihistamines are not as likely to cause these side effects.

Could OTC antihistamines cause problems with any other medicines I take?

Yes. Antihistamines can interact with other drugs you take. If certain drugs are taken at the same time, they can interact with each other and change the way your body processes them. This is called a drug interaction. When this happens, the risk of side effects increases.

If you take any of the following drugs, talk to your doctor before taking a first-generation antihistamine:

- Sleeping pills or sedatives

- Muscle relaxants

- High blood pressure medicine

Antihistamines are often combined with decongestants or pain relievers. If you take one of these combination medicines, it's important to understand each of the active ingredients and the interactions they may have with other drugs you're taking.

Be sure not to "double up" on antihistamine. Many OTC cold and allergy products contain antihistamines, as do some prescription drugs. If you take more than one of these products, you can take much more antihistamine than you intend.

Should I avoid any foods, drinks, or activities while taking antihistamines?

Alcohol can increase the drowsiness caused by antihistamines. Also, be very careful if you drive a car or run machines while taking an antihistamine. Antihistamines may slow your reactions without you even being aware of it.

Who shouldn't take antihistamines?

Talk to your doctor before using a first-generation antihistamine if you have any of the following health problems:

- Glaucoma

- Trouble urinating (from an enlarged prostate gland)
- Breathing problems, such as asthma, emphysema, or chronic bronchitis
- Thyroid disease
- Heart disease
- High blood pressure

Before taking a second-generation antihistamine, tell your doctor if you've ever had kidney or liver disease.

What should I look for on the drug label?

When choosing an OTC antihistamine, check the drug label for possible side effects or interactions with other drugs you're taking. This information will appear in the "warnings" section of the label.

Be sure to check that you're not taking two medicines that contain the same ingredient. You will find this information in the "active ingredient" section.

Always read and follow the directions on the label. Be sure you understand what the label says before taking the medicine. If you have any questions, ask your family doctor or pharmacist.

Chapter 4

Understanding Health Insurance

Chapter Contents

Section 4.1

Health Insurance Basics

"Health Insurance Basics" is reprinted with permission from the State of Michigan Office of Financial and Insurance Services. © 2007 State of Michigan.

What Are My Health Insurance Options?

Health insurance is available to consumers in a variety of plans and coverages. Listed here are some of the most common.

Medical and Hospital Coverage

Major medical: Pays the cost of hospital bills and medical bills. You pay any appropriate co-payments and deductibles. The policy covers only the eligible expenses listed.

Managed care: Provides preventive care and services basic to good health. Out-of-pocket costs are generally less than traditional health insurance. Care is given by the plans network of doctors and hospitals. The managed care plan could be through a traditional health insurance company or a health carrier that provides managed care plans only. Managed care always has a provider network with specific rules to follow if you need care. These plans cover basic care, which is often not included in major medical coverage.

Alternative finance and delivery system (AFDS): Provides limited health services, such as dental, optical, or podiatric care. AFDSs are responsible for the access, availability, and quality of health services provided. AFDSs have a contracted network of providers. Most coverage through an AFDS is available to groups.

Hospital-surgical: Pays only expenses directly related to hospitalization, which usually includes room and board plus doctors' charges.

Short-term: This coverage lasts for only a specified length of time, but for no longer than 180 days in any case. For example, you might buy a six-month policy with major medical coverage for the months that you are between jobs and between group coverage. These policies do not cover pre-existing conditions.

Catastrophic: Has high limits but pays only after you have paid a high deductible, sometimes $2,500 or more.

High-deductible plans: These plans are major medical coverage, but are sold in conjunction with health savings accounts. They pay the cost of hospital and medical bills, but have very high deductibles that you pay from your federally tax exempt health savings account.

Limited Purpose Coverage

Accident only: Pays only when you are treated for accidental injury or if an accident causes death.

Disability income: Pays a fixed amount for a specified period of time when you are unable to work because of an accident or illness.

Hospital indemnity: Pays a flat amount (such as $100 per day) when you are hospitalized.

Long-term care: Pays to take care of you for an extended time in a nursing home or your own home.

Medicare supplement: Pays some medical expenses not paid by Medicare.

Special need: Pays for health care not covered by typical major medical policies (for example, dental or vision care).

Specific disease: Pays only for treatment for a disease or condition specifically named in the policy, such as cancer.

Home health care: Pays for health care delivered to you in your home.

What Is Traditional Health Insurance or Commercial Insurance?

Traditional health insurance or coverage through a commercial insurer are often called "fee-for-service" because the insurer pays the bills after you receive the service. The following are also true:

• You can use any doctor or hospital.

- The medical bills must be sent to the insurance company.

- You will likely have to pay a deductible before the policy begins to pay and co-payments each time you have a claim.

- If the policy pays less than the full bill, you may be responsible for paying the rest.

What Is a Health Maintenance Organization? (HMO)?

HMOs provide preventive care and other services that are basic to good health. Your out-of-pocket costs are generally less than traditional health insurance. Care is likely given by a network of doctors and hospitals under contract with the plan.

Your managed care plan could be through a commercial health insurance company, or you might be covered by a carrier that provides managed care plans only (an HMO).

Regardless, if you have a managed care plan, there is a provider network. Be sure to follow your plan's network rules when you need care.

What Does HIPAA-Eligible Mean and How Does It Apply?

Throughout this chapter, it will be helpful to know if you qualify as a Health Insurance Portability and Accountability Act (HIPAA)–eligible individual. You are a HIPAA-eligible individual only if the following are true:

- You have eighteen months of creditable coverage (see following).

- You were most recently covered by an employer group.

- You were not terminated from your group plan due to nonpayment of premium or fraud.

- You obtained new coverage by midnight of the sixty-third day of your last coverage.

- You are not eligible for Medicare, Medicaid, or any other group coverage.

- You have exhausted all continuation of benefit options such as COBRA (Consolidated Omnibus Reconciliation Act).

- You do not have any other health insurance.

You are not HIPAA eligible unless you meet *all* of these conditions.

What Is Creditable Coverage?

The concept of creditable coverage is that individuals should be given credit for previous health coverage when moving from one employer group health plan to another, from an employer group health plan to an individual policy, or from certain kinds of individual coverage to an employer group health plan.

Most health coverage is creditable coverage, including prior coverage under a group health plan (including a governmental or church plan), health coverage (either group or individual), Medicare, Medicaid, a military-sponsored healthcare program such as TRI-CARE, a program of the Indian Health Service, a state high-risk pool, the Federal Employees Health Benefit Program, a public health plan, a health benefit plan provided for Peace Corps members, a stand-alone prescription drug plan, or a foreign country's government health plan.

How Do I Purchase Health Coverage?

There are two basic ways to buy health coverage: as an individual or through a group. How you buy health coverage affects your rights and responsibilities.

Individual Coverage

- You contract directly with a health carrier just like insuring your home or car.

- You are the policyholder. HMOs call the contract-holder (the person in whose name the contract is written) a subscriber, member, or enrollee.

- Your individual policy can cover your entire family and each family member would be an insured.

- The health carrier needs approval from the Office of Financial and Insurance Services to increase rates.

- Any premium increase affects everyone who has the same kind of policy.

- Unless you have made false statements on your application, filed fraudulent claims, or failed to pay your premiums on time, the company cannot cancel your policy because of your health or claims.

- Coverage must include specific minimum benefits.

Group Coverage

- A group insurance policy may cover two to thousands of people, but it is still only one policy.

- Your employer or trade association is the master policyholder; you and your fellow employees are certificate holders.

- Each family member covered under your certificate is an insured.

- The master policyholder negotiates the terms of a group policy with the insurance company.

- The master policyholder can:

  - Reduce or change the benefits and coverage;

  - Increase your share of the premium;

  - Switch to another insurance company; or

  - Stop providing any coverage.

- In a group contract:

  - Rates for employer groups are negotiable.

  - The contract must include specific minimum benefits required by state law—other benefits are negotiated by the master policyholder.

  - The master policyholder does not need consent of certificate holders to change companies or policies, cancel the policy, or agree to new premiums or benefits.

- Large and small employer group contracts:

  - May cover more conditions than individual contracts;

  - May have more generous benefits; and

  - Cannot reject an application because of poor health as long as the application is made during the eligibility period. Large employer groups are defined as having more than fifty employees. Small employer groups are defined as having two to fifty employees.

Sole-Proprietor Coverage

- Insured must be self-employed.

- You cannot insure employees under this policy.

- This type of coverage may have many of the same benefits as a small group policy.

Section 4.2

How to Make a Health Insurance Claim or Dispute a Denial

Excerpted from "Resolving Health Care Insurance Disputes," © 2007 North Dakota Insurance Department. Reprinted with permission.

Things to Do Before You File a Claim

Review your policy or employee booklet carefully to be sure the service in question is covered.

Follow any managed care rules, including pre-certification requirements and use of network providers.

Give claim forms to the provider, with your policy number and other identifying information.

How to Submit a Claim Properly

Find out if your provider submits the claim for you or if you need to do it. If you need to do it, review the information to be sure it is complete and correct.

File it as soon as you get the bill from the provider.

Send it to the right address.

Keep a copy for your reference.

Allow reasonable time for company to process your claim. The company needs to inform you if it needs any additional information to complete the claim. Sometimes, it will request additional information directly from the providers or return the claim form to you to get more information. After the company has all the information it needs, it has a certain number of working days to process your claim. The company must send you an explanation of benefits that explains its decision.

If Your Claim Is Paid

If you assigned benefits to the provider, the benefit check will be sent directly to the provider.

You will pay any deductibles and co-insurance.

If you did not assign the benefits, the check will come to you and you will need to pay your providers for the entire amount.

If Your Claim Is Denied

The reason for denial should be stated on your explanation of benefits. If you disagree with the basis stated for denial, check your policy or employee booklet for the company's appeal procedures.

The company should be able to answer procedural questions about appeals over the phone.

Your appeal should be in writing and may require information from your doctor.

Filing a Consumer Complaint

If you've tried unsuccessfully to resolve a claim problem with your company or agent, contact your state insurance commission. Very often, companies will resolve disputes after the agency intervenes on a consumer's behalf. If it becomes necessary to file a written complaint with the state insurance department, be sure to do the following things to speed processing of your inquiry:

- Include your name, address, and daytime phone number.

- State your case briefly, giving full explanation of the problem and what type of insurance is involved.

- Include the name of your insurance company, policy number, and the name of the agent or adjuster involved.

- Supply any documentation you have to support your case, including phone notes.

- State what has been done to resolve your problem, including whom you have talked to and what you were told.

- For future reference, keep a copy of your letter to the state insurance department.

If a decision is made that you have a legitimate complaint, your state insurance department will investigate your complaint and keep you advised of what has happened.

If a company insists your complaint or claim is not valid, the state insurance company cannot require the company to make payment unless a state insurance law has been violated. In some cases, legal action is the only way to resolve health insurance disputes. You may want to consult a lawyer if your complaint cannot be resolved and it involves a significant amount of money.

What If You Aren't Protected by Your State?

If the health plan is self-funded and offered by a private-sector employer or bona fide union, take unresolved complaints to the U.S. Department of Labor (DOL) Pension and Welfare Benefits Administration. The DOL does not interpret provisions of any particular health benefit plan or require employers to pay claims, but may investigate your complaint. In certain disputes, the DOL suggests personal legal advice may be your only option.

If the plan is self-funded but offered through a government or church employer, follow the appeals procedures outlined in your benefit booklet and other plan documents. In most cases ultimate responsibility for resolving disputes rests with the governing body of the employer sponsoring the plan, such as a school board.

If you have a disability, you may have certain protections available under the Americans with Disabilities Act (ADA) if your self-funded coverage is dropped or limited. You can reach the ADA Technical Assistance Center at 800-949-4232 or the U.S. Department of Justice at 800-514-0301 (voice) or 800-514-0383 (TDD).

Chapter 5

Your Health Information Privacy Rights

Privacy Is Important to All of Us

You have privacy rights under a federal law that protects your health information. These rights are important for you to know. You can exercise these rights, ask questions about them, and file a complaint if you think your rights are being denied or your health information isn't being protected.

Who must follow this law?

- Most doctors, nurses, pharmacies, hospitals, clinics, nursing homes, and many other healthcare providers

- Health insurance companies, health maintenance organizations (HMOs), and most employer group health plans

- Certain government programs that pay for health care, such as Medicare and Medicaid

Providers and health insurers who are required to follow this law must comply with your right to certain things.

Reprinted from "Your Health Information Privacy Rights," U.S. Department of Health and Human Services Office for Civil Rights, 2006.

You May Ask to See and Get a Copy of Your Health Records

You can ask to see and get a copy of your medical record and other health information. You may not be able to get all of your information in a few special cases. For example, if your doctor decides something in your file might endanger you or someone else, the doctor may not have to give this information to you.

In most cases, your copies must be given to you within thirty days, but this can be extended for another thirty days if you are given a reason.

You may have to pay for the cost of copying and mailing if you request copies and mailing.

You Can Have Corrections Added to Your Health Information

You can ask to change any wrong information in your file or add information to your file if it is incomplete. For example, if you and your hospital agree that your file has the wrong result for a test, the hospital must change it. Even if the hospital believes the test result is correct, you still have the right to have your disagreement noted in your file.

In most cases the file should be changed within sixty days, but the hospital can take an extra thirty days if you are given a reason.

You Should Receive a Notice That Tells You How Your Health Information Is Used and Shared

You can learn how your health information is used and shared by your provider or health insurer. They must give you a notice that tells you how they may use and share your health information and how you can exercise your rights. In most cases, you should get this notice on your first visit to a provider or in the mail from your health insurer, and you can ask for a copy at any time.

You Must Give Your Permission before Your Information Can Be Used or Shared for Certain Purposes

In general, your health information cannot be given to your employer, used or shared for things like sales calls or advertising, or used or shared for many other purposes unless you give your permission by signing an authorization form. This authorization form must tell you who will get your information and what your information will be used for.

You Have the Right to Get a Report on When and Why Your Health Information Was Shared

Under the law, your health information may be used and shared for particular reasons, like making sure doctors give good care, making sure nursing homes are clean and safe, reporting when the flu is in your area, or making required reports to the police, such as reporting gunshot wounds. In many cases, you can ask for and get a list of who your health information has been shared with for these reasons.

You can get this report for free once a year.

In most cases you should get the report within sixty days, but it can take an extra thirty days if you are given a reason.

You Can Ask to Be Reached Somewhere Other Than Home

You can make reasonable requests to be contacted at different places or in a different way. For example, you can have the nurse call you at your office instead of your home, or send mail to you in an envelope instead of on a postcard. If sending information to you at home might put you in danger, your health insurer must talk, call, or write to you where you ask and in the way you ask, if the request is reasonable.

You Can Ask That Your Information Not Be Shared

You can ask your provider or health insurer not to share your health information with certain people, groups, or companies. For example, if you go to a clinic, you could ask the doctor not to share your medical record with other doctors or nurses in the clinic. However, they do not have to agree to do what you ask.

You May File Complaints

If you believe your information was used or shared in a way that is not allowed under the privacy law, or if you were not able to exercise your rights, you can file a complaint with your provider or health insurer. The privacy notice you receive from them will tell you who to talk to and how to file a complaint. You can also file a complaint with the U.S. government.

Other Privacy Rights

You may have other health information rights under your state's laws. When these laws affect how your health information can be used or shared, that should be made clear in the notice you receive.

For More Information

This is a brief summary of your rights and protections under the federal health information privacy law. You can ask your provider or health insurer questions about how your health information is used or shared and about your rights. You also can learn more, including how to file a complaint with the U.S. government, at the website at www.hhs.gov/ocr/hipaa/ or by calling 866-627-7748 (the phone call is free).

Chapter 6

How to Evaluate Health Information on the Internet

Millions of consumers are using the internet to get health information and thousands of websites are offering health information. Some of those sites are reliable and up-to-date; some are not. How can you tell the good from the bad? First, carefully consider the source of information and then discuss the information with your healthcare professional. These questions and answers can help you determine whether the health information you find on the internet or receive by e-mail from a website is likely to be reliable.

Who runs the website?

Any good health website should make it easy to learn who is responsible for the site and its information. On the U.S. Food and Drug Administration's (FDA) website, for example, the FDA is clearly noted on every major page, along with a link to the site's home (main) page, www.fda.gov. Information about who runs the site can often be found in an "About Us" or "About This Website" section, and there's usually a link to that section on the site's home page.

What is the purpose of the website?

Is the purpose of the site to inform? Is it to sell a product? Is it to raise money? If you can tell who runs and pays for the site, this will

Excerpted from "How to Evaluate Health Information on the Internet," U.S. Food and Drug Administration (www.fda.gov), December 2005.

help you evaluate its purpose. Be cautious about sites trying to sell a product or service.

Quackery abounds on the web. Look for these warning signs and remember the adage "If it sounds too good to be true, it probably is":

- Does the site promise quick, dramatic, miraculous results? Is this the only site making these claims?

- Beware of claims that one remedy will cure a variety of illnesses, that it is a "breakthrough," or that it relies on a "secret ingredient."

- Use caution if the site uses a sensational writing style (lots of exclamation points, for example).

- A health website for consumers should use simple language, not technical jargon. Get a second opinion. Check more than one site.

What is the original source of the information?

Always pay close attention to where the information on the site comes from. Many health and medical websites post information collected from other websites or sources. If the person or organization in charge of the site did not write the material, the original source should be clearly identified. Be careful of sites that don't say where the information comes from. Good sources of health information include the following:

- Sites that end in ".gov," sponsored by the federal government, like the U.S. Dept. of Health and Human Services (www.hhs.gov), the FDA (www.fda.gov), the National Institutes of Health (www.nih.gov), the Centers for Disease Control and Prevention (www.cdc.gov), and the National Library of Medicine (www.nlm.nih.gov)

- Sites that end in ".edu," which are run by universities or medical schools, such as Johns Hopkins University School of Medicine and the University of California at Berkeley Hospital, health system, and other healthcare facility sites, like the Mayo Clinic and Cleveland Clinic

- Sites that end in ".org," which are maintained by not-for-profit groups whose focus is research and teaching the public about specific diseases or conditions, such as the American Diabetes Association, the American Cancer Society, and the American Heart Association

- Medical and scientific journals, such as the *New England Journal of Medicine* and the *Journal of the American Medical Association*, although these aren't written for consumers and could be hard to understand

Sites whose addresses end in ".com" are usually commercial sites and are often selling products.

How is the information on the website documented?

In addition to identifying the original source of the material, the site should identify the evidence on which the material is based. Medical facts and figures should have references (such as citations of articles in medical journals). Also, opinions or advice should be clearly set apart from information that is "evidence-based" (that is, based on research results).

How is information reviewed?

Health-related websites should give information about the medical credentials of the people who prepare or review the material on the website.

How current is the information on the website?

Websites should be reviewed and updated on a regular basis. It is particularly important that medical information be current, and that the most recent update or review date be clearly posted. Even if the information has not changed, it is helpful to know that the site owners have reviewed it recently to ensure that the information is still valid. Click on a few links on the site. If there are a lot of broken links, the site may not be kept up-to-date.

How does the website choose links to other sites?

Reliable websites usually have a policy about how they establish links to other sites. Some medical websites take a conservative approach and do not link to any other sites; some link to any site that asks or pays for a link; others link only to sites that have met certain criteria. Look for the website's linking policy.

What information about its visitors does the website collect?

Websites routinely track the path visitors take through their sites to determine what pages are being used. However, many health-related websites ask the visitor to "subscribe" or "become a member." In some cases, this may be done so they can collect a fee or select relevant information for the visitor. In all cases, the subscription or membership will allow the website owners to collect personal information about their visitors.

Many commercial sites sell "aggregate" data about their visitors to other companies—what percentage are women with breast cancer, for example. In some cases, they may collect and reuse information that is personally identifiable, such as a visitor's ZIP code, gender, and birth date.

Any website asking users for personal information should explain exactly what the site will and will not do with the information. Be sure to read and understand any privacy policy on the site.

How does the website manage interactions with visitors?

There should always be a way for visitors to contact the website owners with problems, feedback, and questions. If the site hosts a chat room or other online discussion areas, it should tell its visitors about the terms of using the service. Is the service moderated? If so, by whom, and why? It is always a good idea to spend time reading the discussion without joining in, to feel comfortable with the environment, before becoming a participant.

Can the accuracy of e-mail information be verified?

Carefully evaluate e-mail messages. Consider the origin of the message and its purpose. Some companies or organizations use e-mail to advertise products or attract people to their websites. The accuracy of health information may be influenced by the desire to promote a product or service.

Is the information that's discussed in chat rooms accurate?

Assessing the reliability of health information that you come across in web discussion groups or chat rooms is at least as important as it is for websites. Although these groups can sometimes provide good information about specific diseases or disorders, they can also perpetuate misinformation. Most internet service providers don't verify what is discussed in these groups, and you have no way of knowing the qualifications or credentials of the other people online. Sometimes people use these groups to promote products without letting on that they have a financial stake in the business. It's best to discuss anything you learn from these groups with your healthcare professional.

Part Two

Maintaining Your Health

Chapter 7

Stay Healthy—
Practice Prevention

What can I do to keep myself healthy?

The choices you make about the way you live are important to your health. Here are some choices you can make to help yourself stay healthy:

- Don't use any form of tobacco.
- Eat a healthy diet.
- Exercise regularly.
- Drink alcohol in moderation, if at all.
- Don't use illegal drugs.
- Practice safe sex.
- Use seat belts (and car seats for children) when riding in a car or truck.
- See your doctor regularly for preventive care.

What can my doctor do to help me stay healthy?

In addition to treating you when you are sick, your doctor can follow a program designed to help you stay healthy. This program tells the doctor which preventive services are needed for people at different ages.

What is a "preventive service"?

A preventive service might be a test, or it might be advice from your doctor. Preventive services can include the following:

- Tests (also called screenings) to check your general health or the health of certain parts of your body

- Measurements of weight, cholesterol levels, and blood pressure

- Advice about diet; exercise; tobacco, alcohol, and drug use; stress; and accident prevention

- Immunizations ("shots") for both children and adults

- Special tests at certain times in your life, such as during pregnancy and after age fifty

Will my doctor tell me which preventive services I need?

Yes. Follow your doctor's advice about checkups, about healthy life choices, and about medicines that prevent health problems, such as blood pressure medicine. Preventive services are sometimes offered in your community (for example, blood pressure tests at the local shopping center). If you're not sure you need the service being offered, ask your doctor.

Who pays for preventive services?

Most health insurance companies pay for at least some preventive services. If you aren't sure what your insurance will cover, read your health plan's patient manual or call the health plan's office.

What preventive services do women need?

Adult women should have their weight, blood pressure, and cholesterol levels checked. They also should have a Pap test at least every three years to screen for cervical cancer. After the age of forty, women should have a mammogram every one to two years to screen for breast cancer. They should also be tested for colorectal cancer. These are routine tests that everyone should have. If your doctor orders these tests for you, it does not mean he or she thinks you have cancer. Your doctor will also make sure you have all the shots you need.

Your doctor may give you advice about exercise and diet—for example, how much calcium you need to prevent bone problems, taking folic acid before you get pregnant, and lowering the fat and cholesterol in your diet. Your doctor may also give you advice about alcohol and drug use and sexually transmitted diseases. As you get close to menopause, your doctor will talk to you about hormone replacement therapy. Your doctor may also talk to you about injury prevention practices, such as using seat belts and having smoke detectors in your home.

What preventive services do men need?

Adult men should have their weight, cholesterol levels, and blood pressure checked. Men older than fifty should be tested for colorectal cancer. If your doctor orders this test, it does not mean he or she thinks you have cancer. This is a routine test that everyone should have. Your doctor will also make sure you have all the shots you need.

Your doctor may talk to you about the importance of diet and exercise, testing for prostate cancer, and avoiding alcohol, tobacco, drugs, and sexually transmitted diseases. Your doctor may also talk to you about injury prevention practices, such as using seat belts and having smoke detectors in your home.

Chapter 8

Immunizations: Keys to Disease Prevention

Chapter Contents

Section 8.1

How Vaccines Work

Excerpted from "Understanding Vaccines," National Institute of Allergy
and Infectious Diseases, National Institutes of Health,
NIH Publication No. 03-4219, July 2003.

What Is a Vaccine?

Vaccines take advantage of your body's natural ability to learn how
to eliminate almost any disease-causing germ, or microbe, that attacks
it. What's more, your body "remembers" how to protect itself from the
microbes it has encountered before. Collectively, the parts of your body
that recall and repel diseases are called the immune system. Without the immune system, the simplest illness—even the common cold—
could quickly turn deadly.

On average, your immune system takes more than a week to learn
how to fight off an unfamiliar microbe. Sometimes that isn't soon
enough. Stronger microbes can spread through your body faster than
the immune system can fend them off. Your body often gains the upper hand after a few weeks, but in the meantime you are sick. Certain microbes are so powerful, or virulent, that they can overwhelm
or escape your body's natural defenses. In those situations, vaccines
can make all the difference.

Traditional vaccines contain either parts of microbes or whole microbes that have been killed or weakened so that they don't cause
disease. When your immune system confronts these harmless versions
of the germs, it quickly clears them from your body. In other words,
vaccines fix the fight but at the same time teach your body important
lessons about how to defeat its opponents.

How Do Vaccines Work?

The Immune System

Your immune system is a complex network of cells and organs that
evolved to fight off infectious microbes. Much of the immune system's
work is carried out by an army of various specialized cells, each type

designed to fight disease in a particular way. The invading viruses first run into the vanguard of this army, which includes big, tough, patrolling white blood cells called macrophages (literally, "big eaters"). The macrophages grab onto and gobble up as many of the viruses as they can, engulfing them into their blob-like bodies.

How do the macrophages recognize an invading virus? All cells and microbes wear a "uniform" made up of molecules that cover their surfaces. Each of your cells displays marker molecules unique to you. The invading viruses display different marker molecules unique to them. By "feeling" for these markers, the macrophages and other cells of your immune system can distinguish among the cells that are part of your body, harmless bacteria that reside in your body, and harmful invading microbes that need to be destroyed.

The molecules on a microbe that identify it as foreign and stimulate the immune system to attack it are called antigens. Every microbe carries its own unique set of antigens. As we will see, these molecules are central to creating vaccines.

Antigens Sound the Alarm

The macrophages digest most parts of the invading viruses but save the antigens and carry them back to the immune system's base camps, also known as lymph nodes. Lymph nodes, bean-sized organs scattered throughout your body, are where immune system cells congregate. In these nodes, macrophages sound the alarm by "regurgitating" the antigens, displaying them on their surfaces so other cells can recognize them. In particular, the macrophages show the invading antigens to specialized defensive white blood cells called lymphocytes, spurring them to swing into action.

Lymphocytes: T Cells and B Cells

There are two major kinds of lymphocytes, T cells and B cells, and they do their own jobs in fighting off your virus. T and B cells head up the two main divisions of the immune system army.

T cells: T cells function either offensively or defensively. The offensive T cells don't attack the virus directly, but they use chemical weapons to eliminate the cells of your body already infected with the virus. Because they have been "programmed" by their exposure to the virus antigen, these cytotoxic T cells, also called killer T cells, can "sense" diseased cells that are harboring the virus. The killer T cells latch onto these cells and release chemicals that destroy the infected cells and the viruses inside. The defensive T cells, also called helper T cells, defend the body by secreting chemical signals that direct the activity of other immune system cells. Helper T cells assist in activating killer T cells, and helper T cells also stimulate and work closely with B cells. The work done by T cells is called your cellular or cell-mediated immune response.

B cells: B cells are like weapons factories. They secrete extremely important molecular weapons called antibodies. Antibodies usually work by sticking to and coating microbes, and antibodies use the microbe's antigens to grip them. Antibody molecules fit with antigen molecules like pieces of a jigsaw puzzle fit together—if their shapes are compatible, they bind to each other.

Each antibody can usually fit with only one antigen. So your immune system keeps a supply of millions and possibly billions of different antibodies on hand to be prepared for any foreign invader. Your immune system does this by constantly creating millions of new B cells. About fifty million B cells circulate in each teaspoonful of your blood, and almost every B cell—through random genetic shuffling— produces a unique antibody that it displays on its surface.

Antibodies in Action

The antibodies secreted by B cells circulate throughout your body until they run into the invading virus. Antibodies attack the viruses that have not yet infected a cell but are lurking in the blood or the spaces between cells. When antibodies gather on the surface of a microbe, it is bad news for the microbe. The microbe becomes generally bogged down, gummed up, and unable to function. Antibodies also signal macrophages and other defensive cells to come eat the microbe. Antibodies are like big, bright signs stuck to a microbe saying, "Hey, get rid of this!" Antibodies also work with other defensive molecules that circulate in the blood, called complement proteins, to destroy microbes.

The work of B cells is called the humoral immune response, or simply the antibody response. The goal of most vaccines is to stimulate this response. In fact, many infectious microbes can be defeated by antibodies alone, without any help from killer T cells.

Clearing the Infection: Memory Cells and Natural Immunity

After about a week, your immune system gains the upper hand. Your T cells and antibodies begin to eliminate the virus faster than it can reproduce. Gradually, the virus disappears from your body, and you feel better.

If you are exposed to the virus again, you won't get the disease. You won't even feel slightly sick. You have become immune to it because of another kind of immune system cell: memory cells. After your body eliminated the disease, some of your virus-fighting B cells and T cells converted into memory cells. These cells will circulate through your body for the rest of your life, ever watchful for a return of their enemy. Memory B cells can quickly divide into plasma cells and make more antibody if needed. Memory T cells can divide and grow into a virus-fighting army. If that virus shows up in your body again, your immune system will act swiftly to stop the infection.

How Vaccines Mimic Infection

Vaccines teach your immune system by mimicking a natural infection. The yellow fever vaccine, first widely used in 1938, contains a weakened form of the virus that doesn't cause disease or reproduce very well. This vaccine is injected into your arm. Your macrophages can't tell the vaccine viruses are duds. The macrophages gobble up the viruses as if they were dangerous and, in the lymph nodes, present yellow fever antigen to T and B cells. The alarm is sounded, and your immune system swings into action. Yellow-fever-specific T cells rush out to meet the foe. B cells secrete yellow fever antibodies. But the battle is over quickly. The weakened viruses in the vaccine can't put up much of a fight. The mock infection is cleared, and you are left with a supply of memory T and B cells to protect you against yellow fever, should a mosquito carrying the virus ever bite you.

Different Types of Vaccines

Live, attenuated vaccines: These vaccines contain a version of the living microbe that has been weakened in the lab so it can't cause disease. This weakening of the organism is called attenuation. Because a live, attenuated vaccine is the closest thing to an actual infection, these vaccines are good "teachers" of the immune system: They elicit strong cellular and antibody responses, and often confer lifelong immunity with only one or two doses.

Despite the advantages of live, attenuated vaccines, there is a down side. It is the nature of living things to change, or mutate, and the organisms used in live, attenuated vaccines are no different. The remote possibility exists that the attenuated bacteria in the vaccine could revert to a virulent form and cause disease. For their own protection, people with compromised immune systems—such as people with cancer or people infected with the human immunodeficiency virus (HIV)—usually are not given live vaccines.

Inactivated or "killed" vaccines: Scientists produce inactivated vaccines by killing the disease-causing microbe with chemicals, heat, or radiation. Such vaccines are more stable and safer than live vaccines: The dead microbes can't mutate back to their disease-causing state. Inactivated vaccines usually don't require refrigeration, and they can be easily stored and transported in a freeze-dried form, which makes them accessible to people in developing countries.

Most inactivated vaccines, however, stimulate a weaker immune system response than do live vaccines. So it would likely take several additional doses, so-called booster shots, to maintain a person's immunity to bacteria. This quality could be a drawback in areas where people don't have regular access to health care and can't get their shots on time.

Subunit vaccines: Subunit vaccines dispense with the entire microbe and use just the important parts of it: the antigens that best stimulate the immune system. In some cases, these vaccines use epitopes—the very specific parts of the antigen that antibodies or T cells recognize and bind to. Because subunit vaccines contain only the essential antigens and not all the other molecules that make up the microbe, the chances of adverse reactions to the vaccine are lower.

Toxoid vaccines: These vaccines are used when a bacterial toxin is the main cause of illness. Scientists have found they can inactivate toxins by treating them with formalin, a solution of formaldehyde and sterilized water. Such "detoxified" toxins, called toxoids, are safe for use in vaccines.

When the immune system receives a vaccine containing a harmless toxoid, it learns how to fight off the natural toxin. The immune system produces antibodies that lock on to and block the toxin.

Conjugate vaccines: If a bacteria possesses an outer coating of sugar molecules called polysaccharides, as many harmful bacteria do, a conjugate vaccine is the best bet. Polysaccharide coatings disguise a bacterium's antigens so that the immature immune systems of infants and younger children can't recognize or respond to them. Conjugate vaccines, a special type of subunit vaccine, get around this problem.

When making a conjugate vaccine, scientists link antigens or toxoids from a microbe that an infant's immune system can recognize to the polysaccharides. The linkage helps the immature immune system react to polysaccharide coatings and defend against the disease-causing bacterium.

DNA vaccines: Still in the experimental stages, these vaccines show great promise, and several types are being tested in humans. DNA vaccines take immunization to a new technological level. These vaccines dispense with both the whole organism and its parts and get right down to the essentials: the microbe's genetic material. In particular, DNA vaccines use the genes that code for those all-important antigens.

Researchers have found that when the genes for a microbe's antigens are introduced into the body, some cells will take up that DNA. The DNA then instructs those cells to make the antigen molecules. The cells secrete the antigens and display them on their surfaces. In other words, the body's own cells become vaccine-making factories, creating the antigens necessary to simulate the immune system.

A DNA vaccine against bacterium X would evoke a strong antibody response to the free-floating X antigen secreted by cells, and the vaccine also would stimulate a strong cellular response against the X antigens displayed on cell surfaces. The DNA vaccine couldn't cause the disease because it wouldn't contain bacterium X, just copies of a few of its genes. In addition, DNA vaccines are relatively easy and inexpensive to design and produce.

So-called naked DNA vaccines inject the DNA directly into the body. These vaccines can be administered with a needle and syringe or with a needle-less device that uses high-pressure gas to shoot microscopic gold particles coated with DNA directly into cells. Sometimes, the DNA is mixed with molecules that facilitate its uptake by the body's cells. Naked DNA vaccines being tested in humans include those against malaria, influenza, herpes, and human immunodeficiency virus (HIV).

Recombinant vector vaccines: These experimental vaccines are similar to DNA vaccines, but they use an attenuated virus or bacterium to introduce microbial DNA to cells of the body. "Vector" refers to the virus or bacterium used as the carrier.

In nature, viruses latch on to cells and inject their genetic material into them. In the lab, scientists have taken advantage of this process. They have figured out how to take the roomy genomes of certain benign or attenuated viruses and insert portions of the genetic material from other microbes into them. The carrier viruses then ferry that microbial DNA to cells. Recombinant vector vaccines closely mimic a natural infection and therefore do a good job of stimulating the immune system.

Attenuated bacteria also can be used as vectors. In this case, the inserted genetic material causes the bacterium to display the antigens of other microbes on its surface. In effect, the harmless bacterium mimics a harmful microbe, provoking an immune response.

Researchers are working on both bacterial- and viral-based recombinant vector vaccines for HIV, rabies, and measles.

Adjuvants and Other Vaccine Ingredients

Adjuvants are ingredients added to a vaccine to improve the immune response it produces. Researchers are studying many types of adjuvants, but the only type licensed for human use in the United States so far are the so-called alum adjuvants, which are composed of aluminum salts. These compounds bind to the antigens in the vaccine, help retain antigens at the site of injection, and help deliver antigens to the lymph nodes, where immune responses to the antigens are initiated. The slowed release of antigens to tissue around the injection site and the improved delivery of antigens to the lymph nodes can produce a stronger antibody response than can the antigen alone. Alum adjuvants are also taken up by cells such as macrophages and help these cells better present antigens to lymphocytes.

In addition to adjuvants, vaccines may contain antibiotics to prevent bacterial contamination during manufacturing, preservatives to keep multidose vials of vaccine sterile after they are opened, or stabilizers to maintain a vaccine's potency at less-than-optimal temperatures.

Making Safe Vaccines

No vaccine is perfectly safe or effective. Each person's immune system works differently, so occasionally a person will not respond to a vaccine. Very rarely, a person may have a serious adverse reaction to a vaccine, such as an allergic reaction that causes hives or difficulty breathing. But serious reactions are reported so infrequently—on the order of 1 in 100,000 vaccinations—that they can be difficult to detect and confirm. More commonly, people will experience temporary side effects such as fever, soreness, or redness at the injection site. These side effects are, of course, much preferable to coming down with the illness.

To make vaccines as safe as possible, U.S. Food and Drug Administration (FDA) requires extensive research and testing before allowing a vaccine to be licensed for general use. The time between discovery of a disease agent and production of a widely available vaccine has been as long as fifty years. Today, with improved technology and research methods, the length of time from basic research to availability of a licensed vaccine can sometimes be reduced. If a vaccine is approved, the FDA and other government agencies continue to monitor it for safety.

Conclusion

Vaccines are crucial to maintaining public health. They are a safe, cost-effective, and efficient way to prevent sickness and death from infectious diseases. Vaccines have led to some of the greatest public health triumphs ever, including the eradication of naturally occurring smallpox from the globe and the near-eradication of polio.

In recent years, researchers have increased their understanding of the immune system and how it fights off harmful microbes. Scientists working on vaccines also have advanced technology to draw on, including recombinant DNA technology and the ability to "read" and analyze the genomes of disease-causing organisms. This new knowledge and technology promises to usher in a renaissance in the already vital field of vaccinology. Scientists are hard at work creating improved vaccines, designing new vaccine strategies, and identifying new vaccine candidates to prevent diseases for which no vaccines currently exist.

Section 8.2

Immunizations for Adults

Reprinted from "Vaccinations for Adults," July 2007. Reprinted with permission from the Immunization Action Coalition, www.immunize.org, © 2007.

Getting immunized is a lifelong, life-protecting job. Don't leave your healthcare provider's office without making sure you've had all the vaccinations you need.

Influenza Vaccine

If you are between nineteen and forty-nine years of age, you need a dose yearly if you have a chronic health problem, are a healthcare worker, have close contact with certain individuals (consult your healthcare provider to determine your level of risk for infection and your need for this vaccine), or you simply want to avoid getting influenza or spreading it to others.

If you are aged fifty or older, you need a does every fall or winter.

Pneumococcal Vaccine

Between the ages of nineteen and sixty-four, you need one to two doses of this vaccine if you have certain chronic medical conditions (consult your healthcare provider to determine your level of risk for infection and your need for this vaccine). You need one dose at age sixty-five (or older) if you've never been vaccinated. You may also need a second dose.

Tetanus, Diphtheria, Pertussis (Td, Tdap) Vaccine

If you haven't had at least three tetanus-and-diphtheria-containing shots sometime in your life, you need to get them now. Start with dose number one, followed by dose number two in one month, and dose number three in six months. All adults need Td booster doses every ten years. If you're younger than age sixty-five and haven't had pertussis-containing vaccine as an adult, one of the doses that you receive should have pertussis (whooping cough) vaccine in it—known as Tdap. Be sure to consult your healthcare provider if you have a deep or dirty wound.

Hepatitis B (HepB) Vaccine

You need this vaccine if you have a specific risk factor for hepatitis B virus infection (consult your healthcare provider to determine your level of risk for infection and your need for this vaccine) or you simply wish to be protected from this disease. The vaccine is given as a three-dose series (dose number one now, followed by dose number two in one month, and with dose number three usually given five months later).

Hepatitis A (HepA) Vaccine

You need this vaccine if you have a specific risk factor for hepatitis A virus infection (consult your healthcare provider to determine your level of risk for infection and your need for this vaccine) or you simply wish to be protected from this disease. The vaccine is usually given as two doses, six to eighteen months apart.

Human Papillomavirus (HPV) Vaccine

You need this vaccine if you are a woman who is age twenty-six or younger. The vaccine is given as a three-dose series (dose number one now, followed by dose number two in two months and dose number three four months after that).

Measles, Mumps, Rubella (MMR) Vaccine

You need at least one dose of MMR if you were born in 1957 or later. You may also need a second dose. Consult your healthcare provider to determine your level of risk for infection and your need for this vaccine.

Varicella (Chickenpox) Vaccine

If you've never had chickenpox or you were vaccinated but received only one dose, you should get a second dose or complete a two-dose series now (two doses, one to two months apart).

Meningococcal Vaccine

If you are a young adult going to college and plan to live in a dormitory, you need to get vaccinated against meningococcal disease. People with certain medical conditions should also receive this vaccine (consult your healthcare provider to determine your level of risk for infection and your need for this vaccine).

Zoster (Shingles) Vaccine

If you are age sixty or older, you should get this vaccine now.

Vaccines for Travelers

Do you travel outside the United States? If so, you may need additional vaccines. The Centers for Disease Control and Prevention (CDC) operates an international traveler's health information line. You may also consult a travel clinic or your healthcare provider.

Section 8.3

Vaccine Side Effects

Reprinted from the Centers for Disease Control and Prevention
(www.cdc.gov), July 7, 2005.

Any vaccine can cause side effects. For the most part these are minor (for example, a sore arm or low-grade fever) and go away within a few days. Listed below are some of the vaccines licensed in the United States and side effects that have been associated with each of them.

Hepatitis A Vaccine

Mild problems: Soreness where the shot was given (about 1 out of 2 adults); headache (about 1 out of 6 adults); and tiredness (about 1 out of 14 adults). If these problems occur, they usually last one or two days.

Severe problems: Serious allergic reaction, within a few minutes to a few hours of the shot (very rare).

Hepatitis B Vaccine

Mild problems: Soreness where the shot was given, lasting a day or two (about 1 out of 4 adults); and mild to moderate fever (1 out of 100 adults).

Severe problems: Serious allergic reaction (very rare).

Human Papillomavirus (HPV) Vaccine

HPV vaccine does not appear to cause any serious side effects. However, a vaccine, like any medicine, could possibly cause serious problems, such as severe allergic reactions. The risk of any vaccine causing serious harm, or death, is extremely small.

Several mild problems may occur with HPV vaccine:

- Pain at the injection site (about 8 people in 10)

- Redness or swelling at the injection site (about 1 person in 4)

- Mild fever (100 degrees Fahrenheit) (about 1 person in 10)

- Itching at the injection site (about 1 person in 30)

- Moderate fever, 102 degrees Fahrenheit (about 1 person in 65)

These symptoms do not last long and go away on their own.

Life-threatening allergic reactions from vaccines are very rare. If they do occur, it would be within a few minutes to a few hours after the vaccination.

Like all vaccines, HPV vaccine will continue to be monitored for unusual or severe problems.

Influenza (Inactivated) Vaccine

Serious problems from influenza vaccine are very rare. The viruses in inactivated influenza vaccine have been killed, so you cannot get influenza from the vaccine.

Mild problems: Soreness, redness, or swelling where the shot was given; fever; and aches. If these problems occur, they usually begin soon after the shot and last one to two days.

Severe problems: Life-threatening allergic reactions from vaccines are very rare. If they do occur, it is within a few minutes to a few hours after the shot.

In 1976, a certain type of influenza (swine flu) vaccine was associated with Guillain-Barré syndrome (GBS). Since then, flu vaccines have not been clearly linked to GBS. However, if there is a risk of GBS from current flu vaccines, it would be no more than one or two cases per million people vaccinated. This is much lower than the risk of severe influenza, which can be prevented by vaccination.

Influenza (Live) Vaccine (LAIV)

Live influenza vaccine viruses rarely spread from person to person. Even if they do, they are not likely to cause illness.

LAIV is made from weakened virus and does not cause influenza. The vaccine can cause mild symptoms in people who get it.

Mild problems: Runny nose or nasal congestion; sore throat; cough, chills, tiredness/weakness; and headache. These symptoms did not last long and went away on their own. Although they can occur after vaccination, they may not have been caused by the vaccine.

Severe problems: Life-threatening allergic reactions from vaccines are very rare. If they do occur, it is within a few minutes to a few hours after the vaccination. If rare reactions occur with any new product, they may not be identified until thousands, or millions, of people have used it. Over four million doses of LAIV have been distributed since it was licensed, and no serious problems have been identified. Like all vaccines, LAIV will continue to be monitored for unusual or severe problems.

Measles, Mumps, and Rubella (MMR) Vaccine

Mild problems: Fever (up to 1 person out of 6); mild rash (about 1 person out of 20); and swelling of glands in the cheeks or neck (rare). If these problems occur, it is usually within seven to twelve days after the shot. They occur less often after the second dose.

Moderate problems: Seizure (jerking or staring) caused by fever (about 1 out of 3,000 doses); temporary pain and stiffness in the joints, mostly in teenage or adult women (up to 1 out of 4); and temporary low platelet count, which can cause a bleeding disorder (about 1 out of 30,000 doses).

Severe problems (very rare): Serious allergic reaction (less than 1 out of a million doses).

Several other severe problems have been known to occur after a child gets MMR vaccine. But this happens so rarely that experts cannot be sure whether these problems are caused by the vaccine. These include deafness; long-term seizures, coma, or lowered consciousness; and permanent brain damage.

Meningococcal Vaccine

Mild problems: Up to about half of people who get meningococcal vaccines have mild side effects, such as redness or pain where the shot was given. If these problems occur, they usually last for one or two days. They are more common after meningococcal conjugate vaccine (MCV4) than after meningococcal tetravalent polysaccharide vaccine

(MPSV4). A small percentage of people who receive the vaccine develop a fever.

Severe problems: Serious allergic reactions, within a few minutes to a few hours of the shot, are very rare.

A serious nervous system disorder called Guillain-Barré syndrome (or GBS) has been reported among some people who received MCV4. This happens so rarely that it is currently not possible to tell if the vaccine might be a factor. Even if it is, the risk is very small.

Pneumococcal Polysaccharide Vaccine (PPV23)

PPV is a very safe vaccine. About half of those who get the vaccine have very mild side effects, such as redness or pain where the shot is given. Less than 1 percent develop a fever, muscle aches, or more severe local reactions. Severe allergic reactions have been reported very rarely. As with any medicine, there is a very small risk that serious problems, even death, could occur after getting a vaccine. Getting the disease is much more likely to cause serious problems than getting the vaccine.

Shingles (Herpes Zoster) Vaccine

Mild problems: Redness, soreness, swelling, or itching at the site of the injection (about 1 person in 3); and headache (about 1 person in 70).

Severe problems: No serious problems have been identified with shingles vaccine. Like all vaccines, shingles vaccine is being closely monitored for unusual or severe problems.

Adult Tetanus and Diphtheria (Td) Vaccine

Mild problems: Soreness, redness, or swelling where the shot was given. If these problems occur, they usually start within hours to a day or two after vaccination. They may last one to two days. These problems can be worse in adults who get Td vaccine very often. Acetaminophen or ibuprofen (non-aspirin) may be used to reduce soreness.

Severe problems (these problems happen very rarely): Serious allergic reaction; deep, aching pain and muscle wasting in upper arm(s). This starts two days to four weeks after the shot, and may last many months.

Combined Tetanus, Diphtheria and Pertussis (Tdap) Vaccine

A vaccine, like any medicine, could possibly cause serious problems, such as severe allergic reactions. However, the risk of a vaccine causing serious harm, or death, is extremely small.

If rare reactions occur with any new product, they may not be identified until many thousands, or even millions, of people have used the product. Like all vaccines, Tdap is being closely monitored for unusual or severe problems.

Clinical trials (testing before the vaccine was licensed) involved about 4,200 adolescents and about 1,800 adults. The following problems were reported. These are similar to problems reported after Td vaccine.

Mild problems: Noticeable, but did not interfere with activities:

- Pain (about 2 in 3 adults);

- Redness or swelling (about 1 in 5);

- Mild fever of at least 100.4°F (up to 1 in 100 adults);

- Headache (about 3 in 10 adults);

- Tiredness (about 1 in 4 adults);

- Nausea, vomiting, diarrhea, stomachache (up to 1 in 10 adults);

- Other mild problems reported include chills, body aches, sore joints, rash, and swollen lymph glands.

Moderate problems: Interfered with activities, but did not require medical attention:

- Pain at the injection site (about 1 in 100 adults);

- Redness or swelling (up to about 1 in 25 adults);

- Fever over 102°F (about 1 in 250 adults);

- Nausea, vomiting, diarrhea, stomachache (up to 1 in 100 adults).

Severe problems: Unable to perform usual activities; required medical attention:

- In the adult clinical trial, two adults had nervous system problems after getting the vaccine. These may or may not have been caused by the vaccine. They went away on their own and did not cause any permanent harm.

- A severe allergic reaction could occur after any vaccine. They are estimated to occur less than once in a million doses. A person who gets these diseases is much more likely to have severe complications than a person who gets Tdap vaccine.

Varicella (Chickenpox) Vaccine

Mild problems: Soreness or swelling where the shot was given (up to 1 out of 3 adolescents and adults); fever (1 person out of 10, or less); and mild rash, up to a month after vaccination (1 person out of 20, or less).

It is possible for these people to infect other members of their household, but this is extremely rare.

Note: Measles, mumps, rubella, and varicella (MMRV) vaccine has been associated with higher rates of fever (up to about 1 person in 5) and measles-like rash (about 1 person in 20) compared with MMR and varicella vaccines given separately.

Moderate problems: Seizure (jerking or staring) caused by fever (less than 1 person out of 1,000).

Severe problems: Pneumonia (very rare). Other serious problems, including severe neurological problems (brain reactions) and low blood count, have been reported after chickenpox vaccination. These happen so rarely, however, that experts cannot tell whether they are caused by the vaccine. If they are, it is extremely rare.

What If There Is a Moderate or Severe Reaction?

What Should I Look For?

Look for any unusual condition, such as a high fever, behavior changes, or flu-like symptoms that occur one to thirty days after vaccination. Signs of an allergic reaction can include difficulty breathing, hoarseness or wheezing, hives, paleness, weakness, a fast heartbeat, or dizziness within a few minutes to a few hours after the shot.

What Should I Do?

- Call a doctor, or get the person to a doctor right away.

- Tell your doctor what happened, the date and time it happened, and when the vaccination was given.

- Ask the clinic where you received the vaccine to save any left-over vaccine and the vaccine vial, and record the lot number.

- Ask your doctor, nurse, or health department to report the reaction by filing a Vaccine Adverse Event Reporting System (VAERS) form. Reporting reactions helps experts learn about possible problems with vaccines.

Chapter 9

Lifestyle Changes for a Healthier You

Feel Better Today, Stay Healthy for Tomorrow

The food and physical activity choices you make every day affect your health—how you feel today, tomorrow, and in the future. The science-based advice of the *Dietary Guidelines for Americans, 2005* highlights how make smart choices from every food group, find your balance between food and physical activity, and get the most nutrition out of your calories.

You may be eating plenty of food, but not eating the right foods that give your body the nutrients you need to be healthy. You may not be getting enough physical activity to stay fit and burn those extra calories. This chapter is a starting point for finding your way to a healthier you.

Eating right and being physically active aren't just a "diet" or a "program"—they are keys to a healthy lifestyle. With healthful habits, you may reduce your risk of many chronic diseases such as heart disease, diabetes, osteoporosis, and certain cancers, and increase your chances for a longer life.

The sooner you start, the better for you, your family, and your future.

Make Smart Choices from Every Food Group

The best way to give your body the balanced nutrition it needs is by eating a variety of nutrient-packed foods every day. Just be sure to stay within your daily calorie needs.

Reprinted from "Finding Your Way to a Healthier You," U.S. Department of Agriculture, April 5, 2005.

91

A healthy eating plan is one that does the following:

- Emphasizes fruits, vegetables, whole grains, and fat-free or low-fat milk and milk products

- Includes lean meats, poultry, fish, beans, eggs, and nuts

- Is low in saturated fats, trans fats, cholesterol, salt (sodium), and added sugars

Don't Give in When You Eat Out and Are on the Go

It's important to make smart food choices and watch portion sizes wherever you are—at the grocery store, at work, in your favorite restaurant, or running errands. Try these tips:

- At the store, plan ahead by buying a variety of nutrient-rich foods for meals and snacks throughout the week.

- When grabbing lunch, have a sandwich on whole-grain bread and choose low-fat/fat-free milk, water, or other drinks without added sugars.

- In a restaurant, opt for steamed, grilled, or broiled dishes instead of those that are fried or sautéed.

- On a long commute or shopping trip, pack some fresh fruit, cut-up vegetables, string cheese sticks, or a handful of unsalted nuts—to help you avoid impulsive, less healthful snack choices.

Mix Up Your Choices within Each Food Group

Focus on fruits: Eat a variety of fruits—whether fresh, frozen, canned, or dried—rather than fruit juice for most of your fruit choices. For a two-thousand-calorie diet, you will need two cups of fruit each day (for example, one small banana, one large orange, and 1/4 cup of dried apricots or peaches).

Vary your veggies: Eat more dark green veggies, such as broccoli, kale, and other dark leafy greens; orange veggies, such as carrots, sweet potatoes, pumpkin, and winter squash; and beans and peas, such as pinto beans, kidney beans, black beans, garbanzo beans, split peas, and lentils.

Get your calcium-rich foods: Get three cups of low-fat or fat-free milk—or an equivalent amount of low-fat yogurt and/or low-fat cheese (1½ ounces of cheese equals one cup of milk)—every day. For kids aged two to eight, it's two cups of milk. If you don't or can't consume milk, choose lactose-free milk products or calcium-fortified foods and beverages.

Make half your grains whole: Eat at least 3 ounces of whole-grain cereals, breads, crackers, rice, or pasta every day. One ounce is about 1 slice of bread, 1 cup of breakfast cereal, or ½ cup of cooked rice or pasta. Look to see that grains such as wheat, rice, oats, or corn are referred to as "whole" in the list of ingredients.

Go lean with protein: Choose lean meats and poultry. Bake it, broil it, or grill it. And vary your protein choices—with more fish, beans, peas, nuts, and seeds.

Know the limits on fats, salt, and sugars: Read the Nutrition Facts label on foods. Look for foods low in saturated fats and trans fats. Choose and prepare foods and beverages with little salt (sodium) or added sugars (caloric sweeteners).

Find Your Balance between Food and Physical Activity

Becoming a healthier you isn't just about eating healthy—it's also about physical activity. Regular physical activity is important for your overall health and fitness. It also helps you control body weight by balancing the calories you take in as food with the calories you expend each day. Here are some tips:

- Be physically active for at least thirty minutes most days of the week.

- Increasing the intensity or the amount of time that you are physically active can have even greater health benefits and may be needed to control body weight. About sixty minutes a day may be needed to prevent weight gain.

- Children and teenagers should be physically active for sixty minutes every day, or most every day.

Consider this: If you eat one hundred more food calories a day than you burn, you'll gain about one pound in a month. That's about ten pounds in a year. The bottom line is that to lose weight, it's important to reduce calories and increase physical activity.

Get the Most Nutrition out of Your Calories

There is a right number of calories for you to eat each day. This number depends on your age, activity level, and whether you're trying to gain, maintain, or lose weight. You could use up the entire amount on a few high-calorie items, but chances are you won't get the full range of vitamins and nutrients your body needs to be healthy.

Choose the most nutritionally rich foods you can from each food group each day—those packed with vitamins, minerals, fiber, and other nutrients but lower in calories. Pick foods like fruits, vegetables, whole grains, and fat-free or low-fat milk and milk products more often.

Nutrition: Know the Facts, Use the Label

Most packaged foods have a Nutrition Facts label. For a healthier you, use this tool to make smart food choices quickly and easily. Try these tips:

- **Keep these low:** saturated fats, trans fats, cholesterol, and sodium.

- **Get enough of these:** potassium, fiber, vitamins A and C, calcium, and iron.

- **Use the % Daily Value (DV) column when possible:** 5 percent DV or less is low, 20 percent DV or more is high.

Check servings and calories: Look at the serving size and how many servings you are actually consuming. If you double the servings you eat, you double the calories and nutrients, including the % DVs.

Make your calories count: Look at the calories on the label and compare them with what nutrients you are also getting to decide whether the food is worth eating. When one serving of a single food item has more than 400 calories per serving, it is high in calories.

Don't sugarcoat it: Since sugars contribute calories with few, if any, nutrients, look for foods and beverages low in added sugars. Read the ingredient list and make sure that added sugars are not one of the first few ingredients. Some names for added sugars (caloric sweeteners) include sucrose, glucose, high fructose corn syrup, corn syrup, maple syrup, and fructose.

Know your fats: Look for foods low in saturated fats, trans fats, and cholesterol to help reduce the risk of heart disease (5% DV or less is low, 20% DV or more is high). Most of the fats you eat should be polyunsaturated and monounsaturated fats. Keep total fat intake between 20 percent and 35 percent of calories.

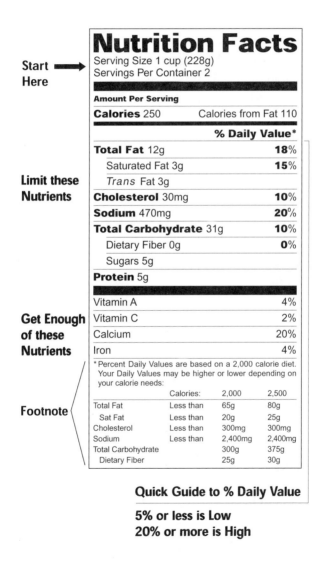

Figure 9.1. Nutrition Facts Label

Reduce sodium (salt), increase potassium: Research shows that eating less than 2,300 milligrams of sodium (about 1 tsp of salt) per day may reduce the risk of high blood pressure. Most of the sodium people eat comes from processed foods, not from the saltshaker. Also look for foods high in potassium, which counteracts some of sodium's effects on blood pressure.

Play It Safe with Food

Know how to prepare, handle, and store food safely to keep you and your family safe:

- Clean hands, food-contact surfaces, fruits, and vegetables. To avoid spreading bacteria to other foods, meat and poultry should not be washed or rinsed.

- Separate raw, cooked, and ready-to-eat foods while shopping, preparing, or storing.

Table 9.1. Safe Cooking and Holding Temperatures for Foods

Temperature	Appropriate For
180° F	Whole poultry
170° F	Poultry breasts
165° F	Stuffing, ground poultry, reheat leftovers
160° F	Meats (medium), egg dishes, pork, and ground meats
145° F	Beef steaks, roasts, veal, lamb (medium rare)
140° F	Hold hot foods
41°–139° F	DANGER ZONE
40° F	Refrigerator temperatures
0° F	Freezer temperatures

- Cook meat, poultry, and fish to safe internal temperatures to kill microorganisms.

- Chill perishable foods promptly and thaw foods properly.

About Alcohol

If you choose to drink alcohol, do so in moderation. Moderate drinking means up to one drink a day for women and up to two drinks for men. Twelve ounces of regular beer, 5 ounces of wine, or 1.5 ounces of 80-proof distilled spirits count as a drink for purposes of explaining moderation. Remember that alcoholic beverages have calories but are low in nutritional value.

Generally, anything more than moderate drinking can be harmful to your health. Some people, or people in certain situations, shouldn't drink at all. If you have questions or concerns, talk to your doctor or healthcare provider.

Chapter 10

A Healthy Diet: Key to Preserving Good Health

Chapter Contents

Section 10.1

Understanding the Food Groups in the Daily Food Guide

Excerpted from "Heart Healthy Diet: Daily Food Guide Food Groups," National Heart, Lung, and Blood Institute, National Institutes of Health. This document is available online at http://nhlbisupport.com/chd1/ Tipsheets/foodgroup.htm; accessed January 18, 2007.

Meat, Poultry, Fish, Dry Beans, Eggs, and Nuts

To keep your blood cholesterol level low, choose only the leanest meats, poultry, fish, and shellfish:

- Choose chicken and turkey without skin or remove skin before eating.

- Some fish, like cod, have less saturated fat than either chicken or meat.

- Since even the leanest meat, chicken, fish, and shellfish have saturated fat and cholesterol, limit the total amount you eat to six ounces or less per day.

Poultry

In general, chicken and turkey are low in saturated fat, especially when the skin is removed. When shopping for poultry remember the following things:

- You can buy chicken and turkey pieces with the skin already removed. Or buy pieces with the skin on and remove it yourself before eating . . . it's easy to do. Remember, the white meat itself always contains less saturated fat than the dark meat.

- Limit goose and duck. They are high in saturated fat, even with the skin removed.

- Try fresh ground turkey or chicken that is made from white meat like the breast.

- Remember that some chicken and turkey hot dogs are lower in saturated fat and total fat than pork and beef hot dogs. There are also "lean" beef hot dogs and vegetarian (made with tofu) franks that are low in fat and saturated fat.

Fish and Shellfish

When shopping for fish and shellfish remember these tips:

- Most fish is lower in saturated fat and cholesterol than meat or poultry.

- Shellfish varies in cholesterol content. Shellfish have little saturated fat and total fat. Even shrimp can be enjoyed occasionally on a heart healthy diet, provided you eat fewer than 300 milligrams of cholesterol a day. For example, three ounces of steamed shrimp has 167 milligrams of cholesterol.

Meat Substitute

Dry peas and beans and tofu (bean curd) are great meat substitutes that are low in saturated fat and cholesterol. Dry peas and beans also have a lot of fiber, which can help to lower blood cholesterol. Try adding one-half cup beans to pasta, soups, casseroles, and vegetable dishes. Tofu takes on the flavor of marinades well. Try marinating tofu in a nonfat dressing or a tangy sauce and grilling or baking for a heart healthy dish.

Eggs

Egg yolks are high in dietary cholesterol—each contains about 213 milligrams. So, egg yolks are limited to no more than four yolks per week. This includes the egg yolks in baked goods and processed foods. Check the label to see how much cholesterol the food contains or ask the bakery if the recipe uses whole eggs. Limit these types of foods for occasional treats.

Egg whites have no cholesterol, and you can substitute them for whole eggs in recipes—two egg whites are equal to one whole egg. You can also use cholesterol-free egg substitute in place of whole eggs. In many baked goods, you can't tell the difference.

Milk, Yogurt, and Cheese Group

Like high-fat meats, regular dairy foods that have fat—such as whole and 2% milk, cheese, and ice cream—are also high in saturated fat and cholesterol. However, dairy products are an important source of nutrients. You should eat two to three servings per day of low-fat or nonfat dairy products. Here is a guide to buying low fat and non-fat dairy foods.

Milk

Buy fat-free and 1% milk rather than whole or 2% milk. Fat-free and 1% milk have just as much or more calcium and other nutrients as whole milk—with much less saturated fat and cholesterol.

Make the Change, Step by Step: If you now drink whole milk, you will probably find it easier to change to fat-free milk in steps so your taste buds can adjust. Drink 2% milk for a few weeks, then 1% milk and finally fat free. You'll get used to the new taste gradually. And, with each step, you'll cut down on the saturated fat and cholesterol.

Cheese

When looking for hard cheeses, go for the versions that are "fat free," "reduced fat," "low fat," or "part skim." Choose varieties that have three grams of fat or less per ounce.

When looking for soft cheeses, choose low-fat (1%) or nonfat cottage cheese, farmer cheese, or part-skim or light ricotta. Some of these cheeses have three grams of fat or less per ounce.

If you are watching your sodium intake, choose lower sodium cheeses. Read the label to compare the sodium content.

Frozen Dairy Desserts

Buy frozen desserts that are lower in saturated fat, like ice milk, low-fat frozen yogurt, low-fat frozen dairy desserts, fruit ices, sorbets, and popsicles.

Other Dairy Foods

Buy low or nonfat yogurt; like many other dairy foods, it is an excellent source of protein and calcium. Eat low-fat or nonfat yogurt alone or as a topping or in recipes. Try topping with fruit.

Try low-fat or nonfat sour cream or cream cheese blends. Many taste as rich as the real thing, but have less fat and calories.

Fats and Oils

You can help keep your blood cholesterol low when you replace saturated fats with unsaturated fat. Just be sure to limit the total amount of fats or oils to keep calories in check.

When buying fats and oils, remember to do the following:

- Choose liquid vegetable oils that are high in unsaturated fats—like canola, corn, olive, peanut, safflower, sesame, soybean, and sunflower oils.

- Buy margarine made with unsaturated liquid vegetable oils as the first ingredient. Choose soft tub or liquid margarine or vegetable oil spreads.

- Limit butter, lard, fatback, and solid shortenings. They are high in saturated fat and cholesterol.

- Buy light or nonfat mayonnaise and salad dressing instead of the regular kind that is high in fat. For example, two tablespoons of regular Italian dressing can add as many as fourteen grams of fat.

A Word about Margarine

You may have heard that margarine has a type of unsaturated fat called "trans" fat. "Trans" fats raise blood cholesterol more than other unsaturated fats, but not as much as saturated fats. "Trans" fats are formed when vegetable oil is hardened to become margarine or shortening, through a process called "hydrogenation." The harder the margarine or shortening, the more likely it is to contain more "trans" fat. Margarines that are free of "trans" fats are now available. Read the ingredient label to choose margarine that is "trans" fat free or contains liquid vegetable oil as the first ingredient rather than hydrogenated or partially hydrogenated oil. Use the food label to choose margarine with the least amount of saturated fat.

Fruits and Vegetables

You should be eating at least three to five servings of fruits and vegetables each day. Fruits and vegetables are very low in saturated fat and total fat, and have no cholesterol. A diet high in fruit and vegetables may also help keep cholesterol levels low. So, fruits and vegetables are great substitutes for foods high in saturated fat and cholesterol.

When shopping, remember to do the following:

• Buy fruits and vegetables to eat as snacks, desserts, salads, side dishes, and main dishes.

• Add a variety of vegetables to meat stews or casseroles or make a vegetarian (meatless) main dish.

• Wash and cut up raw vegetables (carrot, broccoli, cauliflower, lettuce, etc.) and store in the refrigerator for quick and easy use in cooking or snacking.

• Serve fresh fruit for dessert or freeze (banana, berries, melon, grapes) for a delicious frozen treat.

• Display fresh fruit in a bowl in the kitchen to make fruit easier to grab as a snack.

To keep naturally low-fat vegetables low in fat and saturated fat, season with herbs, spices, lemon juice, vinegar, or fat-free or low-fat mayonnaise or salad dressing.

Breads, Cereals, Rice, Pasta, and Other Grains

Breads, cereals, rice, pasta, and other grains, and dry beans and peas are generally high in starch and fiber and low in saturated fat and calories. They also have no dietary cholesterol, except for some bakery breads and sweet bread products made with high-fat, high-cholesterol milk, butter, and eggs.

Like fruits and vegetables, naturally low fat, low cholesterol breads and other foods in this group are also good choices. You should be eating six to eleven servings of foods from this group each day. If you have high triglycerides or low high-density lipoprotein (HDL), you should keep your carbohydrate intake below the maximum of 60 percent of total calories. You can choose a diet up to 35 percent fat, substituting unsaturated fat for saturated fat.

When buying foods from this group, remember to do the following:

• Choose whole-grain breads and rolls often. They have more fiber than white breads.

• Buy dry cereals, as most are low in fat. Limit the high-fat granola, muesli, and oat bran types that are made with coconut or coconut oil and nuts, which increase the saturated fat content. Add fat-free milk or 1% milk instead of whole or low-fat (2%) milk to save saturated fat and cholesterol.

- Buy pasta and rice to use as entrees. Hold the high-fat sauces (butter, cheese, cream, white).

- Limit sweet baked goods that are made with lots of saturated fat, mostly from butter, eggs, and whole milk such as croissants, pastries, muffins, biscuits, butter rolls, and doughnuts. These are also high in cholesterol.

Sweets and Snacks

Some sweets and snacks—like baked goods (cakes and cookies), cheese crackers, and some chips—often are high in saturated fat and cholesterol.

Here are some low-fat sweets and snacks to buy and use only now and then:

- Angel food cake topped with fruit puree or fresh fruit slices

- Fat-free or low-fat brownies, cakes, cheesecake, cupcakes, and pastries

- Fat-free or low-fat cookies like animal crackers, devil's food cookies, fig and other fruit bars, ginger snaps, and vanilla or lemon wafers

- Frozen low-fat or nonfat yogurt, fruit ices, ice milk, sherbet, and sorbet

- Gelatin desserts—watch the whipped cream!

- Graham crackers

- Puddings made with 1% or fat-free milk

Just remember that, while these treats may be low in fat, most are not low in calories. So choose them only every now and then, especially if you are trying to control your weight to improve your blood cholesterol levels.

Not all snack foods are high in saturated fat and cholesterol. Buy some of these low-fat ones and keep them on hand for snack attacks:

- Bagels

- Bread sticks

- Ready-to-eat cereals without added sugar

- Frozen grapes or banana slices or other fresh fruit

- Fruit leather or other dried fruit
- Low-fat or fat-free crackers like melba toast, rice cakes, rye crisp, and soda crackers
- No-oil baked tortilla chips
- Popcorn (air popped or "light")
- Pretzels
- Raw vegetables with nonfat or low-fat dip

If you are watching your sodium intake, be sure to look for low-sodium or unsalted varieties of these items.

Section 10.2

Calcium and Vitamin D: Important at Every Age

Reprinted from the National Institute of Arthritis and Musculoskeletal and Skin Diseases, National Institutes of Health, November 2005.

The foods we eat contain a variety of vitamins, minerals, and other important nutrients that help keep our bodies healthy. Two nutrients in particular, calcium and vitamin D, are needed for strong bones.

The Role of Calcium

Calcium is needed for our heart, muscles, and nerves to function properly and for blood to clot. Inadequate calcium significantly contributes to the development of osteoporosis. Many published studies show that low calcium intake throughout life is associated with low bone mass and high fracture rates. National nutrition surveys have shown that most people are not getting the calcium they need to grow and maintain healthy bones. To find out how much calcium you need, see the recommended calcium intakes chart in Table 10.1.

Table 10.1. Recommended Calcium Intakes

Age	Amount of Calcium
Infants	
Birth–6 months	210 mg
6 months–1 year	270 mg
Children/Young Adults	
1–3 years	500 mg
4–8 years	800 mg
9–18 years	1,300 mg
Adult Women and Men	
19–50 years	1,000 mg
50+ years	1,200 mg
Pregnant or Lactating	
18 years or younger	1,300 mg
19–50 years	1,000 mg

Source: National Academy of Sciences, 1997.

To learn how easily you can include more calcium in your diet without adding much fat, see the Selected Calcium-Rich Foods list in Table 10.2.

You may also increase the calcium in foods by following these suggestions:

1. Add nonfat powdered milk to all soups, casseroles, and drinks.

2. Buy juices, cereals, and breads that are fortified with calcium.

3. Replace whole milk and cream with skim and low-fat milk in recipes.

4. Replace sour cream with yogurt in recipes.

5. Some bottled waters contain calcium, so check the labels for more information.

Table 10.2. Selected Calcium-Rich Foods

Food Item	Serving Size	Calcium (mg)	Fat (g)	Calories
Milk				
Whole	8 oz	290	8.9	156
1% milk	8 oz	300	2.6	102
2% milk	8 oz	297	4.7	121
Skim milk	8 oz	302	0.4	86
Yogurt				
Plain fat-free (with added milk solids)	8 oz	487	0.4	136
Plain low-fat (with added milk solids)	8 oz	447	3.7	155
Fruit, low-fat	8 oz	338	2.8	243
Frozen, vanilla, soft serve	1/2 cup	103	4.0	114
Cheese				
American cheese	1 oz	174	8.9	106
Cheddar cheese	1 oz	204	9.4	114
Cottage cheese, 1% low-fat	1 cup	138	2.3	164
Mozzarella cheese, part skim	1 oz	183	4.5	72
Muenster cheese	1 oz	203	8.5	104
Parmesan cheese, grated	1 tbsp	69	1.5	23
Ricotta cheese, part skim	1/2 cup	337	9.8	171
Ricotta cheese, whole milk	1/2 cup	257	16.1	216
Ice Cream, Vanilla				
Low-fat	1/2 cup	91.7	2.8	91.7
High-fat	1/2 cup	86.6	12	178

Table 10.2. Selected Calcium-Rich Foods, continued

Food Item	Serving Size	Calcium (mg)	Fat (g)	Calories
Fish and Shellfish				
Sardines, canned in oil, drained, including bones	3.75 oz	351	10.5	191
Salmon, pink, canned, including bones	3 oz	181	5.1	118
Shrimp, canned, drained	3 oz	50	1.7	102
Vegetables				
Bok choy, raw (Chinese cabbage)	1 cup	74	0	9
Broccoli, cooked, drained from raw	1 cup	71.6	0.6	23.6
Broccoli, cooked, drained, from frozen	1 cup	94	0.2	50
Soybeans, mature, boiled	1 cup	261	12	254
Collards, cooked, drained, from raw	1 cup	226	0.6	49
Turnip greens, cooked, drained, from raw (leaves and stems)	1 cup	197	0.3	29
Tofu	1/2 cup	204[a]	5.6	97
Orange (navel)	1 whole	56	0.1	65
Orange Juice, fortified with calcium	8 oz	300	0.1	100
Dried figs	10	270	2.2	477
Almonds (dry roasted)	1 oz	75	15	169
Sesame seeds, kernels, toasted	1 oz	37	13.6	161
Sunflower seeds, dried	1 oz	33	14.1	162

Source: USDA Nutrient Data Laboratory, 2000.
[a]The calcium content of tofu may vary depending on processing methods. Tofu processed with calcium salts can have as much as 300 mg (milligrams) for every 4 oz. Often, the label or the manufacturer can provide more specific information.

Calcium Culprits

While a balanced diet aids calcium absorption, high levels of protein and sodium (salt) in the diet are thought to increase calcium excretion through the kidneys. Excessive amounts of these substances should be avoided, especially in those whose calcium intake is low.

Lactose intolerance also can lead to inadequate calcium intake. Those who are lactose intolerant have insufficient amounts of the enzyme lactase, which is needed to break down the lactose found in dairy products. In order to include dairy products in the diet, dairy foods can be taken in small quantities or treated with lactase drops, or lactase can be taken as a pill. There are even some milk products on the market that already have been treated with lactase.

Calcium Supplements

If you have trouble getting enough calcium in your diet, you may need to take a calcium supplement. The amount of calcium you will need from a supplement depends on how much calcium you obtain from food sources. There are several different calcium compounds from which to choose, such as calcium carbonate and calcium citrate, among others. Except in people with gastrointestinal disease, all major forms of calcium supplements are absorbed equally well when taken with food.

Calcium supplements are better absorbed when taken in small doses (500 mg or less) several times throughout the day. In many individuals, calcium supplements are better absorbed when taken with food. It is important to check supplement labels to ensure that the product meets United States Pharmacopeia (USP) standards.

Vitamin D

The body needs vitamin D to absorb calcium. Without enough vitamin D, we can't form enough of the hormone calcitriol (known as the "active vitamin D"). This, in turn, leads to insufficient calcium absorption from the diet. In this situation, the body must take calcium from its stores in the skeleton, which weakens existing bone and prevents the formation of strong, new bone.

You can get vitamin D in three ways: through the skin, from the diet, and from supplements. Vitamin D is formed naturally by the body after exposure to sunlight. Fifteen minutes in the sun a few times a week without sunscreen is plenty for many people to manufacture and store all of the vitamin D they need. Experts recommend a daily intake of between 400 and 800 International Units (IU) of vitamin D, which also can be obtained from supplements or vitamin D-rich foods such as egg yolks, saltwater fish, liver, and fortified milk. The Institute of Medicine recommends no more than 2,000 IU per day. However, sometimes doctors prescribe higher doses for people who are deficient in vitamin D.

A Complete Osteoporosis Program

Remember, a balanced diet rich in calcium and vitamin D is only one part of an osteoporosis prevention or treatment program. Like exercise, getting enough calcium is a strategy that helps strengthen bones at any age. But these strategies may not be enough to stop bone loss caused by lifestyle, medications, or menopause. It is important to speak to your doctor to determine the need for an osteoporosis medication in addition to diet and exercise.

Section 10.3

Diet and Disease

Excerpted from "Diet and Disease," © 2007 A.D.A.M., Inc.
Reprinted with permission.

There are nutritional and dietary elements that have proven relationships to certain diseases or conditions.

Calcium and Osteoporosis

Calcium is one of the most important minerals for human life. The body uses it to form and maintain healthy bones and teeth. Calcium also plays a vital role in nerve conduction, muscle contraction, and blood clotting.

Osteoporosis is a disease in which the calcium content of bones is very low. In this disease, calcium and phosphorus, which are normally present in the bones, become reabsorbed back into the body. This process results in brittle, fragile bones that are easily broken.

Getting enough calcium in the diet throughout childhood and puberty is one key to preventing osteoporosis. A person who does not get enough calcium growing up will not have sturdy bones. An older person who is on a low-calcium diet is also at great risk for osteoporosis.

The recommended dietary allowances (RDA) for calcium are based on age, gender, and hormonal factors. Many foods, such as some vegetables, contain calcium. However, milk and dairy products are some of the best food sources. Calcium may also be obtained by taking supplements.

Fiber and Cancer

Dietary fiber is found in plant foods, where it occurs in two forms: soluble and insoluble. Soluble fiber attracts water and turns to gel during digestion. This process slows digestion and the rate of nutrient absorption from the stomach and intestine.

Soluble fiber is found in oat bran, barley, nuts, seeds, dried beans and legumes, lentils, peas, and some fruits and vegetables. Insoluble fiber also adds bulk (fiber) to the stool. It is found in wheat bran, vegetables, and whole grains.

A diet high in fiber is thought to reduce the risk of cancers of the rectum and colon.

Fruits, Vegetables, and Cancer

Eating more fruits and vegetables helps provide a good supply of fiber, vitamin A, vitamin C, beta carotene and other carotenoids, and valuable substances called phytochemicals. Studies have shown that a diet high in these nutrients and fiber can reduce the risk of developing cancers of the stomach, colon, rectum, esophagus, larynx, and lung.

Vitamin C and beta carotene, which forms vitamin A, are antioxidants. As such, they protect body cells from oxidation, a process that can lead to cell damage and may play a role in cancer.

In addition to nutrients that are needed for normal metabolism, plant foods also contain phytochemicals, plant chemicals that may affect human health. There are hundreds of phytochemicals, and their exact role in promoting health is still uncertain. However, a growing body of evidence indicates that phytochemicals may help protect against cancer.

To get these benefits, eat more fruits and vegetables that contain vitamins A and C and beta carotene. These include dark-green leafy vegetables such as spinach, kale, collards, and turnip greens. Citrus fruits, such as oranges, grapefruit, and tangerines are also high in antioxidants. Other red, yellow, and orange fruits and vegetables or their juices are also healthful choices. Note: Juicing removes the fiber.

Fiber and Coronary Heart Disease

Some fiber, especially soluble fiber, binds to lipids such as choles-terol. The fiber then carries the lipids out of the body through the stool. This lowers the concentration of lipids in the blood and may reduce the risk of coronary heart disease.

Fat and Cancer

A diet high in fat has been shown to increase the risk of cancers of the breast, colon, and prostate. A high-fat diet does not necessarily cause cancer. Rather, it may promote the development of cancer in people who are exposed to cancer-causing agents.

A diet high in fat may promote cancer by causing the body to se-crete more of certain hormones that create a favorable environment for certain types of cancer. Breast cancer is one of these hormone-influenced cancers. High-fat diets also may change the characteristics of the cells to make them more vulnerable to cancer-causing agents.

To reduce fat in the diet, choose lean cuts of beef, lamb, and pork as well as skinless poultry and fish. Baking, broiling, poaching, and steaming are recommended cooking methods. Choose skim or low-fat milk and dairy products, as well as low-fat salad dressings.

Saturated Fat, Cholesterol, and Coronary Heart Disease

Eating too much saturated fat is one of the major risk factors for heart disease. A diet high in saturated fat causes cholesterol, a soft, waxy substance, to build up in the arteries. Eventually, the arteries harden and narrow. The result is an increased pressure in the arter-ies as well as strain on the heart to maintain adequate blood flow throughout the body.

Because of its high calorie content, too much dietary fat also increases the risk of heart disease in that it increases the likelihood that a person will become obese. Obesity is another risk factor for heart disease.

Sodium and Hypertension

Sodium is a mineral that helps the body regulate blood pressure. Sodium is also commonly known as salt. It also plays a role in the proper functioning of cell membranes, muscles, and nerves. Sodium concentration in the body is mainly controlled by the kidneys, adre-nal glands, and the pituitary gland in the brain.

The balance between dietary intake and kidney excretion through urine determines the amount of sodium in the body. Only a small amount of sodium is lost through the stool or sweat. The amount of sodium in urine is controlled by the steroid hormone aldosterone. Water and sodium are also related. Retention of more sodium is followed by retention of more fluid, and vice versa.

Sodium-sensitive individuals may experience high blood pressure from too much sodium in the diet. The American Heart Association has developed specific guidelines for sodium intake. Dietary changes may be helpful. Sodium intake may have little effect in persons without high blood pressure, but it may have a profound effect in sodium-sensitive individuals. Blood pressure is often controlled by diuretics that cause sodium excretion in the urine.

Alcohol

Alcohol use increases the risk of liver cancer. When combined with smoking, alcohol intake also increases the risk of cancers of the mouth, throat, larynx, and esophagus. In addition, alcohol intake is associated with an increased risk of breast cancer in women.

Alcohol is processed by the liver into energy for the body. Continued and excessive use of alcohol can damage the liver in various ways, including the development of a fatty liver. A fatty liver can lead to cirrhosis of the liver.

Alcohol can damage the lining of the small intestine and stomach, where most nutrients are digested. As a result, alcohol can impair the absorption of essential nutrients. Alcohol also increases the body's need for some nutrients, and interferes with the absorption and storage of other nutrients.

Continued and excessive use of alcohol can result in an increase in blood pressure. Chronic heavy drinking also can cause damage to the heart muscle (cardiomyopathy). In addition, stroke is associated with both chronic heavy drinking and binge drinking.

If you choose to drink alcohol, do so in moderation—no more than two drinks per day for a man, one per day for a woman.

Nitrates and Cancer

Countries in which people eat a lot of salt-cured, smoked, and nitrite-cured foods have a high rate of cancer of the stomach and esophagus. Examples of such foods include bacon, ham, hot dogs, and salt-cured fish.

Eat salted, smoked, or cured foods only on occasion.

Chapter 11

Physical Activity Can Keep You Healthy

Chapter Contents

Section 11.1

Physical Activity and Health

Excerpted from "Physical Activity and Health At-a-Glance," National Center for Chronic Disease Prevention and Health Promotion, Centers for Disease Control and Prevention, November 17, 1999. Reviewed by David A. Cooke, M.D., May 2007.

A New View of Physical Activity

This section brings together what has been learned about physical activity and health from decades of research. Major findings are as follows:

- People who are usually inactive can improve their health and well-being by becoming even moderately active on a regular basis.

- Physical activity need not be strenuous to achieve health benefits.

- Greater health benefits can be achieved by increasing the amount (duration, frequency, or intensity) of physical activity.

The Benefits of Regular Physical Activity

Regular physical activity that is performed on most days of the week reduces the risk of developing or dying from some of the leading causes of illness and death in the United States. Regular physical activity improves health in the following ways:

- It reduces the risk of dying prematurely.

- It reduces the risk of dying from heart disease.

- It reduces the risk of developing diabetes.

- It reduces the risk of developing high blood pressure.

- It helps reduce blood pressure in people who already have high blood pressure.

- It reduces the risk of developing colon cancer.

- It reduces feelings of depression and anxiety.

- It helps control weight.

- It helps build and maintain healthy bones, muscles, and joints.

- It helps older adults become stronger and better able to move about without falling.

- It promotes psychological well-being.

A Major Public Health Concern

Given the numerous health benefits of physical activity, the hazards of being inactive are clear. Physical inactivity is a serious, nationwide problem. Its scope poses a public health challenge for reducing the national burden of unnecessary illness and premature death.

What Is a Moderate Amount of Physical Activity?

As the following list shows, a moderate amount of physical activity (roughly equivalent to physical activity that uses approximately 150 calories [kcal] of energy per day, or 1,000 calories per week) can be achieved in a variety of ways. People can select activities that they enjoy and that fit into their daily lives. Because amount of activity is a function of duration, intensity, and frequency, the same amount of activity can be obtained in longer sessions of moderately intense activities (such as brisk walking) as in shorter sessions of more strenuous activities (such as running). Some activities can be performed at various intensities; the suggested durations correspond to expected intensity of effort.

Examples of Moderate Amounts of Activity

The following activities are listed in order from those that are less vigorous and take more time to those that are more vigorous and take less time:

- Washing and waxing a car for 45–60 minutes

- Washing windows or floors for 45–60 minutes

- Playing volleyball for 45 minutes

- Playing touch football for 30–45 minutes

- Gardening for 30–45 minutes
- Wheeling self in wheelchair for 30–40 minutes
- Walking 1.75 miles in 35 minutes (20 minutes/mile)
- Basketball (shooting baskets) for 30 minutes
- Bicycling 5 miles in 30 minutes
- Dancing fast (social) for 30 minutes
- Pushing a stroller 1.5 miles in 30 minutes
- Raking leaves for 30 minutes
- Walking 2 miles in 30 minutes (15 minutes/mile)
- Water aerobics for 30 minutes
- Swimming laps for 20 minutes
- Wheelchair basketball for 20 minutes
- Basketball (playing a game) for 15–20 minutes
- Bicycling 4 miles in 15 minutes
- Jumping rope for 15 minutes
- Running 1.5 miles in 15 minutes (10 minutes/mile)
- Shoveling snow for 15 minutes
- Stair walking for 15 minutes

Precautions for a Healthy Start

To avoid soreness and injury, individuals contemplating an increase in physical activity should start out slowly and gradually build up to the desired amount to give the body time to adjust. People with chronic health problems, such as heart disease, diabetes, or obesity, or who are at high risk for these problems should first consult a physician before beginning a new program of physical activity. Also, men over age forty and women over age fifty who plan to begin a new vigorous physical activity program should consult a physician first to be sure they do not have heart disease or other health problems.

Section 11.2

Physical Activity and Chronic Disease Prevention

The benefits of regular physical activity in preventing chronic disease have been reported widely. Regular physical activity can also help manage the symptoms of chronic disease and improve quality of life. For example, swimming can reduce pain in people with arthritis.

The Surgeon General of the United States, the National Institutes of Health, the Centers for Disease Control and Prevention, the American College of Sports Medicine, and the American Heart Association have all written reports about these important health benefits.

What are the chronic diseases that regular physical activity can help prevent or manage?

- Heart disease
- High blood pressure
- Colon cancer
- Type 2 diabetes
- Osteoarthritis
- Depression and anxiety

What are other benefits to regular physical activity?

- Greater sense of well-being
- Maintain proper body weight
- Improve strength and flexibility
- Increase energy
- Improve balance

- Improve sleep
- Prevent falls and fractures

How much physical activity does a person need?

According to the groups named previously, to maintain good health every person should accumulate thirty minutes or more of moderate-intensity physical activity throughout the day, on five or more days of the week. Please be aware that this is a goal to set for yourself, not something you have to be doing today. If you have a chronic disease or are inactive, consult your healthcare provider before you begin an exercise program.

What is considered moderate physical activity?

Moderate physical activity can be almost any activity that makes you feel the way you do when you walk briskly for thirty minutes. These include the following:

- Dancing
- Riding a bike
- Gardening
- Vacuuming
- Swimming
- Hiking
- Wheeling oneself in a wheelchair

Also, these activities can be done ten minutes at a time over the course of the day, instead of thirty minutes at one time.

What if I'm not currently physically active?

Even small increases in light to moderate activity will improve your health if you are not currently active. It is important to start slowly and check with your healthcare provider before getting started. Keep in mind that the recommendations listed above are goals to try to reach over a period of time. For people who are inactive or who have a chronic disease, try starting with five minutes a day and find something you like to do. Then gradually increase your activity level. Find something that you enjoy doing and stick with it.

What if I have a chronic disease?

As mentioned previously, physical activity can be extremely helpful for people with chronic disease. The following are some specific recommendations for those with certain chronic diseases.

Heart disease: Exercise is important in the prevention and management of heart disease. According to the National Institute of Health, it can reduce symptoms, improve ability and capacity to exercise, improve psychological well-being, and reduce the chance of dying from heart disease. You need to work very closely with your healthcare provider to design an exercise program that is safe for you. Many hospitals have rehabilitation programs specifically designed for people who have heart disease. Do not begin an exercise program on your own.

Asthma and other lung diseases: Lung diseases include asthma, chronic obstructive pulmonary disease, emphysema, and other conditions that decrease your ability to breathe. Physical activity can help increase the length of time you are able to do things (like walking), reduce your symptoms, and decrease the number of hospital visits. Begin with low-intensity exercise and gradually increase as your shortness of breath begins to decrease. Work with your healthcare provider to determine the best exercise program for you.

Some things to keep in mind:

- Use your medicine, particularly your inhaler, before your exercise to help you exercise longer with less shortness of breath.

- If you become severely short of breath with only minimal exertion, check with your healthcare provider about changing your medicines. He or she may even suggest having you use supplemental oxygen before you begin your activities.

- It is important to take plenty of time to warm up and cool down before and after exercise. For those with exercise-induced asthma, a six- to ten-minute warm-up period before exercising is recommended.

- Keep your level of exercise well below those levels that cause severe shortness of breath.

- Swimming can be quite helpful for those with chronic lung disease, since cold and dry air can make breathing and exercising more difficult.

- Strengthening exercises such as light weightlifting and rowing may be helpful, particularly for people who have become weakened or deconditioned from medications such as steroids.

Diabetes: Regular physical activity can help a person with diabetes control the disease in several ways. Physical activity can:

- control blood glucose levels;

- decrease the need for insulin;

- improve circulation; and

- help with weight loss.

Mild to moderate aerobic exercise for no more than forty minutes as part of a general conditioning program can help control diabetes. Again, consult with your healthcare provider before starting an exercise program if you have diabetes. It's important to have your diabetes under good control and to work with your provider to coordinate changes in other parts of your diabetes management plan.

Section 11.3

Exercise and Weight Control

Reprinted from the President's Council on Physical Fitness and Sports,
October 15, 2004.

Just about everybody seems to be interested in weight control.
Some of us weigh just the right amount, others need to gain a few
pounds. Most of us "battle the bulge" at some time in our life. Whatever our goals, we should understand and take advantage of the important role of exercise in keeping our weight under control.

Carrying around too much body fat is a major nuisance. Yet excess
body fat is common in modern-day living. Few of today's occupations
require vigorous physical activity, and much of our leisure time is
spent in sedentary pursuits.

Recent estimates indicate that thirty-four million adults are considered obese (20 percent above desirable weight). Also, there has been
an increase in body fat levels in children and youth over the past
twenty years. After infancy and early childhood, the earlier the onset
of obesity, the greater the likelihood of remaining obese.

Excess body fat has been linked to such health problems as coronary heart disease, high blood pressure, osteoporosis, diabetes, arthritis, and certain forms of cancer. Some evidence now exists showing
that obesity has a negative effect on both health and longevity.

Exercise is associated with the loss of body fat in both obese and normal weight persons. A regular program of exercise is an important component of any plan to help individuals lose, gain, or maintain their weight.

Overweight or Overfat?

Overweight and overfat do not always mean the same thing. Some
people are quite muscular and weigh more than the average for their
age and height. However, their body composition, the amount of fat
versus lean body mass (muscle, bone, organs, and tissue), is within a
desirable range. This is true for many athletes. Others weigh an average amount yet carry around too much fat. In our society, however,
overweight often implies overfat because excess weight is commonly

121

distributed as excess fat. The addition of exercise to a weight control program helps control both body weight and body fat levels.

A certain amount of body fat is necessary for everyone. Experts say that body fat for women should be about 20 percent, 15 percent for men. Women with more than 30 percent fat and men with more than 25 percent fat are considered obese.

How much of your weight is fat can be assessed by a variety of methods including underwater (hydrostatic) weighing, skin fold thickness measurements, and circumference measurements. Each requires a specially trained person to administer the test and perform the correct calculations. From the numbers obtained, a body fat percentage is determined. Assessing body composition has an advantage over the standard height-weight tables because it can help distinguish between "overweight" and "overfat."

An easy self-test you can do is to pinch the thickness of the fat folds at your waist and abdomen. If you can pinch an inch or more of fat (make sure no muscle is included), chances are you have too much body fat.

People who exercise appropriately increase lean body mass while decreasing their overall fat level. Depending on the amount of fat loss, this can result in a loss of inches without a loss of weight, since muscle weighs more than fat. However, with the proper combination of diet and exercise, both body fat and overall weight can be reduced.

Energy Balance: A Weighty Concept

Losing weight, gaining weight, or maintaining your weight depends on the amount of calories you take in and use up during the day, otherwise referred to as energy balance. Learning how to balance energy intake (calories in food) with energy output (calories expended through physical activity) will help you achieve your desired weight.

Although the underlying causes and the treatments of obesity are complex, the concept of energy balance is relatively simple. If you eat more calories than your body needs to perform your day's activities, the extra calories are stored as fat. If you do not take in enough calories to meet your body's energy needs, your body will go to the stored fat to make up the difference. (Exercise helps ensure that stored fat, rather than muscle tissue, is used to meet your energy needs.) If you eat just about the same amount of calories as is needed to meet your body's energy needs, your weight will stay the same.

On the average, a person consumes between 800,000 and 900,000 calories each year! An active person needs more calories than a sedentary person, as physically active people require energy above and beyond the day's basic needs. All too often, people who want to lose weight concentrate on counting calorie intake while neglecting calorie output. The most powerful formula is the combination of dietary modification with exercise. By increasing your daily physical activity and decreasing your caloric input you can lose excess weight in the most efficient and healthful way.

Counting Calories

Each pound of fat your body stores represents 3,500 calories of unused energy. In order to lose one pound, you would have to create a calorie deficit of 3,500 calories by either taking in 3,500 fewer calories over a period of time than you need or doing 3,500 calories worth of exercise. It is recommended that no more than two pounds (7,000 calories) be lost per week for lasting weight loss.

Adding fifteen minutes of moderate exercise, say walking one mile, to your daily schedule will use up 100 extra calories per day. (Your body uses approximately 100 calories of energy to walk one mile, depending on your body weight.) Maintaining this schedule would result in an extra 700 calories per week used up, or a loss of about 10 pounds in one year, assuming your food intake stays the same. To look at energy balance another way, just one extra slice of bread or one extra soft drink a day—or any other food that contains approximately 100 calories—can add up to ten extra pounds in a year if the amount of physical activity you do does not increase.

If you already have a lean figure and want to keep it you should exercise regularly and eat a balanced diet that provides enough calories to make up for the energy you expend. If you wish to gain weight you should exercise regularly and increase the number of calories you consume until you reach your desired weight. Exercise will help ensure that the weight you gain will be lean muscle mass, not extra fat.

The Diet Connection

A balanced diet should be part of any weight control plan. A diet high in complex carbohydrates and moderate in protein and fat will complement an exercise program. It should include enough calories to satisfy your daily nutrient requirements and include the proper number of servings per day from the "basic four food groups": vegetables and fruits (four servings), breads and cereals (four servings), milk and milk products (two to four servings, depending on age) and meats and fish (two servings).

Experts recommend that your daily intake not fall below 1200 calories unless you are under a doctor's supervision. Also, weekly weight loss should not exceed two pounds.

Remarkable claims have been made for a variety of "crash" diets and diet pills. Some of these very restricted diets do result in noticeable weight loss in a short time. Much of this loss is water and such a loss is quickly regained when normal food and liquid intake is resumed. These diet plans are often expensive and may be dangerous. Moreover, they do not emphasize lifestyle changes that will help you maintain your desired weight. Dieting alone will result in a loss of valuable body tissue such as muscle mass in addition to a loss in fat.

How Many Calories

The estimates for number of calories (energy) used during a physical activity are based on experiments that measure the amount of oxygen consumed during a specific bout of exercise for a certain body weight.

The energy costs of activities that require you to move your own body weight, such as walking or jogging, are greater for heavier people since they have more weight to move. For example, a person weighing 150 pounds would use more calories jogging one mile than a person jogging alongside who weighs 115 pounds. Always check to see what body weight is referred to in caloric expenditure charts you use.

Exercise and Modern Living

One thing is certain. Most people do not get enough exercise in their ordinary routines. All of the advances of modern technology—from electric can openers to power steering—have made life easier, more comfortable, and much less physically demanding. Yet our bodies need activity, especially if they are carrying around too much fat. Satisfying this need requires a definite plan, and a commitment. There are two main ways to increase the number of calories you expend:

1. Start a regular exercise program if you do not have one already.

2. Increase the amount of physical activity in your daily routine.

The best way to control your weight is a combination of the above. The sum total of calories used over time will help regulate your weight as well as keep you physically fit.

Table 11.1. Energy Expenditure Chart

Sedentary Activities	Energy Costs (Cals/Hour)[a]
Lying down or sleeping	90
Sitting quietly	84
Sitting and writing, card playing, etc.	114
Moderate Activities	**150–350**
Bicycling (5 mph)	174
Canoeing (2.5 mph)	174
Dancing (Ballroom)	210
Golf (twosome, carrying clubs)	324
Horseback riding (sitting to trot)	246
Light housework, cleaning, etc.	246
Swimming (crawl, 20 yards/min)	288
Tennis (recreational doubles)	312
Volleyball (recreational)	264
Walking (2 mph)	198
Vigorous Activities	**More than 350**
Aerobic Dancing	546
Basketball (recreational)	450
Bicycling (13 mph)	612
Circuit weight training	756
Cross-Country Skiing (5 mph)	690
Football (touch, vigorous)	498
Ice Skating (9 mph)	384
Racquetball	588
Roller Skating (9 mph)	384
Jogging (10 minute mile, 6 mph)	654
Scrubbing Floors	440
Swimming (crawl, 45 yards/min)	522
Tennis (recreational singles)	450

[a] Hourly estimates based on values calculated for calories burned per minute for a 150 pound (68 kg) person.

Sources: William D. McArdle, Frank I. Katch, Victor L. Katch, *Exercise Physiology: Energy, Nutrition and Human Performance* (2nd edition), Lea & Febiger, Philadelphia, 1986; Melvin H. Williams, *Nutrition for Fitness and Sport*, William C. Brown Company Publishers, Dubuque, 1983.

Active Lifestyles

Before looking at what kind of regular exercise program is best, let's look at how you can increase the amount of physical activity in your daily routine to supplement your exercise program:

- Recreational pursuits such as gardening on weekends, bowling in the office league, family outings, an evening of social dancing, and many other activities provide added exercise. They are fun and can be considered an extra bonus in your weight control campaign.

- Add more "action" to your day. Walk to the neighborhood grocery store instead of using the car. Park several blocks from the office and walk the rest of the way. Walk up the stairs instead of using the elevator; start with one flight of steps and gradually increase.

- Change your attitude toward movement. Instead of considering an extra little walk or trip to the files an annoyance, look upon it as an added fitness boost. Look for opportunities to use your body. Bend, stretch, reach, move, lift and carry. Time-saving devices and gadgets eliminate drudgery and are a bonus to mankind, but when they substitute too often for physical activity they can demand a high cost in health, vigor, and fitness.

These little bits of action are cumulative in their effects. Alone, each does not burn a huge number of calories. When added together, however, they can result in a sizable amount of energy used over the course of the day. And they will help improve your muscle tone and flexibility at the same time.

What Kind of Exercise?

Although any kind of physical movement requires energy (calories), the type of exercise that uses the most energy is aerobic exercise. The term "aerobic" is derived from the Greek word meaning "with oxygen." Jogging, brisk walking, swimming, biking, cross-country skiing, and aerobic dancing are some popular forms of aerobic exercise.

Aerobic exercises use the body's large muscle groups in continuous, rhythmic, sustained movement and require oxygen for the production of energy. When oxygen is combined with food (which can come from stored fat) energy is produced to power the body's musculature. The longer you move aerobically, the more energy needed and the more calories used. Regular aerobic exercise will improve your cardiorespiratory endurance, the ability of your heart, lungs, blood vessels, and associated tissues to use oxygen to produce energy needed for activity. You'll build a healthier body while getting rid of excess body fat.

In addition to the aerobic exercise, supplement your program with muscle-strengthening and stretching exercises. The stronger your muscles, the longer you will be able to keep going during aerobic activity, and the less chance of injury.

How Much? How Often?

Experts recommend that you do some form of aerobic exercise at least three times a week for a minimum of twenty continuous minutes. Of course, if that is too much, start with a shorter time span and gradually build up to the minimum. Then gradually progress until you are able to work aerobically for twenty to forty minutes. If you need to lose a large amount of weight, you may want to do your aerobic workout five times a week.

It is important to exercise at an intensity vigorous enough to cause your heart rate and breathing to increase. How hard you should exercise depends to a certain degree on your age, and is determined by measuring your heart rate in beats per minute.

The heart rate you should maintain is called your target heart rate, and there are several ways you can arrive at this figure. The simplest is to subtract your age from 220 and then calculate 60 to 80 percent of that figure. Beginners should maintain the 60 percent level, more advanced can work up to the 80 percent level. This is just a guide however, and people with any medical limitations should discuss this formula with their physician.

You can do different types of aerobic activities, say walking one day, riding a bike the next. Make sure you choose an activity that can be done regularly and is enjoyable for you. The important thing to remember is not to skip too many days between workouts or fitness benefits will be lost. If you must lose a few days, gradually work back into your routine.

The Benefits of Exercise in a Weight Control Program

The benefits of exercise are many, from producing physically fit bodies to providing an outlet for fun and socialization. When added to a weight control program these benefits take on increased significance.

We already have noted that proper exercise can help control weight by burning excess body fat. It also has two other body-trimming advantages: exercise builds muscle tissue and muscle uses calories up at a faster rate than body fat; and exercise helps reduce inches and a firm, lean body looks slimmer even if your weight remains the same.

Remember, fat does not "turn into" muscle, as is often believed. Fat and muscle are two entirely different substances and one cannot become the other. However, muscle does use calories at a faster rate than fat, which directly affects your body's metabolic rate or energy requirement. Your basal metabolic rate (BMR) is the amount of energy required to sustain the body's functions at rest and it depends on your age, sex, body size, genes, and body composition. People with high levels of muscle tend to have higher BMRs and use more calories in the resting stage.

Some studies have even shown that your metabolic rate stays elevated for some time after vigorous exercise, causing you to use even more calories throughout your day. Additional benefits may be seen in how exercise affects appetite. A lean person in good shape may eat more following increased activity, but the regular exercise will burn up the extra calories consumed. On the other hand, vigorous exercise has been reported to suppress appetite. And physical activity can be used as a positive substitute for between-meal snacking.

Better Mental Health

The psychological benefits of exercise are equally important to the weight-conscious person. Exercise decreases stress and relieves tensions that might otherwise lead to overeating. Exercise builds physical fitness, which, in turn, builds self-confidence, enhanced self-image, and a positive outlook. When you start to feel good about yourself, you are more likely to want to make other positive changes in your lifestyle that will help keep your weight under control.

In addition, exercise can be fun, provide recreation, and offer opportunities for companionship. The exhilaration and emotional release of participating in sports or other activities are a boost to mental and physical health. Pent-up anxieties and frustrations seem to disappear when you're concentrating on returning a serve, sinking a putt, or going that extra mile.

Tips to Get You Started

Hopefully, you are now convinced that in order to successfully manage your weight you must include exercise in your daily routine. Here are some tips to get you started:

- Check with your doctor first. Since you are carrying around some extra "baggage," it is wise to get your doctor's "OK" before embarking on an exercise program.

- Choose activities that you think you'll enjoy. Most people will stick to their exercise program if they are having fun, even though they are working hard.

- Set aside a regular exercise time. Whether this means joining an exercise class or getting up a little earlier every day, make time for this addition to your routine and don't let anything get in your way. Planning ahead will help you get around interruptions in your workout schedule, such as bad weather and vacations.

- Set short-term goals. Don't expect to lose twenty pounds in two weeks. It has taken awhile for you to gain the weight, it will take time to lose it. Keep a record of your progress and tell your friends and family about your achievements.

- Vary your exercise program. Change exercises or invite friends to join you to make your workout more enjoyable. There is no "best" exercise—just the one that works best for you. It won't be easy, especially at the start. But as you begin to feel better, look better, and enjoy a new zest for life, you will be rewarded many times over for your efforts.

Tips to Keep You Going

- Adopt a specific plan and write it down.

- Keep setting realistic goals as you go along, and remind yourself of them often.

- Keep a log to record your progress and make sure to keep it up-to-date.

- Include weight and/or percent body fat measures in your log. Extra pounds can easily creep back.

- Upgrade your fitness program as you progress.

- Enlist the support and company of your family and friends.

- Update others on your successes.

- Avoid injuries by pacing yourself and including a warm-up and cool down period as part of every workout.

- Reward yourself periodically for a job well done!

Section 11.4

Tips to Help You Get Active

Reprinted from Weight-control Information Network, National Institute of Diabetes and Digestive and Kidney Diseases, National Institutes of Health, NIH Publication No. 06-5578, January 2006.

You know that physical activity is good for you. So what is stopping you from getting out there and getting at it? Maybe you think that working out is boring, joining a gym is costly, or doing one more thing during your busy day is impossible. Physical activity can be part of your daily life. This section can help you get moving by offering ideas to beat your roadblocks to getting active.

Why Should I Be Physically Active?

You may know that regular physical activity can help you control your weight. But do you know why? Physical activity burns calories. When you burn more calories than you eat each day, you will take off pounds. You can also avoid gaining weight by balancing the number of calories you burn with the number of calories you eat.

Regular physical activity may also help prevent or delay the onset of chronic diseases like type 2 diabetes, heart disease, high blood pressure, stroke, and colon cancer. If you have one of these health problems, physical activity may improve your condition. (If you are a man and over age forty or a woman and over age fifty, or have a chronic health problem, talk to your healthcare provider before starting a vigorous physical activity program. You do not need to talk to your provider before starting an activity like walking.) Regular physical activity may also increase your energy and boost your mood.

What Is Standing in My Way?

Would you like to do more physical activity but do not know how to make it a part of your life? The following text describes some common barriers to physical activity and ways to overcome them. After you read them, try writing down the top two or three barriers that you face. Then write down solutions that you think will work for you. You can make regular physical activity a part of your life!

Personal Barriers

Barrier: Between work, family, and other demands, I am too busy to exercise.

Solutions

- Make physical activity a priority. Carve out some time each week to be active and put it on your calendar. Try waking up a half-hour earlier to walk, scheduling lunchtime workouts, or taking an evening fitness class.

- Build physical activity into your routine chores. Rake the yard, wash the car, or do energetic housework. That way you do what needs to get done and move around too.

- Make family time physically active. Plan a weekend hike through a park, a family softball game, or an evening walk around the block.

Barrier: By the end of a long day, I am just too tired to work out.

Solutions

- Break your workout into three ten-minute segments each day: Taking three short walks during the day may seem easier and less tiring than one thirty-minute workout, and is just as good for you.

- Find another time during the day to work out. If evening workouts are not for you, then try a bike ride before breakfast or a walk at lunchtime.

- Sneak physical activity into your days. Take stairs instead of elevators, park further away in parking lots, and walk in place while watching TV.

Barrier: I think my weight is fine, so I am not motivated to exercise.

Solutions

- Think about the other health benefits of physical activity. Regular physical activity may help lower cholesterol and blood pressure, and lower your odds of having heart disease, type 2 diabetes, or cancer. Research shows that people who are overweight, active, and fit live longer than people who are not overweight but are inactive and unfit. Also, physical activity may lift your mood and increase your energy level.

- Do it just for fun. Play a team sport, work in a garden, or learn a new dance and make getting fit something fun.

- Train for a charity event. You can work to help others while you work out.

Barrier: Getting on a treadmill or stationary bike is boring.

Solutions

- Meet a friend for workouts. If your buddy is on the next bike or treadmill, your workout will be less boring.

- Watch TV or listen to music or a book on tape while you walk or pedal indoors. Check out music or books on tape from your local library.

- Get outside. A change in scenery can relieve your boredom. If you are riding a bike outside, be sure to wear a helmet and learn safe rules of the road.

Mac in Tucson, Arizona, says, "I would take walks in the morning and see a lot of birds. Now I bring my camera along and get some great shots of birds. Taking pictures makes walking more fun. I don't get bored. I mail my pictures to my grandson and he enjoys them."

Barrier: I am afraid I will hurt myself.

Solutions

- Start slowly. If you are starting a new physical activity program, go slow at the start. Even if you are doing an activity that you once did well, start up again slowly to lower your risk of injury or burnout.

- Choose moderate-intensity physical activities. You are not likely to hurt yourself by walking thirty minutes per day. Doing vigorous physical activities may increase your risk for injury, but moderate-intensity physical activity is low risk.

- Take a class. A knowledgeable group fitness instructor should be able to teach you how to move with proper form and lower risk for injury. The instructor can watch your actions during class and let you know if you are doing things right.

- Choose water workouts. Whether you swim laps or try water aerobics, working out in the water is easy on your joints and helps reduce sore muscles and injury.

- Work with a personal trainer. A certified personal trainer should be able to show you how to warm up, cool down, use fitness equipment like treadmills and weight-training machines, and use proper form to help lower your risk for injury. Personal training sessions may be cheap or costly, so find out about fees before making an appointment.

Barrier: I have never been into sports.

Solutions

- Find a physical activity that you enjoy. You do not have to be an athlete to benefit from physical activity. Try yoga, hiking, or planting a garden.

- Choose an activity that you can stick with, like walking. Just put one foot in front of the other. Use the time you spend walking to relax, talk with a friend or family member, or just enjoy the scenery.

Barrier: I do not want to spend a lot of money to join a gym or buy workout gear.

Solutions

- Choose free activities. Garden, take your children to the park to play, lift plastic milk jugs filled with water or sand, or take a walk.

- Find out if your job offers any discounts on memberships. Some companies get lower membership rates at fitness or community centers. Other companies will even pay for part of an employee's membership fee.

- Check out your local recreation or community center. These centers may cost less than other gyms, fitness centers, or health clubs.

- Choose physical activities that do not require any special gear. Walking requires only a pair of sturdy shoes. To dance, just turn on some music.

Barrier: I do not have anyone to watch my kids while I work out.

Solutions

- Do something physically active with your kids. Kids need physical activity too. No matter what age your kids are, you can find an activity you can do together. Dance to music, take a walk, run around the park, or play basketball or soccer together.

- Take turns with another parent to watch the kids. One of you minds the kids while the other one works out.

- Hire a baby-sitter.

- Look for a fitness or community center that offers childcare. Centers that have childcare are becoming more popular. Cost and quality vary, so get all the information up front.

Barrier: My family and friends are not physically active.

Solutions

- Do not let that stop you. Do it for yourself. Enjoy the rewards— such as better sleep, a happier mood, more energy, and a stronger body—you get from working out.

- Join a class or sports league where people count on you to show up. If your basketball team or dance partner counts on you, you will not want to miss a workout, even if your family and friends are not involved.

John from Chicago says, "When I moved to Chicago, I joined a basketball team that some people in my office put together. It's been great for building relationships with co-workers and getting rid of stress. We are all of different ages and abilities, but we are competitive too. It is social and fun."

Barrier: I would be embarrassed if my neighbors or friends saw me exercising.

Solutions

- Ask yourself if it really matters. You are doing something positive for your health and that is something to be proud of. You may even inspire others to get physically active too.

- Invite a friend or neighbor to join you. You may feel less self-conscious if you are not alone.

- Go to a park, nature trail, or fitness or community center to be physically active.

Place Barriers

Barrier: My neighborhood does not have sidewalks.

Solutions

- Find a safe place to walk. Instead of walking in the street, walk in a friend or family member's neighborhood that has sidewalks. Walk during your lunch break at work. Find out if you can walk at a local school track.

- Work out in the yard. Do yard work or wash the car. These count as physical activity too.

Barrier: The winter is too cold/summer is too hot to be active outdoors.

Solutions

- Walk around the mall.

- Join a fitness or community center. Find one that lets you pay for only the months or classes you want, instead of the whole year.

- Exercise at home. Work out to fitness videos or DVDs. Check a different one out from the library each week for variety.

Jennifer from Detroit says, "I needed to find something to do to keep off the extra five pounds I gain every winter. I didn't feel like doing anything after work, when it is already dark. So, I started working out at a fitness center near my office at lunchtime. I do the treadmill and lift weights three days a week. It makes me feel great. Also, I don't pay for my membership during the summer, when I'd rather be outside."

Barrier: I do not feel safe exercising by myself.

Solutions

- Join or start a walking group. You can enjoy added safety and company as you walk.

- Take an exercise class at a nearby fitness or community center.

- Work out at home. You don't need a lot of space. Turn on the radio and dance or follow along with a fitness show on TV.

Health Barriers

Barrier: I have a health problem (diabetes, heart disease, asthma, arthritis) that I do not want to make worse.

Solutions

- Talk with your healthcare professional. Most health problems are helped by physical activity. Find out what physical activities you can safely do and follow advice about length and intensity of workouts.

- Start slowly. Take it easy at first and see how you feel before trying more challenging workouts. Stop if you feel out of breath, dizzy, faint, or nauseated, or if you have pain.

Barrier: I have an injury and do not know what physical activities, if any, I can do.

Solutions

- Talk with your healthcare professional. Ask your physician or physical therapist about what physical activities you can safely perform. Follow advice about length and intensity of workouts.

- Start slowly. Take it easy at first and see how you feel before trying more challenging workouts. Stop if you feel pain.

- Work with a personal trainer. A knowledgeable personal trainer should be able to help you design a fitness plan around your injury.

What Can I Do to Break through My Roadblocks?

What are the top two or three roadblocks to physical activity that you face? What can you do to break through these barriers? Write down a list of the barriers you face and solutions you can use to overcome them.

What's Next?

You have thought about ways to beat your roadblocks to physical activity. Now, create your road map for adding physical activity to your days in the following three steps.

- **Know your goal:** Set up short-term goals, like walking ten minutes a day, three days a week, and try to build up to at least thirty minutes of moderate-intensity physical activity on most days of the week—or preferably, every day of the week. Moderate-intensity physical activity makes you breathe harder, but you should still have enough breath to carry on a conversation. You may need to be physically active for more than thirty minutes a day to help you lose and keep off extra weight. Track your progress by writing down your goals and what you have done each day, including the type of activity and how long you spent doing it. Seeing your progress in black and white can help keep you motivated.

- **See your healthcare provider if necessary:** If you are a man and over age forty or a woman and over age fifty, or have a chronic health problem such as heart disease, high blood pressure, diabetes, osteoporosis, or obesity, talk to your healthcare provider before starting a vigorous physical activity program. You do not need to talk to your provider before starting an activity like walking.

- **Answer questions about how physical activity will fit into your life:** Think about answers to the following four questions. You can write your answers down on a sheet of paper. Your answers will be your road map to your physical activity program.

  - *What physical activities will you do?* List the activities you would like to do, such as walking, energetic yard work or housework, joining a sports league, exercising with a video, dancing, swimming, bicycling, or taking a class at a fitness or community center. Think about sports or other activities that you enjoyed doing when you were younger. Could you enjoy one of these activities again?

  - *When will you be physically active?* List the days and times you could do each activity on your list, such as first thing in the morning, during lunch break from work, after dinner, or on Saturday afternoon. Look at your calendar or planner to find the days and times that work best.

  - *Who will remind you to get off the couch?* List the people—your spouse, sibling, parent, or friends—who can support your efforts to become physically active. Give them ideas about how they could be supportive, like offering encouraging words, watching your kids, or working out with you.

- *When will you start your physical activity program?* Set a date when you will start getting active. The date might be the first meeting of an exercise class you have signed up for, or a date you will meet a friend for a walk. Write the date on your calendar. Then stick to it. Before you know it, physical activity will become a regular part of your life.

Chapter 12

Maintaining a Healthy Weight

Chapter Contents

Section 12.1

Are You Overweight?

Reprinted from "Weight and Waist Measurement: Tools for Adults," Weight-Control Information Network, National Institute of Diabetes and Digestive and Kidney Diseases, National Institutes of Health, NIH Publication No. 04-5283, June 2004.

Healthcare providers use body mass index (BMI) and waist circumference measures to assess a person's risk of developing diabetes, heart disease, or other health problems. This section tells you how to measure your BMI and waist circumference, and what these measures mean for your health.

Body Mass Index

Today, 64.5 percent of adults in the United States are overweight or obese. How do you know if you are among them? Two simple measures, body mass index (BMI) and waist circumference, provide useful estimates of overweight, obesity, and body fat distribution.

BMI measures your weight in relation to your height, and is closely associated with measures of body fat. You can calculate your BMI using the formula in Figure 12.1.

$$BMI = \frac{weight \ (pounds) \ x \ 703}{height \ squared \ (inches^2)}$$

Figure 12.1. How to calculate body mass index.

For example, for someone who is 5 feet, 7 inches tall and weighs 220 pounds, the calculation would look like this: (220 pounds x 703) / (67 inches x 67 inches) = 154,660 / 4,489 = 34.45.

A BMI of 18.5 to 24.9 is considered healthy. A person with a BMI of 25 to 29.9 is considered overweight, and a person with a BMI of 30 or more is considered obese.

You can also find your weight group in Figure 12.2. The chart applies to all adults. The higher weights in the healthy range apply to people with more muscle and bone, such as men. Even within the healthy range, weight gain could increase your risk for health problems.

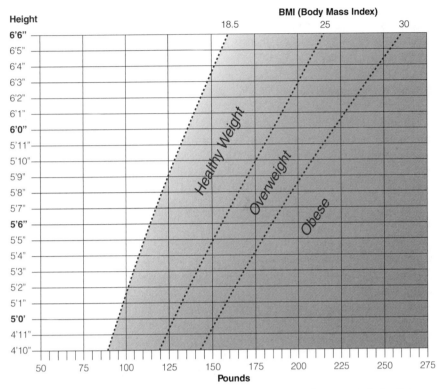

Find your weight on the bottom of the graph. Go straight up from that point until you come to the line that matches your height. Then look to find your weight group. The higher your BMI is over 25, the greater chance you may have of developing health problems.

Figure 12.2. Body mass index chart (Height is figured without shoes and weight is figured without clothes.)

Find your weight on the bottom of the graph. Go straight up from that point until you come to the line that matches your height. Then look to find your weight group. The more your BMI is over 25, the greater chance you may have of developing health problems.

Because BMI does not show the difference between fat and muscle, it does not always accurately predict when weight could lead to health problems. For example, someone with a lot of muscle (such as a body builder) may have a BMI in the unhealthy range, but still be healthy and have little risk of developing diabetes or having a heart attack.

BMI also may not accurately reflect body fatness in people who are very short (under five feet tall) and in older people, who tend to lose muscle mass as they age. And it may not be the best predictor of weight-related health problems among some racial and ethnic groups such as African American and Hispanic/Latino American women. But for most people, BMI is a reliable way to tell if your weight is putting your health at risk.

Waist Circumference

Excess weight, as measured by BMI, is not the only risk to your health. So is the location of fat on your body. If you carry fat mainly around your waist, you are more likely to develop health problems than if you carry fat mainly in your hips and thighs. This is true even if your BMI falls within the normal range. Women with a waist measurement of more than thirty-five inches or men with a waist measurement of more than forty inches may have a higher disease risk than people with smaller waist measurements because of where their fat lies.

To measure your waist circumference, place a tape measure around your bare abdomen just above your hip bone. Be sure that the tape is snug, but does not compress your skin, and is parallel to the floor. Relax, exhale, and measure your waist.

How Does Overweight or Obesity Affect My Health?

Extra weight can put you at higher risk for these health problems:

- Type 2 diabetes (high blood sugar)
- High blood pressure
- Heart disease and stroke
- Some types of cancer
- Sleep apnea (when breathing stops for short periods during sleep)
- Osteoarthritis (wearing away of the joints)
- Gallbladder disease
- Liver disease
- Irregular menstrual periods

What Should I Do If My BMI or Waist Measurement Is Too High?

If your BMI is between 25 and 30 and you are otherwise healthy, try to avoid gaining more weight, and look into healthy ways to lose weight and increase physical activity. Talk to your healthcare provider about losing weight if any of the following are true:

- Your BMI is 30 or above, or

- Your BMI is between 25 and 30 and you have either of the following:

  - Two or more of the health problems listed previously

  - A family history of heart disease or diabetes

- Your waist measures over thirty-five inches (women) or forty inches (men)—even if your BMI is less than 25—and you have either of the following:

  - Two or more of the health problems listed previously

  - A family history of heart disease or diabetes

Section 12.2

Do You Know the Health Risks of Being Overweight?

Reprinted from the Weight-control Information Network, National Institute of Diabetes and Digestive and Kidney Diseases, National Institutes of Health, NIH Publication No. 04-4098, November 2004.

Weighing too much may increase your risk for developing many health problems. If you are overweight or obese on a body mass index (BMI) chart (see Table 12.1), you may be at risk for one or more of the following:

- Type 2 diabetes

- Heart disease and stroke

- Cancer

- Sleep apnea

- Osteoarthritis

- Gallbladder disease
- Fatty liver disease

You can lower your health risks by losing as little as ten to twenty pounds.

BMI	19	20	21	22	23	24	25	26	27	28	29	30	31	32	33	34	35
Height (inches)	Body Weight (pounds)																
58	91	96	100	105	110	115	119	124	129	134	138	143	148	153	158	162	167
59	94	99	104	109	114	119	124	128	133	138	143	148	153	158	163	168	173
60	97	102	107	112	118	123	128	133	138	143	148	153	158	163	168	174	179
61	100	106	111	116	122	127	132	137	143	148	153	158	164	169	174	180	185
62	104	109	115	120	126	131	136	142	147	153	158	164	169	175	180	186	191
63	107	113	118	124	130	135	141	146	152	158	163	169	175	180	186	191	197
64	110	116	122	128	134	140	145	151	157	163	169	174	180	186	192	197	204
65	114	120	126	132	138	144	150	156	162	168	174	180	186	192	198	204	210
66	118	124	130	136	142	148	155	161	167	173	179	186	192	198	204	210	216
67	121	127	134	140	146	153	159	166	172	178	185	191	198	204	211	217	223
68	125	131	138	144	151	158	164	171	177	184	190	197	203	210	216	223	230
69	128	135	142	149	155	162	169	176	182	189	196	203	209	216	223	230	236
70	132	139	146	153	160	167	174	181	188	195	202	209	216	222	229	236	243
71	136	143	150	157	165	172	179	186	193	200	208	215	222	229	236	243	250
72	140	147	154	162	169	177	184	191	199	206	213	221	228	235	242	250	258
73	144	151	159	166	174	182	189	197	204	212	219	227	235	242	250	257	265
74	148	155	163	171	179	186	194	202	210	218	225	233	241	249	256	264	272
75	152	160	168	176	184	192	200	208	216	224	232	240	248	256	264	272	279
76	156	164	172	180	189	197	205	213	221	230	238	246	254	263	271	279	287

BMI	36	37	38	39	40	41	42	43	44	45	46	47	48	49	50	51	52	53	54
58	172	177	181	186	191	196	201	205	210	215	220	224	229	234	239	244	248	253	258
59	178	183	188	193	198	203	208	212	217	222	227	232	237	242	247	252	257	262	267
60	184	189	194	199	204	209	215	220	225	230	235	240	245	250	255	261	266	271	276
61	190	195	201	206	211	217	222	227	232	238	243	248	254	259	264	269	275	280	285
62	196	202	207	213	218	224	229	235	240	246	251	256	262	267	273	278	284	289	295
63	203	208	214	220	225	231	237	242	248	254	259	265	270	278	282	287	293	299	304
64	209	215	221	227	232	238	244	250	256	262	267	273	279	285	291	296	302	308	314
65	216	222	228	234	240	246	252	258	264	270	276	282	288	294	300	306	312	318	324
66	223	229	235	241	247	253	260	266	272	278	284	291	297	303	309	315	322	328	334
67	230	236	242	249	255	261	268	274	280	287	293	299	306	312	319	325	331	338	344
68	236	243	249	256	262	269	276	282	289	295	302	308	315	322	328	335	341	348	354
69	243	250	257	263	270	277	284	291	297	304	311	318	324	331	338	345	351	358	365
70	250	257	264	271	278	285	292	299	306	313	320	327	334	341	348	355	362	369	376
71	257	265	272	279	286	293	301	308	315	322	329	338	343	351	358	365	372	379	386
72	265	272	279	287	294	302	309	316	324	331	338	346	353	361	368	375	383	390	397
73	272	280	288	295	302	310	318	325	333	340	348	355	363	371	378	386	393	401	408
74	280	287	295	303	311	319	326	334	342	350	358	365	373	381	389	396	404	412	420
75	287	295	303	311	319	327	335	343	351	359	367	375	383	391	399	407	415	423	431
76	295	304	312	320	328	336	344	353	361	369	377	385	394	402	410	418	426	435	443

Table 12.1. Body Mass Index Table. To use the table, find the appropriate height in the left-hand column labeled Height. Move across to a given weight. The number at the top of the column is the BMI at that height and weight. Pounds have been rounded off. (Source: Excerpted from "Am I at Risk for Type 2 Diabetes? Taking Steps to Lower the Risk of Getting Diabetes," a brochure produced by the National Institute of Diabetes and Digestive and Kidney Diseases (NIDDK), NIH Publication Number 02-4805.)

Type 2 Diabetes

What it is: Type 2 diabetes used to be called adult-onset diabetes or non-insulin-dependent diabetes. It is the most common type of diabetes in the United States. Type 2 diabetes is a disease in which blood sugar levels are above normal. High blood sugar is a major cause of early death, heart disease, kidney disease, stroke, and blindness.

How it is linked to being overweight: More than 80 percent of people with type 2 diabetes are overweight. It is not known exactly why people who are overweight are more likely to suffer from this disease. It may be that being overweight causes cells to change, making them less effective at using sugar from the blood. This then puts stress on the cells that produce insulin (a hormone that carries sugar from the blood to cells) and makes them gradually fail.

What weight loss can do: You can lower your risk for developing type 2 diabetes by losing weight and increasing the amount of physical activity you do. If you have type 2 diabetes, losing weight and becoming more physically active can help you control your blood sugar levels. Losing weight and exercising more may also allow you to reduce the amount of diabetes medication you take.

Heart Disease and Stroke

What it is: Heart disease means that the heart and circulation (blood flow) are not functioning normally. If you have heart disease, you may suffer from a heart attack, congestive heart failure, sudden cardiac death, angina (chest pain), or abnormal heart rhythm. During a stroke, blood and oxygen do not flow normally to the brain, possibly causing paralysis or death. Heart disease is the leading cause of death in the United States, and stroke is the third leading cause.

How it is linked to being overweight: People who are overweight are more likely to suffer from high blood pressure, high levels of triglycerides (blood fats) and low-density lipoprotein (LDL) cholesterol (a fat-like substance often called the "bad cholesterol"), and low levels of high-density lipoprotein (HDL) cholesterol (the "good cholesterol"). These are all risk factors for heart disease and stroke. In addition, people with more body fat have higher blood levels of substances that cause inflammation. Inflammation in blood vessels and throughout the body may raise heart disease risk.

What weight loss can do: Losing 5 to 15 percent of your weight can lower your chances for developing heart disease or having a stroke. If you weigh two hundred pounds, this means losing as little as ten pounds. Weight loss may improve your blood pressure, triglyceride, and cholesterol levels; improve how your heart works and your blood flows; and decrease inflammation throughout your body.

Cancer

What it is: Cancer occurs when cells in one part of the body, such as the colon, grow abnormally or out of control and possibly spread to other parts of the body, such as the liver. Cancer is the second leading cause of death in the United States.

How it is linked to being overweight: Being overweight may increase the risk of developing several types of cancer, including cancers of the colon, esophagus, and kidney. Being overweight is also linked with uterine and postmenopausal breast cancer in women. Gaining weight during adult life increases the risk for several of these cancers. Being overweight also may increase the risk of dying from some cancers. It is not known exactly how being overweight increases cancer risk. It may be that fat cells make hormones that affect cell growth and lead to cancer. Also, eating or physical activity habits that may lead to being overweight may also contribute to cancer risk.

What weight loss can do: Avoiding weight gain may prevent a rise in cancer risk. Weight loss, and healthy eating and physical activity habits, may lower cancer risk.

Sleep Apnea

What it is: Sleep apnea is a condition in which a person stops breathing for short periods during the night. A person who has sleep apnea may suffer from daytime sleepiness, difficulty concentrating, and even heart failure.

How it is linked to being overweight: The risk for sleep apnea is higher for people who are overweight. A person who is overweight may have more fat stored around his or her neck. This may make the airway smaller. A smaller airway can make breathing difficult, loud (snoring), or stop altogether. In addition, fat stored in the neck and throughout the body can produce substances that cause inflammation. Inflammation in the neck may be a risk factor for sleep apnea.

What weight loss can do: Weight loss usually improves sleep apnea. Weight loss may help to decrease neck size and lessen inflammation.

Osteoarthritis

What it is: Osteoarthritis is a common joint disorder. With osteoarthritis, the joint bone and cartilage (tissue that protects joints) wear away. Osteoarthritis most often affects the joints of the knees, hips, and lower back.

How it is linked to being overweight: Extra weight may place extra pressure on joints and cartilage, causing them to wear away. In addition, people with more body fat may have higher blood levels of substances that cause inflammation. Inflammation at the joints may raise the risk for osteoarthritis.

What weight loss can do: Weight loss can decrease stress on your knees, hips, and lower back, and lessen inflammation in your body. If you have osteoarthritis, losing weight may help improve your symptoms.

Gallbladder Disease

What it is: Gallstones are clusters of solid material that form in the gallbladder. They are made mostly of cholesterol and can sometimes cause abdominal or back pain.

How it is linked to being overweight: People who are overweight have a higher risk for developing gallbladder disease and gallstones. They may produce more cholesterol, a risk factor for gallstones. Also, people who are overweight may have an enlarged gallbladder, which may not work properly.

What weight loss can do: Weight loss—especially fast weight loss (more than three pounds per week) or loss of a large amount of weight—can actually increase your chance of developing gallstones. Modest, slow weight loss of about one-half to two pounds a week is less likely to cause gallstones.

Fatty Liver Disease

What it is: Fatty liver disease occurs when fat builds up in the liver cells and causes injury and inflammation in the liver. It can sometimes lead to severe liver damage, cirrhosis (buildup of scar tissue that blocks proper blood flow in the liver), or even liver failure. Fatty liver disease is like alcoholic liver damage, but it is not caused by alcohol and can occur in people who drink little or no alcohol.

How it is linked to being overweight: People who have diabetes or "pre-diabetes" (when blood sugar levels are higher than normal but not yet in the diabetic range) are more likely to have fatty liver disease than people without these conditions. And people who are overweight are more likely to have diabetes (see preceding discussion of type 2 diabetes). It is not known why some people who are overweight or diabetic get fatty liver and others do not.

What weight loss can do: Losing weight can help you control your blood sugar levels. It can also reduce the buildup of fat in your liver and prevent further injury. People with fatty liver disease should avoid drinking alcohol.

How Can I Lower My Health Risks?

If you are overweight, losing as little as 5 percent of your body weight may lower your risk for several diseases, including heart disease and diabetes. If you weigh two hundred pounds, this means losing ten pounds. Slow and steady weight loss of one-half to two pounds per week, and not more than three pounds per week, is the safest way to lose weight.

To lose weight and keep it off over time, try to make long-term changes in your eating and physical activity habits. Choose healthy foods, such as vegetables, fruits, whole grains, and low-fat meat and dairy products, more often and eat just enough food to satisfy you. Try to do at least thirty minutes of moderate-intensity physical activity— like walking— on most days of the week, preferably every day. To lose weight, or to maintain weight loss, you may need to do more than thirty minutes of moderate physical activity daily.

Section 12.3

Guide to Safe Weight Loss

Excerpted from "Weight Loss for Life," Weight-control Information Network, National Institute of Diabetes and Digestive and Kidney Diseases, National Institutes of Health, NIH Publication No. 04-3700, July 2006.

There are many ways to lose weight, but it is not always easy to keep the weight off. The key to successful weight loss is making changes in your eating and physical activity habits that you can keep up for the rest of your life. The information presented here may help put you on the road to healthy habits.

Can I Benefit from Weight Loss?

Health experts agree that you may gain health benefits from even a small weight loss if any of the following are true:

- You are obese based on your body mass index (BMI)

- You are overweight based on your BMI and have weight-related health problems or a family history of such problems

- You have a waist that measures more than forty inches if you are a man or more than thirty-five inches if you are a woman

A weight loss of 5 to 15 percent of body weight may improve your health and quality of life, and prevent these health problems. For a person who weighs two hundred pounds, that means losing ten to thirty pounds.

Even if you do not need to lose weight, you still should follow healthy eating and physical activity habits to help prevent weight gain and stay healthy as you age.

How Can I Lose Weight?

Your body weight is controlled by the number of calories you eat and the number of calories you use each day. To lose weight you need to take

149

in fewer calories than you use. You can do this by creating and following a plan for healthy eating and a plan for regular physical activity.

You may also choose to follow a formal weight-loss program that can help you make lifelong changes in your eating and physical activity habits.

Your Plan for Healthy Eating

A weight-loss "diet" that limits your portions to a very small size or that excludes certain foods may be hard to stick to. It may not work over the long term. Instead, a healthy eating plan takes into account your likes and dislikes and includes a variety of foods that give you enough calories and nutrients for good health.

Make sure your healthy eating plan is one that does all of the following:

- Emphasizes fruits, vegetables, whole grains, and fat-free or low-fat milk and milk products
- Includes lean meats, poultry, fish, beans, eggs, and nuts
- Is low in saturated fats, trans fats, cholesterol, salt (sodium), and added sugars

Your Plan for Regular Physical Activity

Regular physical activity may help you lose weight and keep weight off. It may also improve your energy level and mood and lower your risk for developing diseases like heart disease, diabetes, and some cancers.

Any amount of physical activity is better than none. Experts recommend doing at least thirty minutes of moderate-intensity physical activity on most or all days of the week for good health. To lose weight or maintain a weight loss, you may need to do more than thirty minutes of physical activity a day, as well as follow your healthy eating plan.

You can get your daily thirty minutes or more all at once, or break it up into shorter sessions of twenty, fifteen, or even ten minutes. Try some of these moderate-intensity physical activities:

- Walking (fifteen minutes per mile or four miles per hour)
- Biking
- Tennis
- Aerobic exercise classes (step aerobics, kick boxing, dancing)
- Energetic house or yard work (gardening, raking, mopping, vacuuming)

What Types of Weight-Loss Programs Are Available?

There are two different types of weight-loss programs—clinical and nonclinical. Knowing what a good program will offer and what to watch out for may help you choose a weight-loss program that will work for you.

Nonclinical Programs

What it is: A nonclinical program may be commercially operated, such as a privately owned weight-loss chain. You can follow a nonclinical program on your own by using a counselor, book, website, or weight-loss product. You can also join others in a support group, worksite program, or community-based program. Nonclinical weight-loss programs may require you to use the program's foods or supplements.

What a safe and effective program will offer: A safe and effective weight-loss program should offer all of the following:

- Books, pamphlets, and websites that are written or reviewed by a licensed health professional such as a medical doctor (M.D.) or registered dietitian (R.D.)

- Balanced information about following a healthy eating plan and getting regular physical activity

- Leaders or counselors who show you their training credentials (program leaders or counselors may not be licensed health professionals)

Program cautions: Here are some things to watch out for in evaluating a nonclinical weight-loss program:

- If a program requires you to buy prepackaged meals, find out how much the meals will cost—they may be expensive. Also, eating prepackaged meals does not let you learn the food selection and cooking skills you will need to maintain weight loss over the long term.

- Avoid any diet that suggests you eat a certain formula, food, or combination of foods for easy weight loss. Some of these diets may work in the short term because they are low in calories. But they may not give you all the nutrients your body needs and they do not teach healthy eating habits.

- Avoid programs that do not include a physical activity plan.

- Talk to your healthcare provider before using any weight-loss product, such as a supplement, herb, or over-the-counter medication.

Clinical Programs

What it is: A clinical program provides services in a healthcare setting, such as a hospital. One or more licensed health professionals, such as medical doctors, nurses, registered dietitians, and/or psychologists, provide care. A clinical program may or may not be commercially owned.

Clinical programs may offer services such as nutrition education, physical activity, and behavior change therapy. Some programs offer prescription weight-loss drugs or gastrointestinal surgery.

Prescription weight-loss drugs: If your BMI is 30 or more, or your BMI is 27 or more and you have weight-related health problems, you may consider using prescription weight-loss drugs. Drugs should be used as part of an overall program that includes long-term changes in eating and physical activity habits. Only a licensed healthcare provider can prescribe these drugs.

Gastrointestinal surgery: If your BMI is 40 or more, or your BMI is 35 or more and you have weight-related health problems such as diabetes or heart disease, you may consider gastrointestinal surgery (also called bariatric surgery). Most patients lose weight quickly, and many keep off most of their weight with a healthy eating plan and regular physical activity. Still, surgery can lead to problems that require more operations. Surgery may also reduce the amount of vitamins and minerals in your body and cause gallstones.

What a safe and effective program will offer: A safe and effective clinical weight-loss program should offer all of the following:

• A team of licensed health professionals

• A plan to help you keep weight off after you have lost it

Program cautions: There may be side effects or health risks involved in the program that can be serious. Discuss these with your healthcare provider.

It is not always easy to change your eating and physical activity habits. You may have setbacks along the way. But keep trying—you can do it!

Section 12.4

Prescription Medications for the Treatment of Obesity

Reprinted from the Weight-control Information Network, National Institute of Diabetes and Digestive and Kidney Diseases, National Institutes of Health, NIH Publication No. 04-4191, November 2004.

Obesity is a chronic disease that affects many people and often requires long-term treatment to promote and sustain weight loss. As in other chronic conditions, such as diabetes or high blood pressure, long-term use of prescription medications may be appropriate for some people.

Prescription weight-loss medications should be used only by patients who are at increased medical risk because of their weight. They should not be used for "cosmetic" weight loss. Prescription weight-loss drugs are approved only for those with a body mass index (BMI) of 30 and above, or 27 and above if they have obesity-related conditions, such as high blood pressure, dyslipidemia (abnormal amounts of fat in the blood), or type 2 diabetes. BMI is a measure of weight in relation to height. A BMI of 18.5 to 24.9 is considered healthy.

Although most side effects of prescription medications for obesity are mild, serious complications have been reported. Also, there are few studies lasting more than two years evaluating the safety or effectiveness of weight-loss medications. Weight-loss medications should always be combined with a program of healthy eating and regular physical activity.

The information in this section may help you decide if and what kind of weight-loss medication may help you in your efforts to reach and stay at a healthy weight. It does not replace medical advice from your doctor.

Weight-loss medications should always be combined with a program of healthy eating and regular physical activity.

Medications That Promote Weight Loss

Until more information on their safety or effectiveness is available, using combinations of medications for weight loss is not recommended, except as part of a research study.

Appetite suppressants: Most available weight-loss medications approved by the Food and Drug Administration (FDA) are appetite-suppressant medications. Appetite-suppressant medications promote weight loss by decreasing appetite or increasing the feeling of being full. These medications make you feel less hungry by increasing one or more brain chemicals that affect mood and appetite. Phentermine and sibutramine are the most commonly prescribed appetite-suppressants in the United States. Note: Amphetamines are a type of appetite suppressant. However, amphetamines are not recommended for use in the treatment of obesity due to their strong potential for abuse and dependence.

Lipase inhibitors: One drug works in a different way. Orlistat works by reducing the body's ability to absorb dietary fat by about one third. It does this by blocking the enzyme lipase, which is responsible for breaking down dietary fat. When fat is not broken down, the body cannot absorb it, so fewer calories are taken in.

Other medications: These are not FDA-approved for the treatment of obesity. They include the following:

- *Drugs to treat depression:* Some antidepressant medications have been studied as appetite-suppressant medications. While these medications are FDA-approved for the treatment of depression, their use in weight loss is an "off-label" use (see "What Is 'Off-Label' Use?" below for more information). Studies of these medications generally have found that patients lose modest amounts of weight for up to six months, and tend to regain weight while they are still on the drug. One exception is bupropion. In one study, patients taking bupropion maintained weight loss for up to one year.

- *Drugs to treat seizures:* Two medications used to treat seizures, topiramate and zonisamide, have been shown to cause weight loss. Whether these drugs will be useful in treating obesity is being studied.

- *Drugs to treat diabetes:* The diabetes medication metformin may promote small amounts of weight loss in people with obesity and type 2 diabetes. How this medication promotes weight loss is not clear, although research has shown reduced hunger and food intake in people taking the drug.

- *Drug combinations:* The combined drug treatment using fenfluramine and phentermine ("fen/phen") is no longer available due to the withdrawal of fenfluramine from the market after some patients experienced serious heart and lung disorders. (See "Potential Risks and Concerns" below for more information.) Little information is available about the safety or effectiveness of other drug combinations for weight loss, including fluoxetine/ phentermine, phendimetrazine/phentermine, orlistat/sibutramine, herbal combinations, or others. Until more information on their safety or effectiveness is available, using combinations of medications for weight loss is not recommended, except as part of a research study.

- *Drugs in development:* Many medications are being tested as potential treatments for obesity. Two are being studied with patients in clinical trials. Rimonabant affects brain chemicals and ciliary neurotrophic factor affects hormones to control appetite. Currently, these medications are available only in clinical trials. Clinical trials are research studies with human volunteers so that specific health questions can be answered.

Table 12.2. FDA-Approved Prescription Weight-Loss Medications

Approved for Long-Term Use

Generic Name	Trade Name(s)	Drug Type	FDA Approval Date
orlistat	Xenical	lipase inhibitor	1999
sibutramine	Meridia	appetite suppressant	1997

Approved for Short-Term Use

Generic Name	Trade Name(s)	Drug Type	FDA Approval Date
diethylpropion	Tenuate, Tenuate Dospan	appetite suppressant	1959
phendimetrazine	Bontril, Plegine, Prelu-2, X-Trozine, Adipost	appetite suppressant	1982
phentermine	Adipex-P, Fastin, Ionamin, Oby-trim, Pro-Fast, Zantryl	appetite suppressant	1959

Most currently available weight-loss medications are FDA-approved for short-term use, meaning a few weeks, but doctors may prescribe them for longer periods of time—a practice called "off-label use" (as described in the following). Sibutramine and orlistat are the only weight-loss medications approved for longer-term use in patients who are significantly obese. Their safety and effectiveness have not been established for use beyond two years, however.

What Is "Off-Label" Use?

Although the FDA regulates how a medication can be advertised or promoted by the manufacturer, these regulations do not restrict a doctor's ability to prescribe the medication for different conditions, in different doses, or for different lengths of time. The practice of prescribing medication for periods of time or for conditions not FDA-approved is known as "off-label" use. While such use often occurs in the treatment of many conditions, you should feel comfortable about asking your doctor if he or she is using a medication or combination of medications in a manner that is not approved by the FDA. The use of more than one weight-loss medication at a time (combined drug treatment) is an example of an off-label use. Using weight-loss medications other than sibutramine or orlistat for more than a short period of time (i.e., more than a few weeks) is also considered off-label use.

Potential Benefits of Medication Treatment

People respond differently to weight-loss medications, and some people experience more weight loss than others. Weight-loss medications lead to an average weight loss of five to twenty-two pounds more than what you might lose with non-drug obesity treatments. Some patients using medication lose more than 10 percent of their starting body weight. Maximum weight loss usually occurs within six months of starting medication treatment. Weight then tends to level off or increase during the remainder of treatment.

Over the short term, weight loss in individuals who are obese may reduce a number of health risks. Studies have found that weight loss with some medications improves blood pressure, blood cholesterol, triglycerides (fats), and insulin resistance (the body's inability to use blood sugar). New research suggests that long-term use of weight-loss medications may help individuals keep off the weight they have lost. However, more studies are needed to determine the long-term effects of weight-loss medications on weight and health.

Potential Risks and Concerns

When considering long-term weight-loss medication treatment for obesity, you should consider the following areas of concern and potential risks:

- **Potential for abuse or dependence:** Currently, all prescription medications to treat obesity except orlistat are controlled substances, meaning doctors need to follow certain restrictions when prescribing them. Although abuse and dependence are not common with nonamphetamine appetite-suppressant medications, doctors should be cautious when they prescribe these medications for patients with a history of alcohol or other drug abuse.

- **Development of tolerance:** Most studies of weight-loss medications show that a patient's weight tends to level off after six months while still on medication. Although some patients and doctors may be concerned that this shows tolerance to the medications, the leveling off may mean that the medication has reached its limit of effectiveness. Based on the currently available studies, it is not clear if weight gain with continuing treatment is due to drug tolerance. It is clear, however, that weight gain would be much faster if the patient stopped taking the drug.

- **Reluctance to view obesity as a chronic disease:** Obesity often is viewed as the result of a lack of willpower, weakness, or a lifestyle "choice"—the choice to overeat and under-exercise. Such social views on obesity should not prevent patients from seeking medical treatment to prevent health risks that can cause serious illness and death. Weight-loss medications, however, are not "magic bullets" or a one-shot fix for this chronic disease. They should be combined with a healthy eating plan and increased physical activity.

- **Side effects:** Because weight-loss medications are used to treat a condition that affects millions of people, many of whom are basically healthy, the possibility that side effects may outweigh benefits is of great concern. Most side effects of these medications are mild and usually improve with continued treatment. Rarely, serious and even fatal outcomes have been reported. Side effects of medications are explained below.

  - *Orlistat:* Some side effects of orlistat include cramping, intestinal discomfort, passing gas, diarrhea, and leakage of

157

oily stool. These side effects are generally mild and temporary, but may be worsened by eating foods that are high in fat. Also, because orlistat reduces the absorption of some vitamins, patients should take a multivitamin at least two hours before or after taking orlistat.

- *Sibutramine:* The main side effects of sibutramine are increases in blood pressure and heart rate, which are usually small but may be of concern in some patients. Other side effects include headache, dry mouth, constipation, and insomnia. People with poorly controlled high blood pressure, heart disease, irregular heartbeat, or history of stroke should not take sibutramine, and all patients taking the medication should have their blood pressure monitored on a regular basis.

- *Other appetite suppressants:* Phentermine, phendimetrazine, and diethylpropion may cause symptoms of sleeplessness, nervousness, and euphoria (feeling of well-being). People with heart disease, high blood pressure, an overactive thyroid gland, or glaucoma should not use these drugs. Two appetite-suppressant medications, fenfluramine and dexfenfluramine, were withdrawn from the market in 1997. These drugs, used alone and in combination with phentermine ("fen/phen"), were linked to the development of valvular heart disease and primary pulmonary hypertension (PPH), a rare but potentially fatal disorder that affects the blood vessels in the lungs. There have been only a few case reports of PPH in patients taking phentermine alone, but the possibility that phentermine use is associated with PPH cannot be ruled out.

Commonly Asked Questions about Weight-Loss Medications

Can medications replace physical activity or changes in eating habits as a way to lose weight?

No. Studies show that weight-loss medications work best when combined with a weight-control program that helps you improve your eating and physical activity habits. Ask your doctor about ways you can improve your eating plan and become more physically active.

What medical conditions or medications might influence my decision to take a weight-loss drug?

Let your doctor know if you have any of the following medical conditions, which may affect which weight-loss drugs you can take, if any:

- Pregnancy or breast-feeding
- History of drug or alcohol abuse
- History of anorexia or bulimia
- History of depression or manic depressive disorder
- Use of monoamine oxidase (MAO) inhibitors or antidepressant medications
- Migraine headaches requiring medication
- Glaucoma
- Diabetes
- Heart disease or heart condition, such as an irregular heartbeat
- High blood pressure
- Plan to have surgery that requires general anesthesia.

How long will I need to take weight-loss medications to treat obesity?

The answer depends upon whether the medication helps you to lose and maintain weight and whether you have any side effects. Because obesity is a chronic disease, any treatment, whether drug or nondrug, may need to be continued for years, and perhaps a lifetime, to improve health and maintain a healthy weight. However, like many other types of drugs, there is still little information on how safe and effective weight-loss medications are for many years of use. At least one study has shown that intermittent use (one month on medication and one month off medication) may help some people lose and maintain weight, but more research is needed.

Will I regain some weight after I stop taking weight-loss medications?

Probably. Most studies show that the majority of patients who stop taking weight-loss medications regain the weight they lost. Maintaining healthy eating and physical activity habits may help you regain less weight.

159

Can children or teens use weight-loss medications?

Orlistat is currently approved for use in teens age twelve or above. Other weight-loss medications are not approved for use in children under the age of sixteen, although studies in children and teens are ongoing.

Will insurance cover the cost of weight-loss medication?

Many insurance companies currently will not pay for weight-loss prescriptions, but this is changing as insurers begin to recognize obesity as a chronic disease. Contact your insurance company to find out if prescription weight-loss medication is covered under your plan. The cost of one month of a prescription can cost from sixty dollars to more than twice this amount. Ask a staff member at your pharmacy the cost of a one-month supply of the medication you are considering taking.

Most patients should not expect to reach an "ideal" body weight using currently available medications. However, even a modest weight loss of 5 to 10 percent of your starting body weight can improve your health.

Together, you and your doctor can make an informed choice as to whether medication can be a useful part of your weight-control program.

Section 12.5

Gastrointestinal Surgery for Severe Obesity

Excerpted from the Weight-control Information Network, National Institute of Diabetes and Digestive and Kidney Diseases, National Institutes of Health, NIH Publication No. 04-4006, December 2004.

Severe obesity is a chronic condition that is difficult to treat through diet and exercise alone. Gastrointestinal surgery is an option for people who are severely obese and cannot lose weight by traditional means or who suffer from serious obesity-related health problems. The operation promotes weight loss by restricting food intake and, in some operations, interrupting the digestive process. As in other treatments for obesity, the best results are achieved with healthy eating behaviors and regular physical activity.

You may be a candidate for surgery if you have the following:

- A body mass index (BMI) of 40 or more—about one hundred pounds overweight for men and eighty pounds for women

- A BMI between 35 and 39.9 and a serious obesity-related health problem such as type 2 diabetes, heart disease, or severe sleep apnea (when breathing stops for short periods during sleep)

- An understanding of the operation and the lifestyle changes you will need to make

The Normal Digestive Process

Normally, as food moves along the digestive tract, digestive juices and enzymes digest and absorb calories and nutrients (see Figure 12.3). After we chew and swallow our food, it moves down the esophagus to the stomach, where a strong acid continues the digestive process. The stomach can hold about three pints of food at one time.

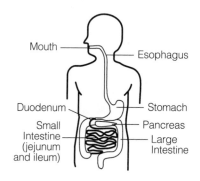

Figure 12.3. *The body's digestive organs*

161

When the stomach contents move to the duodenum, the first segment of the small intestine, bile and pancreatic juice speed up digestion. Most of the iron and calcium in the foods we eat is absorbed in the duodenum. The jejunum and ileum, the remaining two segments of the nearly twenty feet of small intestine, complete the absorption of almost all calories and nutrients. The food particles that cannot be digested in the small intestine are stored in the large intestine until eliminated.

How Does Surgery Promote Weight Loss?

Gastrointestinal surgery for obesity, also called bariatric surgery, alters the digestive process. The operations can be divided into three types: restrictive, malabsorptive, and combined restrictive/malabsorptive. Restrictive operations limit food intake by creating a narrow passage from the upper part of the stomach into the larger lower part, reducing the amount of food the stomach can hold and slowing the passage of food through the stomach. Malabsorptive operations do not limit food intake, but instead exclude most of the small intestine from the digestive tract so fewer calories and nutrients are absorbed. Malabsorptive operations, also called intestinal bypasses, are no longer recommended because they result in severe nutritional deficiencies. Combined operations use stomach restriction and a partial bypass of the small intestine.

What Are the Surgical Options?

There are several types of restrictive and combined operations. Each one has its own benefits and risks.

Restrictive Operations

Purely restrictive operations only limit food intake and do not interfere with the normal digestive process. To perform the operation, doctors create a small pouch at the top of the stomach where food enters from the esophagus. At first, the pouch holds about one ounce of food and later may stretch to two to three ounces. The lower outlet of the pouch is usually about one-half inch in diameter or smaller. This small outlet delays the emptying of food from the pouch into the larger part of the stomach and causes a feeling of fullness.

After the operation, patients can no longer eat large amounts of food at one time. Most patients can eat about one-half to one cup of food without discomfort or nausea, but the food has to be soft, moist, and well chewed. Patients who undergo restrictive procedures generally are not able to eat as much as those who have combined operations.

Purely restrictive operations for obesity include adjustable gastric banding (AGB) and vertical banded gastroplasty (VBG).

Adjustable gastric banding: In this procedure, a hollow band made of silicone rubber is placed around the stomach near its upper end, creating a small pouch and a narrow passage into the rest of the stomach (see Figure 12.4). The band is then inflated with a salt solution through a tube that connects the band to an access port placed under the skin. It can be tightened or loosened over time to change the size of the passage by increasing or decreasing the amount of salt solution.

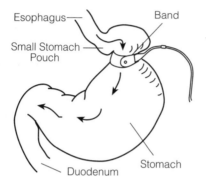

Figure 12.4. *Adjustable gastric banding*

Vertical banded gastroplasty: VBG uses both a band and staples to create a small stomach pouch, as illustrated in Figure 12.5. Once the most common restrictive operation, VBG is not often used today.

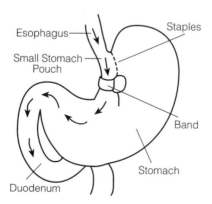

Figure 12.5. *Vertical banded gastroplasty*

There are some advantages to restrictive operations. Restrictive operations are easier to perform and are generally safer than malabsorptive operations. AGB is usually done via laparoscopy, which uses smaller incisions, creates less tissue damage, and involves shorter operating time and hospital stays than open procedures. (See following for more information on laparoscopy.) Restrictive operations can be reversed if necessary, and result in few nutritional deficiencies.

There are also a few disadvantages. Patients who undergo restrictive operations generally lose less weight than patients who have malabsorptive operations, and are less likely to maintain weight loss over the long term. Patients generally lose about half of their excess body weight in the first year after restrictive procedures. However, in the first three to five years after VBG patients may regain some of the weight they lost. By ten years after surgery, as few as 20 percent of patients have kept the weight off. (Although there is less information about long-term results with AGB, there is some evidence that weight loss results are better than with VBG.) Some patients regain weight by eating high-calorie soft foods that easily pass through the opening to the stomach. Others are unable to change their eating habits and do not lose much weight to begin with. Successful results depend on the patient's willingness to adopt a long-term plan of healthy eating and regular physical activity.

There are also a few risks to this type of surgery. One of the most common risks of restrictive operations is vomiting, which occurs when the patient eats too much or the narrow passage into the larger part of the stomach is blocked. Another is slippage or wearing away of the band. A common risk of AGB is a break in the tubing between the band and the access port. This can cause the salt solution to leak, requiring another operation to repair. Some patients experience infections and bleeding, but this is much less common than other risks. Between 15 and 20 percent of VBG patients may have to undergo a second operation for a problem related to the procedure. Although restrictive operations are the safest of the bariatric procedures, they still carry risk—in less than 1 percent of all cases, complications can result in death.

Combined Restrictive/Malabsorptive Operations

Combined operations are the most common bariatric procedures. They restrict both food intake and the amount of calories and nutrients the body absorbs.

Roux-en-Y gastric bypass (RGB): This operation, illustrated in Figure 12.6, is the most common and successful combined procedure in the United States. First, the surgeon creates a small stomach pouch to restrict food intake. Next, a Y-shaped section of the small intestine is attached to the pouch to allow food to bypass the lower stomach, the duodenum (the first segment of the small intestine), and the first portion of the jejunum (the second segment of the small intestine). This reduces the amount of calories and nutrients the body absorbs. Rarely, a cholecystectomy (gall bladder removal) is performed to avoid the gallstones that may result from rapid weight loss. More commonly, patients take medication after the operation to dissolve gallstones.

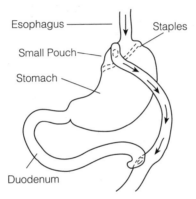

Figure 12.6. Roux-en-Y gastric bypass

Biliopancreatic diversion (BPD): In this more complicated combined operation, the lower portion of the stomach is removed (see Figure 12.7). The small pouch that remains is connected directly to the final segment of the small intestine, completely bypassing the duodenum and the jejunum. Although this procedure leads to weight loss, it is used less often than other types of operations because of the high risk for nutritional deficiencies. A variation of BPD includes a "duodenal switch" (see Figure 12.8), which leaves a larger portion of the stomach intact, including the pyloric valve that regulates the release of stomach contents into the small intestine. It also keeps a small part of the duodenum in the digestive pathway. The larger stomach allows patients to eat more after the surgery than patients who have other types of procedures.

There are a number of advantages to combined procedures. Most patients lose weight quickly and continue to lose for eighteen to twenty-four months after the procedure. With the Roux-en-Y gastric bypass, many patients maintain a weight loss of 60 to 70 percent of their excess weight for ten years or more. With BPD, most studies report an average weight loss of 75 to 80 percent of excess weight. Because combined operations result in greater weight loss than restrictive operations, they may also be more effective in improving the health problems associated with severe obesity, such as hypertension (high blood pressure), sleep apnea, type 2 diabetes, and osteoarthritis.

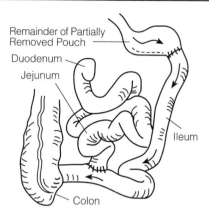

Figure 12.7. Biliopancreatic diversion

There are also some disadvantages. Combined procedures are more difficult to perform than the restrictive procedures. They are also more likely to result in long-term nutritional deficiencies. This is because the operation causes food to bypass the duodenum and jejunum, where most iron and calcium are absorbed. Menstruating women may develop anemia because not enough vitamin B_{12} and iron are absorbed.

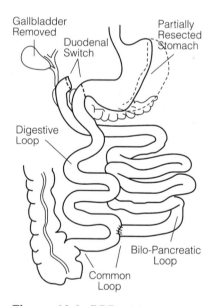

Figure 12.8. BPD with duodenal switch

Decreased absorption of calcium may also bring on osteoporosis and related bone diseases. Patients must take nutritional supplements that usually prevent these deficiencies. Patients who have the biliopancreatic diversion procedure must also take fat-soluble (dissolved by fat) vitamins A, D, E, and K supplements, and require lifelong use of special foods and medications.

166

RGB and BPD operations may also cause "dumping syndrome," an unpleasant reaction that can occur after a meal high in simple carbohydrates, which contain sugars that are rapidly absorbed by the body. Stomach contents move too quickly through the small intestine, causing symptoms such as nausea, bloating, abdominal pain, weakness, sweating, faintness, and sometimes diarrhea after eating. Because the duodenal switch operation keeps the pyloric valve intact, it may reduce the likelihood of dumping syndrome.

In addition to risks associated with restrictive procedures such as infection, combined operations are more likely to lead to complications. The risk of death associated with these types of procedures is lower for the gastric bypass (less than 1 percent of patients) than for the biliopancreatic diversion with duodenal switch (2.5 to 5 percent). Combined operations carry a greater risk than restrictive operations for abdominal hernias (up to 28 percent), which require a follow-up operation to correct. The risk of hernia, however, is lower (about 3 percent) when laparoscopic techniques are used.

Laparoscopic Bariatric Surgery

In laparoscopy, the surgeon makes one or more small incisions through which slender surgical instruments are passed. This technique eliminates the need for a large incision and creates less tissue damage. Patients who are super-obese (more than 350 pounds) or have had previous abdominal operations may not be good candidates for laparoscopy, however. Adjustable gastric banding is routinely performed via laparoscopy.

This technique is often used for Roux-en-Y gastric bypass, and although less common, biliopancreatic diversion can also be performed laparoscopic ally. The small incisions result in less blood loss, shorter hospitalization, a faster recovery, and fewer complications than open operations. However, combined laparoscopic procedures are more difficult to perform than open procedures and can create serious problems if done incorrectly.

Bariatric Surgery for Adolescents

With rates of obesity among youth on the rise, bariatric surgery is sometimes considered as a treatment option for adolescents who are severely overweight. However, there are many concerns about the long-term effects of this type of operation on adolescents' developing bodies and minds. Experts in pediatric obesity and bariatric surgery

167

recommend that surgical treatment be considered only when adolescents have tried for at least six months to lose weight and have not been successful. Candidates should be severely overweight (BMI of 40 or more), have reached their adult height (usually thirteen or older for girls, fifteen or older for boys), and have serious weight-related health problems such as type 2 diabetes or heart disease. In addition, potential patients and their parents should be evaluated to see how emotionally prepared they are for the operation and the lifestyle changes they will need to make. Patients should also be referred to a team of experts in adolescent medicine and bariatric surgery who are qualified to meet their unique needs.

Chapter 13

Managing Stress

Chapter Contents

Section 13.1

Stress and the Body

Reprinted from "Stressed Out? Stress Affects Both Body and Mind," *News in Health*, National Institutes of Health, January 2007.

Maybe it's money trouble or the burden of caring for a sick relative. Maybe it's your job. Maybe it's the traffic. Whatever the cause, everyone seems stressed out these days. People once hotly debated the idea that stress can affect your body, but we now know that stress can cause both short- and long-term changes to your body and mind. The more we understand how stress affects us, the more we learn about how to cope better.

Long before we humans learned how to drive cars to work and check in with the office on handheld computers, our bodies evolved to be finely attuned to a predator's attack. When we sense danger, our bodies quickly release hormones like adrenaline into our bloodstream that increase our heart rate, focus our attention, and cause other changes to quickly prepare us for coming danger. Stress was—and still is—crucial to our survival.

The stress that we're adapted to deal with, however, is the short, intense kind—like running away before a bear can make a lunch of us. Modern life frequently gives us little time between periods of stress for our body to recuperate. This chronic stress eventually takes both a mental and a physical toll.

It's long been known that blood pressure and cholesterol levels go up in people who are stressed. Studies have now linked chronic stress with cardiovascular problems like hypertension, coronary heart disease, and stroke.

The immune system is also affected by stress. Dr. Esther M. Sternberg at the National Institute of Health's (NIH's) National Institute of Mental Health says it makes sense for the immune system to gear up and get ready to heal potential wounds. But chronic stress can cause the system to backfire. Research has shown that wounds in people under chronic stress heal more slowly. Caregivers of people with Alzheimer disease, who are often under great stress, are more likely to get the flu or a cold—and when they take vaccines to protect their loved ones from getting flu, their bodies don't respond as well.

Certain hormones that are released when you're stressed out, such as cortisol and catecholamines, have been tied to these long-term effects of stress. Sternberg says, "If you're pumping out a lot of cortisol and your immune cells are bathed in high levels of stress hormones, they're going to be tuned down."

Animal studies and brain imaging studies in people have shown that chronic stress can have a similar effect on the brain. Dr. Bruce S. McEwen of Rockefeller University explains, "Hyperactivity of the stress response results in changes over time in the circuitry of the brain."

Brain cells bombarded by stress signals have little recovery time and eventually start to shrink and cut connections to other brain cells. The network that coordinates our thoughts, emotions, and reactions thus starts to rearrange. Over time, entire regions of the brain can grow or shrink. That may explain why studies have linked higher levels of stress hormones with lower memory, focus, and problem-solving skills.

Not everyone deals with stress the same way, however, and why some people seem to cope better is a major area of research. McEwen says studies in animals show that early life experiences and the quality of maternal care affect how curious an animal is when it's older and how stressed it gets in a new environment.

Dr. Teresa Seeman of the University of California at Los Angeles School of Medicine points out that studies have also linked poverty and deprivation in childhood with how well people deal with stress. "There does appear to be a lingering impact," Seeman says, but adds that it's difficult to know the exact cause.

Two things that affect how much stress people feel are self-esteem and a sense of control. Workers who feel more in control at their jobs tend to feel less stress. People with low self-esteem produce more cortisol when they're asked to do something that's not easy for them, like speak in front of other people. They also don't become accustomed to the stress even after doing something several times and continue to produce high levels of cortisol.

It's not easy to change things like self-esteem and your sense of control at work, but there are things you can do to help you cope with the stresses of modern life.

"Sleep deprivation is a major issue," McEwen says. People who are stressed out tend to get less quality sleep. And sleep deprivation affects your ability to control your mood and make good decisions. It also throws the stress hormones in your body off balance.

"If you're sleep deprived," McEwen explains, "blood pressure and cortisol don't go down at night like they should." McEwen sees people who work night shifts as a window into what chronic stress does to the body over time. "They're more likely to become obese and to have diabetes, cardiovascular disease, and depression," he says.

People who are stressed out tend to do other things that make their bodies less healthy and more vulnerable to the effects of stress. Many eat more fatty comfort foods, which can lead to obesity and diabetes. They may smoke or drink more, raising the risk for cancer and other diseases. And they often feel they're just too busy to exercise.

Seeman says, "Being physically active helps keep the body's systems in better shape and thus better able to deal with any demands from other stressful conditions."

Another factor affecting how we deal with stress is the isolation of modern life. Sometimes it seems like the only time we interact with our family or co-workers is when we're having a conflict. Seeman says it's important to develop a network of people you can go to and talk with when you're confronted with difficulties in your life.

"Large studies have clearly shown," she says, "that people who have more social relationships, a larger network of people they interact with on a regular basis, live longer. Research suggests they're less likely to show declines as they're older."

All this research highlights the fact that healthy practices can complement mainstream medicine to help treat and prevent disease. Do things that make you feel good about yourself, mentally and physically. Get enough sleep. Eat a healthy diet and exercise regularly. Develop a network of people you can turn to in difficult times.

If you still find yourself too stressed out, talk to your healthcare professional. There are many therapies they may recommend to help you deal with stress and its consequences. The effects of being chronically stressed are too serious to simply accept as a fact of modern life.

Ways of Reducing Stress

Here are some tips for reducing stress:

- Get enough sleep.
- Exercise and control your diet.
- Build a social support network.
- Create peaceful times in your day.
- Try different relaxation methods until you find one that works for you.
- Don't smoke.
- Don't drink too much or abuse any other substances.

Section 13.2

Identifying Stress

Although it is natural to feel anxious or "stressed out" sometimes, anxiety and prolonged stress, or stress that goes ignored, can be unhealthy. However, you can learn how to recognize both the physical and the emotional signs of stress and anxiety. Once you learn to recognize stress, then you will be much better able to use coping strategies to relieve your stress and ease your tension.

What are some physical signs of a stress response?

- Increased or irregular blood pressure
- Headache
- Insomnia
- Digestive upset
- Tight muscles
- Weight change
- Restlessness
- Lack of energy
- Shallow, rapid breathing
- Back or neck ache
- Blurred vision
- Knot in stomach
- High voice
- Rapid pulse
- Cold extremities

- Breathing difficulties
- Tight throat
- Sweating
- Change in blood sugar
- Elevated cholesterol

What are some emotional signs of a stress response?

- Irritability
- Anger
- Forgetfulness
- Confusion
- Boredom
- Worrying
- Feeling of "emptiness"
- Lack of concentration
- Anxiety
- Fear
- Feeling hopeless or helpless
- Discouragement
- Decreased libido
- Lowered psychological resistance

What types of things are common causes of stress?

- People
- Money
- Work
- Body
- Mind
- Leisure
- Perceived loss
- Other fears

Section 13.3

Relaxation Techniques

There are many techniques for relaxing; and no one method is better than another. Experiment with the following relaxation techniques and discover what is rewarding for you!

Visualization

Through visualization you can achieve a focused awareness while minimizing thoughts, emotions, and physical pain. It will be useful to tape each exercise and play it back while you are resting in a comfortable position.

Push Your Tension Away

Close your eyes. Give your tension or pain a color and a shape. Pause. Now change the shape and color of your tension or pain. Pause. Push this second shape and color away until it is out of your awareness.

Colors

Close your eyes. Imagine your body filled with lights. For example, red lights for tension or pain, and blue lights for relaxation. Pause. Imagine the lights changing from red to blue, or from blue to red, and be aware of any physical sensation you may experience while this is taking place. Pause. Change all of the lights in your body to blue and experience the overall relaxation.

Mountain Path

Close your eyes. Imagine yourself leaving the area where you live. Leave the daily hassles and the fast pace behind. Imagine yourself going across a valley and moving closer and closer to a mountain range.

Imagine yourself in a mountain range. You are going up a winding road. Find a place on the winding road to stop. Find a path to walk up. Start walking up the path. Find a comfortable place to stop on the path. At this place, take some time to examine all the tension and stress in your life. Give the tension and stress shapes and colors. Look at them very carefully and after you have done this, put them down on the side of the path. Continue walking up the path until you come to the top of a hill. Look out over the hill. What do you see? Find an inviting, comfortable place and go there. Be aware of your surroundings. What is your "special" place like? Be aware of the sights, smells, and sounds. Be aware of how you are feeling. Get settled and gradually start to relax. You are now feeling totally relaxed. Experience being relaxed totally and completely. Look around at your special place once more. Remember this is your special place to relax, and you can come here anytime you want to. Come back to the room and tell yourself that this imagery is something you have created, and you can use it whenever you want to feel relaxed.

Meditation

Here is a short meditation (5–10 minutes):

- First, scan your body. See what your muscles feel like. Attempt to relax and loosen up. Allow yourself to feel body sensations. Stay with this body scanning for a couple of minutes. Allow the muscles to feel as heavy and warm as possible. Focus on warmth in your arms and hands.

- Focus now on your thoughts. What are you thinking of? What kinds of thoughts have you had today, and which ones come to mind now? Are these upsetting thoughts or comforting ones? Dwell on the comforting or pleasant thoughts.

Table 13.1. Meditation Phrases

On the Inhaling Breath	On the Exhaling Breath
I close my eyes	I bring my awareness inside
I deepen my breathing	I quiet my thoughts
I allow my body to be still	I relax my muscles
I focus into my center	I release my tensions (frustration, anxiety, fear, expectations)

- Focus now on your emotions or feelings. What do you feel? Content? Angry? Annoyed? Sad? Excited? Peaceful? Allow yourself to feel.

- Take three deep breaths (easy and slow) and return to your activities.

Progressive Muscular Relaxation

Whether you're performing an athletic feat or merely doing your job, the quality of your efforts depends in part on your ability to relax. There are a variety of relaxation techniques to choose from. Progressive relaxation yields a variety of benefits, including the development of a feeling of well-being, lowered blood pressure, and decreased muscle tension, thereby reducing the body's need for oxygen and reducing fatigue and anxiety.

To profit fully from progressive relaxation, you have to create a habit of the process, which means you have to set aside time three to five times a week for relaxing. The nice thing about establishing a routine of relaxation is that it requires only twenty minutes and it can be done almost anywhere.

There are two basic parts to progressive relaxation: (1) the recognition of tension in muscles, and (2) the relaxation of each muscle group.

The process for muscle tension recognition begins by assuming a comfortable position of lying down, sitting, or leaning back. You should be in a quiet area, away from distractions. Check for tension in each muscle group in your body: major tension areas include the shoulders, jaw, and forehead. Since there is tension in every muscle group, progression in a logical order is required to recognize and alleviate tension.

As you focus on a muscle group, begin the relaxation process by tensing the muscle group; hold that tension for five seconds. Then relax your muscles slowly for twenty to thirty seconds so that the tension feels like it's draining from your body. As you perform the process, tell yourself to "feel the tension go," and "let all the tension drain slowly from the muscle." Tension of a muscle group followed by a relaxation of those muscles can be repeated several times before moving on to the next muscle group. The progression is as follows:

1. **Chest:** Take a deep breath. Beginning with the abdominal area, fill the lungs with air while feeling the tension in the chest area from the expanded lungs. Expire from the top of your lungs to your abdomen while relaxing.

2. **Right foot and lower leg:** Keeping the heel down, curl the toes back until tension can be felt in the ankle and calf muscle.

3. **Right upper leg:** Tense the top of the upper leg (quadriceps) and the bottom of the upper leg (hamstring).

4. **Left foot, lower leg, and upper leg:** Repeat the process identified in numbers 2 and 3.

5. **Right hand and forearm:** With the palm down, lift the hand until tension can be felt in the top of the hand, the wrist, and the forearm.

6. **Right upper arm:** Tense the biceps and triceps.

7. **Right shoulder:** Shrug the shoulder toward the ear and roll the head toward the shoulder so that shoulder and ear are touching.

8. **Left hand and forearm, upper arm, and shoulder:** Repeat the process identified in numbers 5, 6, and 7.

9. **Jaw area:** Without damaging the teeth, bite down until tension can be felt in the jaw area.

10. **Mouth:** Purse the lips as if whistling.

11. **Chin:** Place the bottom of the tongue on the roof of the mouth and push upward.

12. **Forehead:** Wrinkle the brow.

13. **Breathing:** Throughout the full exercise, breathe at a steady rate.

As you begin the relaxation process, your body should feel heavy and warm. The feeling of heaviness will turn into a sensation of weightlessness as your body begins to relax. Typically, a cool band forms across the forehead as relaxation occurs. The feelings of weightlessness, warmness, and a cool band across the forehead are all natural responses in the relaxation process. You will feel a sense of well-being if relaxation is achieved.

It takes several weeks to attain a full relaxation response, but you'll make progress daily as you acquire the skill of relaxing. There will be days where there are setbacks followed by days of great gains. Eventually, relaxation can be achieved in short period of time in any location.

Chapter 14

Smoking and Your Health

Chapter Contents

Section 14.1

Effects of Smoking on Your Health

"Why It's Important to Quit Smoking" is reprinted from "Independence from Smoking: A Breath of Fresh Air! Why It's Important to Quit," and "The Effects of Quitting" is reprinted from "Independence from Smoking: A Breath of Fresh Air! The Effects of Quitting," National Women's Health Information Center, November 2005.

Why It's Important to Quit Smoking

People smoke for different reasons. Some people smoke to deal with stress or control weight. Younger people may start smoking as a way of rebelling, being independent, or being accepted among their peers. But there is never a good reason to smoke. Smoking causes serious health problems:

- Lung cancer and other lung diseases, such as emphysema and chronic bronchitis

- Cancer of the throat, mouth, larynx, lungs, esophagus, pancreas, kidneys, bladder, cervix, and stomach

- Leukemia, or cancer of the blood

- Aortic aneurysms, which happen when an artery near your stomach weakens and swells

- Bronchitis and pneumonia more often than for nonsmokers

- Gum disease

- Increased risk of cataracts, which cause blindness

- Ulcers in smokers who have the *Helicobacter pylori* bacteria

- Atherosclerosis or hardening and narrowing of the arteries

- Greatly increased risk for heart disease and stroke

- Greatly increased risk of dying from chronic obstructive lung disease

- Early menopause, which is the stopping of menstrual periods, in women
- Increased risk of hip fracture
- Increased tendency to form blood clots
- Additional health problems related to diabetes
- Increased wound infections after surgery
- Increased difficulty in women in becoming pregnant
- Stained teeth, fingers, and fingernails
- Bad breath
- Wrinkling skin
- Illnesses that last longer

Pregnant women who smoke are more likely to have these problems:

- Placenta previa, which is when the placenta grows too close to the opening of the uterus or womb. This can lead to delivery by cesarean section.
- Placental abruption, which is when the placenta separates too early from the wall of the uterus. This can lead to preterm delivery, stillbirth, and early infant death.
- Early rupture of membranes, or water breaking, before labor begins, so the baby is carried for a shorter amount of time.
- A baby with a low birth weight.
- Damage to an infant's developing lungs.

Infants exposed to secondhand smoke after birth have an increased risk of these health problems:

- Having harmful chemicals from tobacco passed to them through breast milk
- Sudden infant death syndrome (SIDS)
- Asthma, pneumonia, bronchitis, and fluid in the middle ear, or ear infections

The good news is that you can quit smoking, no matter how old you are or how long you have smoked. Quitting smoking has immediate as well as long-term benefits. Within minutes and hours after you inhale that last cigarette, your body begins a series of positive changes that continue for years. Among these health improvements are a drop in heart rate, improved circulation, and reduced risk of heart attack, lung cancer, and stroke. By quitting smoking today, you can have many healthier tomorrows.

All Forms of Tobacco Are Dangerous

People view other forms of tobacco as less harmful than cigarettes, but all tobacco is dangerous to your health.

The Effects of Quitting

When you quit smoking, there will be many positive affects on your body:

- Twenty minutes after quitting, your blood pressure drops. The temperature in your hands and feet rises.

- Eight hours after quitting, the carbon monoxide (a gas that can be toxic) in your blood drops to normal.

- Twenty-four hours after quitting, your chance of having a heart attack goes down.

- Two days after quitting, you can taste and smell things better.

- Two weeks to three months after quitting, you have better circulation. Your lungs are working better.

- One to nine months after quitting, coughing, sinus congestion, fatigue, and shortness of breath decrease. Your lungs start to function better, lowering your risk of lung infections.

- One year after quitting, your risk for heart disease is half that of a smoker's.

- Five years after quitting, your risk of having a stroke is the same as that of someone who doesn't smoke.

- Ten years after quitting, your risk of dying from lung cancer is half that of a smoker's. Your risk of cancer of the mouth, throat, esophagus, bladder, kidney, and pancreas also decreases.

- Fifteen years after quitting, your risk of heart disease is now the same as that of someone who doesn't smoke.

Section 14.2

Tips to Help You Quit Smoking

Reprinted from "Independence from Smoking: A Breath of Fresh Air! How to Quit," National Women's Health Information Center, November 2005.

Here are some steps that research has shown will help you to quit smoking for good.

Get ready to quit by picking a date to stop smoking: Before that day, get rid of all cigarettes, ashtrays, and lighters in your home, car, and workplace. Make it a rule never to let anyone smoke in your home. Write down why you want to quit and keep this list as a handy reminder.

Get support and encouragement from your family, friends, and co-workers: Studies have shown you will be more successful when you have help. Let the people important to you in your life know the date you will be quitting and ask them for their support. Ask them not to smoke around you or leave cigarettes out around you.

Learn new skills and do things differently: When you get the urge to smoke, try to do something that's different—talk to a friend, go for a walk, or do something you enjoy like gardening or going to the movies. Try to reduce your stress with exercise, meditation, hot baths, or reading. It's helpful to plan ahead for how you will deal with situations or triggers that will make you want to smoke. Have sugar-free gum or candy around to help handle your cravings. Drinking lots of water or other fluids also helps. You might want to change your daily routine as well—try drinking tea instead of coffee, eating your breakfast in a different place, or taking a different route to work.

Talk to your doctor or nurse about medicines to help you quit: Some people have symptoms of withdrawal when they quit smoking, such as depression; not being able to sleep; feeling cranky, frustrated, nervous, or restless; and trouble thinking clearly. Even though smoking doesn't suppress appetite, you may also feel hungry.

There are medicines to help relieve these symptoms. Most medicines help you quit smoking by giving you small, steady doses of nicotine, the drug in cigarettes that causes addiction. Talk to your doctor or nurse about which of these medicines is right for you:

- *Nicotine patch:* worn on the skin, through which it supplies a steady amount of nicotine to the body

- *Nicotine gum:* releases nicotine into the bloodstream through the lining in your mouth

- *Nicotine nasal spray:* inhaled through your nose, through which it passes into your bloodstream

- *Nicotine inhaler:* inhaled through the mouth and absorbed in the mouth and throat, but not in the lungs

- *Bupropion SR:* an antidepressant medicine that helps relieve nicotine withdrawal and the urge to smoke

Be prepared for relapse: Most people relapse, or start smoking again, within the first three months after quitting. Don't get discouraged if this happens to you or has happened to you before when you've tried to quit. Remember, many people try to quit several times before quitting for good. Think of what helped you and what didn't the last time you tried to quit—figuring these out before you try to quit again will increase your chances for success. Certain things or situations can increase your chances of smoking again, such as drinking alcohol, being around other smokers, gaining weight, stress, becoming depressed, or having more bad moods than usual. Talk to your doctor or nurse for ways to cope with these situations.

Section 14.3

Nicotine Replacement Therapy and Other Medications to Help You Stop Smoking

"Nicotine Replacement Therapy and Other Medication Which Aid Smoking Cessation," © 2006 American Lung Association. Reprinted with permission. For more information about the American Lung Association or to support the work it does, call 1-800-LUNG-USA (1-800-586-4872) or log on to http://www.lungusa.org.

Nicotine replacement products help relieve some of the withdrawal symptoms people experience when they quit smoking. There are several nicotine replacement products currently available over the counter in the United States, including two nicotine patches, nicotine gum, and nicotine lozenges. A nicotine nasal spray, inhaler (Zyban), and the recently approved nicotine-free tablet (Chantix®) are available only by prescription. To be most effective, nicotine replacement products should be used in conjunction with a behavior change program. The U.S. Food and Drug Administration (FDA) has approved all of the following medications to help you quit smoking.[1]

Over the Counter

Nicotine Patch (Also Available by Prescription)[2]

The nicotine patch releases a constant amount of nicotine in the body. Unlike the nicotine in tobacco smoke, which passes almost instantaneously into the blood through the lining of the lungs, the nicotine in the patch takes up to three hours to pass through the layers of skin and into the user's blood.

The patches are similar to adhesive bandages and are available in different shapes and sizes. A larger patch delivers more nicotine through the skin.

The patch must be worn all day, and cannot be put on and removed as a substitute for a cigarette. Most of the patch products are changed once every twenty-four hours. One particular patch is worn only during the waking hours and is removed during sleep.

Wearing the nicotine patch lessens chances of suffering from several of the major smoking withdrawal symptoms such as tenseness, irritability, drowsiness, and lack of concentration.

Some side effects from wearing the patch may include:[3]

- Skin irritation;

- Dizziness;

- Racing heartbeat;

- Sleep problems;

- Headache;

- Nausea;

- Vomiting, muscle aches, and stiffness.

Average retail price for over-the-counter transdermal nicotine patches (starter box) is approximately $4 a day.[4]

Nicotine Gum[5]

Nicotine gum delivers nicotine to the brain more quickly than the patch; however, unlike smoke, which passes almost instantaneously into the blood through the lining of the lung; the nicotine in the gum takes several minutes to reach the brain. This makes the "hit" less intense with the gum than with a cigarette.

Nicotine gum is not designed to be chewed like normal gum. Rather it is used in the "chew and park" method. When you insert a piece of gum into your mouth, chew it a few times to break it down, then park it between your gum and cheek and leave it there. The nicotine from the gum will make its way into your system via the blood vessels just under the lining of the oral cavity. If you continue chewing without parking, the nicotine will be released directly into the saliva in your mouth, which will eventually be swallowed, leaving you with a nasty stomachache and a craving for a cigarette.

Nicotine gum contains enough nicotine to reduce the urge to smoke. The over-the-counter gum is available in 2 mg doses (for smokers of twenty-four or fewer cigarettes each day) and 4 mg doses (for smokers of twenty-five or more cigarettes each day). One piece of gum is one dose; maximum dosage should not exceed twenty-four pieces per day.

Nicotine gum helps take the edge off cigarette cravings without providing the tars and poisonous gases found in cigarettes. It is a temporary aid that reduces symptoms of nicotine withdrawal after quitting smoking.

Nicotine gum must be used properly in order to be effective. Steps for nicotine gum users include:

- Stop all smoking when beginning the nicotine gum therapy.

- Do not eat or drink for fifteen minutes before using, or while chewing the gum (some beverages can reduce its effectiveness).

- Chew the gum slowly on and off for thirty minutes to release most of the nicotine. Parking the gum between the cheek and gum allows the absorption of nicotine into the lining of the cheek.

- Chew enough gum to reduce withdrawal symptoms (ten to fifteen pieces a day but no more than thirty a day).

- Use the gum every day for about a month or so, then start to reduce the number of pieces you chew a day, chewing only what you need to avoid withdrawal symptoms.

- Discontinue use of gum after three months.

- If the gum sticks to your dental work, stop using it and check with your medical healthcare professional or dentist. Dentures or other dental work may be damaged because nicotine gum is stickier and harder to chew than ordinary gum.

The average retail price for nicotine gum is approximately $4.50 (ten pieces) a day for average usage during the first six weeks of use.[6]

Nicotine Lozenge[7]

In 2002, the first and only over-the-counter nicotine lozenge meant to help smokers kick the habit was introduced to the market.

Nicotine lozenge comes in the form of a hard candy and releases nicotine as it slowly dissolves in the mouth. Eventually, the quitter will use fewer and fewer lozenges during the twelve-week program until he or she is completely nicotine-free. Biting or chewing the lozenge will cause more nicotine to be swallowed quickly and result in indigestion and/or heartburn.

Nicotine lozenge is available in 2 mg or 4 mg doses. One lozenge is one dose; maximum dosage should not exceed twenty lozenges per day.

Each lozenge will last about twenty to thirty minutes and nicotine will continue to leach through the lining of the mouth for a short time after the lozenge has disappeared. Do not eat or drink fifteen minutes before using the lozenge or while it is in your mouth.

Do not use nicotine lozenges for longer than twelve weeks. If you feel the need to continue using the lozenges after twelve weeks, contact your healthcare professional.

The most common side effects of lozenge use are:

- Soreness of the teeth and gums;
- Indigestion;
- Throat irritation.

The average retail price for nicotine lozenge is approximately $6 a day for average usage (twelve doses) and up to $12 a day for maximum usage (twenty doses) during the first six weeks of use.

By Prescription Only

Nicotine Nasal Spray[8]

Nicotine nasal spray, dispensed from a pump bottle similar to over-the-counter decongestant sprays, relieves cravings for a cigarette.

Nicotine is rapidly absorbed through the nasal membranes and reaches the bloodstream faster than any other nicotine replacement therapy (NRT) product, giving a rapid nicotine "hit." This feature makes it attractive to some highly dependent smokers.

The most common side effects due to the nasal spray are nose and throat irritations.

A usual single dose is two sprays, one in each nostril. The maximum recommended dose is five doses per hour or forty doses total per day.

The average retail price for nicotine nasal spray is approximately $5 a day for average use (thirteen doses) and up to $15 a day for maximum usage (forty doses).[9]

Nicotine Inhaler[10]

The nicotine inhaler consists of a plastic cylinder containing a cartridge that delivers nicotine when you puff on it. Use the inhaler when you have a craving for a cigarette. Use no more than sixteen cartridges a day for up to twelve weeks.

Although similar in appearance to a cigarette, the inhaler delivers nicotine into the mouth, not the lung, and it enters the body much more slowly than the nicotine in cigarettes. The nicotine inhaler is available only by prescription.

Each cartridge delivers up to four hundred puffs of nicotine vapor. It takes at least eighty puffs to obtain the equivalent amount of nicotine delivered by one cigarette.

The initial dosage is individualized. The best effect is achieved by frequent, continuous puffing for twenty minutes. One cartridge will last for twenty minutes of continuous puffing and deliver 4 mg of nicotine; only 2 mg are actually absorbed. This is the equivalent of about two cigarettes. The maximum suggested dose is sixteen cartridges per day.

Side effects include irritation of the throat and mouth in the beginning. You may also start to cough but you should get over this after a while; if not make sure to consult with your doctor.

The average retail cost of the nicotine inhaler is approximately $45.00 for a package (forty-two cartridges).[11]

Non-Nicotine Pill—Zyban[12]

Bupropion hydrochloride (Zyban®) was approved in 1997 to help smokers quit. The drug, available by prescription only, is also sold as an antidepressant under the name Wellbutrin®.

Common side effects include insomnia, dry mouth, and dizziness.

Treatment with bupropion begins while the user is still smoking, one week prior to the quit date. Treatment is then continued for seven to twelve weeks. Length of treatment is individualized.

Dosing should begin at 150 mg/day given every day for the first three days, followed by a dose increase for most people to the recommended dose of 300 mg/day, starting on the fourth day of treatment. The maximum recommended dose is 300 mg/day, given as 150 mg twice daily. An interval of at least eight hours between successive doses is advised.

People who have not made significant progress toward abstinence by the seventh week of therapy are unlikely to successfully quit during this attempt, and bupropion treatment should be discontinued.

The average wholesale price for bupropion is approximately $2 per day.[13]

Chantix Tablets[14]

The newest prescription drug Chantix, varenicline tartrate, is only the second nicotine-free smoking-cessation drug to gain FDA approval. The active ingredient varenicline works in two ways—by cutting the pleasure of smoking and reducing the withdrawal symptoms that lead smokers to light up again and again.

The tablet will be taken twice daily for twelve weeks, a period that can be doubled in patients who successfully quit to increase the likelihood they remain smoke-free.

The most common adverse side effects include nausea, headache, vomiting, gas, insomnia, abnormal dreams, and a change in taste perception.

It is necessary with all types of medication to follow the doctor's orders and use the products only as prescribed and according to labeling.

Studies suggest that everyone can quit smoking. Your situation or condition can give you a special reason to quit:

- **Pregnant women/new mothers:** By quitting, you protect your baby's health and your own.

- **Hospitalized patients:** By quitting, you reduce health problems and help healing.

- **Heart attack patients:** By quitting, you reduce your risk of a second heart attack.

- **Lung, head, and neck cancer patients:** By quitting, you reduce your chance of a second cancer.

- **Parents of children and adolescents:** By quitting, you protect your children and adolescents from illnesses caused by secondhand smoke.[15]

The goal in using nicotine replacement therapy is to stop smoking completely. If you plan to take nicotine medications, begin using them on the day you quit. If you continue to have strong urges to smoke or are struggling to stop smoking completely, ask your healthcare provider about additional help.

Notes

1. Nicotine: A Powerful Addiction: Available at: http://www.cdc.gov/tobacco/quit/canquit.htm. Accessed on 5/15/06.

2. American Caner Society: Quitting Smoking. Prevention and Early Detection; Available at: http://www.cancer.org/docroot/PED_10_13xGuide_for_Qutting_Smoking.acs.htm. Accessed on 5/4/05.

3. Ibid.

4. *The Wall Street Journal Online*: Case Grows to Cover Quitting, April 26, 2005; D1

5. American Caner Society: Quitting Smoking. Prevention and Early Detection; Available at: http://www.cancer.org/docroot/PED_10_13xGuide_for_Qutting_Smoking.acs.htm. Accessed on 5/4/05.

6. *The Wall Street Journal Online*: Case Grows to Cover Quitting, April 26, 2005; D1

7. American Caner Society: Quitting Smoking. Prevention and Early Detection; Available at: http://www.cancer.org/docroot/PED_10_13xGuide_for_Qutting_Smoking.acs.htm. Accessed on 5/4/05.

8. FDA Approves Novel Medication for Smoking Cessation. Available at: http://www.fda.gov/cder/foi/label/2001/20066s8lbl.pdf. Accessed on 4/6/06.

9. American Caner Society: Quitting Smoking. Prevention and Early Detection; Available at: http://www.cancer.org/docroot/PED_10_13xGuide_for_Qutting_Smoking.acs.htm. Accessed on 5/4/05.

10. *The Wall Street Journal Online*: Case Grows to Cover Quitting, April 26, 2005; D1

11. American Caner Society: Quitting Smoking. Prevention and Early Detection; Available at: http://www.cancer.org/docroot/PED_10_13xGuide_for_Qutting_Smoking.acs.htm. Accessed on 5/4/05.

12. FDA Approves Novel Medication for Smoking Cessation. Available at: http://www.fda.gov/cder/foi/label/2001/20066s8lbl.pdf. Accessed on 4/6/06.

13. *The Wall Street Journal Online*: Case Grows to Cover Quitting, April 26, 2005; D1

14. Ibid.

15. Nicotine: A Powerful Addiction: Available at: http://www.cdc.gov/tobacco/quit/canquit.htm. Accessed on 5/15/06.

Chapter 15

Alcohol:
Too Much Can Be Harmful

Chapter Contents

Section 15.1

Alcohol: What You Don't Know Can Harm You

Reprinted from National Institute on Alcohol Abuse and Alcoholism,
National Institutes of Health, NIH Publication No. 99-4323, 2004.

If you are like many Americans, you may drink alcohol occasionally. Or, like others, you may drink moderate amounts of alcohol on a more regular basis. If you are a woman or someone over the age of sixty-five, this means you have no more than one drink per day; if you are a man, this means you have no more than two drinks per day. Drinking at these levels usually is not associated with health risks and may help prevent certain forms of heart disease.

But did you know that even moderate drinking, under certain circumstances, can be risky? If you drink at more than moderate levels, you may be putting yourself at risk for serious problems with your health as well as problems with family, friends, and co-workers. This booklet explains some of the problems that can be caused by drinking that you may not have considered.

What Is a Drink?

A standard drink is:

- One 12-ounce bottle of beer[1] or wine cooler;
- One 5-ounce glass of wine;
- 1.5 ounces of 80-proof distilled spirits.

Drinking and Driving

It may surprise you to learn that you don't need to drink much alcohol before your driving ability is affected. For example, certain driving skills can be impaired by blood alcohol concentrations (BACs) as low as 0.02 percent. (The BAC refers to the amount of alcohol in the blood.) A 160-pound man will have a BAC of about 0.04 percent one hour after drinking two twelve-ounce beers or two other standard drinks on an empty stomach. And the more alcohol you drink, the more impaired your driving skills will be. Although most states set the BAC limit for adults who drive after drinking at 0.08 percent, driving skills are affected at much lower levels.

Interactions with Medications

Drinking alcohol while taking certain medications can cause problems. In fact, there are more than 150 medications that should not be mixed with alcohol. For example, if you are taking antihistamines for a cold or allergy and drink alcohol, the alcohol will increase the drowsiness that the medicine alone can cause, making driving or operating machinery even more dangerous. If you are taking large doses of the painkiller acetaminophen (Tylenol®) and drinking alcohol, you are risking serious liver damage. Check with your doctor or pharmacist before drinking any amount of alcohol if you are taking any over-the-counter or prescription medicines.

Social and Legal Problems

The more heavily you drink, the greater the potential for problems at home, at work, with friends, and even with strangers. These problems may include the following:

- Arguments with or separation from your spouse and other family members
- Strained relationships with co-workers
- Absence from or lateness to work with increasing frequency
- Loss of employment due to decreased productivity
- Committing or being the victim of violence

Alcohol-Related Birth Defects

If you are pregnant or trying to get pregnant, you should not drink alcohol. Drinking alcohol while you are pregnant can cause a range of birth defects, and children exposed to alcohol before birth can have lifelong learning and behavioral problems. The most serious problem that can be caused by drinking during pregnancy is fetal alcohol syndrome (FAS). Children born with FAS have severe physical, mental, and behavioral problems. Because scientists do not know exactly how much alcohol it takes to cause alcohol-related birth defects, it is best not to drink any alcohol during this time.

Long-Term Health Problems

Some problems, like those mentioned previously, can occur after drinking over a relatively short period of time. But other problems—such as liver disease, heart disease, certain forms of cancer, and pancreatitis—often develop more gradually and may become evident only after many years of heavy drinking. Women may develop alcohol-related health problems sooner than men, and from drinking less alcohol than men. Because alcohol affects nearly every organ in the body, long-term heavy drinking increases the risk for many serious health problems, some of which are described here.

Alcohol-related liver disease: More than two million Americans suffer from alcohol-related liver disease. Some drinkers develop alcoholic hepatitis, or inflammation of the liver, as a result of heavy drinking over a long period of time. Its symptoms include fever, jaundice (abnormal yellowing of the skin, eyeballs, and urine), and abdominal pain. Alcoholic hepatitis can cause death if drinking continues. If drinking stops, the condition may be reversible. About 10 to 20 percent of heavy drinkers develop alcoholic cirrhosis, or scarring of the liver. People with cirrhosis should not drink alcohol. Although treatment for the complications of cirrhosis is available, a liver transplant may be needed for someone with life-threatening cirrhosis. Alcoholic cirrhosis can cause death if drinking continues. Cirrhosis is not reversible, but if a person with cirrhosis stops drinking, the chances of survival improve considerably. People with cirrhosis often feel better, and liver function may improve, after they stop drinking. About four million Americans are infected with hepatitis C virus (HCV), which can cause liver cirrhosis and liver cancer. Some heavy drinkers also have HCV infection. As a result, their livers may be damaged not only by alcohol but by HCV-related problems as well. People with HCV infection are more susceptible to alcohol-related liver damage and should think carefully about the risks when considering whether to drink alcohol.

Heart disease: Moderate drinking can have beneficial effects on the heart, especially among those at greatest risk for heart attacks, such as men over the age of forty-five and women after menopause. However, heavy drinking over a long period of time increases the risk for heart disease, high blood pressure, and some kinds of stroke.

Cancer: Long-term heavy drinking increases the risk of certain forms of cancer, especially cancer of the esophagus, mouth, throat, and larynx (voice box). Research suggests that, in some women, as little as one drink per day can slightly raise the risk of breast cancer. Drinking may also increase the risk for developing cancer of the colon and rectum.

Pancreatitis: The pancreas helps regulate the body's blood sugar levels by producing insulin. The pancreas also has a role in digesting the food we eat. Long-term heavy drinking can lead to pancreatitis, or inflammation of the pancreas. Acute pancreatitis can cause severe abdominal pain and can be fatal. Chronic pancreatitis is associated with chronic pain, diarrhea, and weight loss.

If you or someone you know has been drinking heavily, there is a risk of developing serious health problems. Because some of these health problems can be treated, it is important to see a doctor for help. Your doctor will be able to advise you about your health and your drinking.

Research Directions

The National Institute on Alcohol Abuse and Alcoholism (NIAAA), National Institutes of Health, supports about 90 percent of the nation's research on alcohol use and its related consequences. Today, alcohol researchers are working on the cutting edge of medical science to answer questions such as:

- Who is at greatest risk for developing alcohol problems?

- What are the effects of binge drinking, particularly among young people?

- When does alcohol use increase the risk of violent behavior?

- Why are women more vulnerable to alcohol's effects?

Each new research discovery leads us to better ways to prevent and treat the alcohol-related problems that harm individuals, families, and society.

Notes

1. Different beers have different alcohol content. Malt liquor has a higher alcohol content than most other brewed beverages.

Section 15.2

Alcoholism: Get the Facts

Reprinted from "Alcoholism: Getting the Facts," National Institute on Alcohol Abuse and Alcoholism, National Institutes of Health, NIH Publication No. 96-4153, 2001. Reviewed by David A. Cooke, M.D., May 2007.

For many people, the facts about alcoholism are not clear. What is alcoholism, exactly? How does it differ from alcohol abuse? When should a person seek help for a problem related to his or her drinking?

A Widespread Problem

For most people who drink, alcohol is a pleasant accompaniment to social activities. Moderate alcohol use—up to two drinks per day for men and one drink per day for women and older people—is not harmful for most adults. (A standard drink is one 12-ounce bottle or can of either beer or wine cooler, one 5-ounce glass of wine, or 1.5 ounces of 80-proof distilled spirits.) Nonetheless, a large number of people get into serious trouble because of their drinking. Currently, nearly 17.6 million adult Americans abuse alcohol or are alcoholic. Several million more adults engage in risky drinking that could lead to alcohol problems. These patterns include binge drinking and heavy drinking on a regular basis. In addition, 53 percent of men and women in the United States report that one or more of their close relatives have a drinking problem.

The consequences of alcohol misuse are serious—in many cases, life threatening. Heavy drinking can increase the risk for certain cancers, especially those of the liver, esophagus, throat, and larynx (voice box). Heavy drinking can also cause liver cirrhosis, immune system problems, brain damage, and harm to the fetus during pregnancy. In addition, drinking increases the risk of death from automobile crashes as well as recreational and on-the-job injuries. Furthermore, both homicides and suicides are more likely to be committed by persons who have been drinking. In purely economic terms, alcohol-related problems cost society approximately $185 billion per year. In human terms, the costs cannot be calculated.

What Is Alcoholism?

Alcoholism, also known as "alcohol dependence," is a disease that includes four symptoms:

• **Craving:** A strong need, or compulsion, to drink.

• **Loss of control:** The inability to limit one's drinking on any given occasion.

• **Physical dependence:** Withdrawal symptoms, such as nausea, sweating, shakiness, and anxiety, occur when alcohol use is stopped after a period of heavy drinking.

• **Tolerance:** The need to drink greater amounts of alcohol in order to "get high."

People who are not alcoholic sometimes do not understand why an alcoholic can't just "use a little willpower" to stop drinking. However, alcoholism has little to do with willpower. Alcoholics are in the grip of a powerful "craving," or uncontrollable need, for alcohol that overrides their ability to stop drinking. This need can be as strong as the need for food or water.

Although some people are able to recover from alcoholism without help, the majority of alcoholics need assistance. With treatment and support, many individuals are able to stop drinking and rebuild their lives.

Many people wonder why some individuals can use alcohol without problems but others cannot. One important reason has to do with genetics. Scientists have found that having an alcoholic family member makes it more likely that if you choose to drink you too may develop alcoholism. Genes, however, are not the whole story. In fact, scientists now believe that certain factors in a person's environment influence whether a person with a genetic risk for alcoholism ever develops the disease. A person's risk for developing alcoholism can increase based on the person's environment, including where and how he or she lives; family, friends, and culture; peer pressure; and even how easy it is to get alcohol.

What Is Alcohol Abuse?

Alcohol abuse differs from alcoholism in that it does not include an extremely strong craving for alcohol, loss of control over drinking, or physical dependence. Alcohol abuse is defined as a pattern of drinking that results in one or more of the following situations within a twelve-month period:

- Failure to fulfill major work, school, or home responsibilities
- Drinking in situations that are physically dangerous, such as while driving a car or operating machinery
- Having recurring alcohol-related legal problems, such as being arrested for driving under the influence of alcohol or for physically hurting someone while drunk
- Continued drinking despite having ongoing relationship problems that are caused or worsened by the drinking

Although alcohol abuse is basically different from alcoholism, many effects of alcohol abuse are also experienced by alcoholics.

What Are the Signs of a Problem?

How can you tell whether you may have a drinking problem? Answering the following four questions can help you find out:

- Have you ever felt you should cut down on your drinking?
- Have people annoyed you by criticizing your drinking?
- Have you ever felt bad or guilty about your drinking?
- Have you ever had a drink first thing in the morning (as an "eye opener") to steady your nerves or get rid of a hangover?

One "yes" answer suggests a possible alcohol problem. If you answered "yes" to more than one question, it is highly likely that a problem exists. In either case, it is important that you see your doctor or other healthcare provider right away to discuss your answers to these questions. He or she can help you determine whether you have a drinking problem and, if so, recommend the best course of action.

Even if you answered "no" to all of the above questions, if you encounter drinking-related problems with your job, relationships, health, or the law, you should seek professional help. The effects of alcohol abuse can be extremely serious—even fatal—both to you and to others.

The Decision to Get Help

Accepting the fact that help is needed for an alcohol problem may not be easy. Keep in mind, however, that the sooner you get help, the better your chances are for a successful recovery.

Any concerns you may have about discussing drinking-related problems with your healthcare provider may stem from common misconceptions about alcoholism and alcoholic people. In our society, the myth prevails that an alcohol problem is a sign of moral weakness.

As a result, you may feel that to seek help is to admit some type of shameful defect in yourself. In fact, alcoholism is a disease that is no more a sign of weakness than is asthma. Moreover, taking steps to identify a possible drinking problem has an enormous payoff—a chance for a healthier, more rewarding life.

When you visit your healthcare provider, he or she will ask you a number of questions about your alcohol use to determine whether you are having problems related to your drinking. Try to answer these questions as fully and honestly as you can. You also will be given a physical examination. If your healthcare provider concludes that you may be dependent on alcohol, he or she may recommend that you see a specialist in treating alcoholism. You should be involved in any referral decisions and have all treatment choices explained to you.

Getting Well

Alcoholism Treatment

The type of treatment you receive depends on the severity of your alcoholism and the resources that are available in your community. Treatment may include detoxification (the process of safely getting alcohol out of your system); taking doctor-prescribed medications, such as disulfiram (Antabuse®), naltrexone (ReVia™), or acamprosate (Campral®) to help prevent a return (or relapse) to drinking once drinking has stopped; and individual or group counseling. There are promising types of counseling that teach alcoholics to identify situations and feelings that trigger the urge to drink and to find new ways to cope that do not include alcohol use. These treatments are often provided on an outpatient basis.

Because the support of family members is important to the recovery process, many programs also offer brief marital counseling and family therapy as part of the treatment process. Programs may also link individuals with vital community resources, such as legal assistance, job training, childcare, and parenting classes.

Alcoholics Anonymous

Virtually all alcoholism treatment programs also include Alcoholics Anonymous (AA) meetings. AA describes itself as a "worldwide fellowship of men and women who help each other to stay sober." Although AA is generally recognized as an effective mutual help program for recovering alcoholics, not everyone responds to AA's style or message, and other recovery approaches are available. Even people who are helped by AA usually find that AA works best in combination with other forms of treatment, including counseling and medical care.

Can Alcoholism Be Cured?

Although alcoholism can be treated, a cure is not yet available. In other words, even if an alcoholic has been sober for a long time and has regained health, he or she remains susceptible to relapse and must continue to avoid all alcoholic beverages. "Cutting down" on drinking doesn't work; cutting out alcohol is necessary for a successful recovery.

However, even individuals who are determined to stay sober may suffer one or several "slips," or relapses, before achieving long-term sobriety. Relapses are very common and do not mean that a person has failed or cannot recover from alcoholism. Keep in mind, too, that every day that a recovering alcoholic has stayed sober prior to a relapse is extremely valuable time, both to the individual and to his or her family. If a relapse occurs, it is very important to try to stop drinking once again and to get whatever additional support you need to abstain from drinking.

Help for Alcohol Abuse

If your healthcare provider determines that you are not alcohol dependent but are nonetheless involved in a pattern of alcohol abuse, he or she can help you to take the following steps:

- Examine the benefits of stopping an unhealthy drinking pattern.
- Set a drinking goal for yourself. Some people choose to abstain from alcohol. Others prefer to limit the amount they drink.
- Examine the situations that trigger your unhealthy drinking patterns, and develop new ways of handling those situations so that you can maintain your drinking goal.

Some individuals who have stopped drinking after experiencing alcohol-related problems choose to attend AA meetings for information and support, even though they have not been diagnosed as alcoholic.

New Directions

With the support of the National Institute on Alcohol Abuse and Alcoholism (NIAAA), scientists at medical centers and universities throughout the country are studying alcoholism. The goal of this research is to develop better ways of treating and preventing alcohol problems. Today, NIAAA funds approximately 90 percent of all alcoholism research in the United States. Some of the more exciting investigations focus on the causes, consequences, treatment, and prevention of alcoholism:

- **Genetics:** Alcoholism is a complex disease. Therefore, there are likely to be many genes involved in increasing a person's risk for alcoholism. Scientists are searching for these genes and have found areas on chromosomes where they are probably located. Powerful new techniques may permit researchers to identify and measure the specific contribution of each gene to the complex behaviors associated with heavy drinking. This research will provide the basis for new medications to treat alcohol-related problems.

- **Treatment:** NIAAA-supported researchers have made considerable progress in evaluating commonly used therapies and in developing new types of therapies to treat alcohol-related problems. One large-scale study sponsored by NIAAA found that each of three commonly used behavioral treatments for alcohol abuse and alcoholism—motivation enhancement therapy, cognitive-behavioral therapy, and twelve-step facilitation therapy— significantly reduced drinking in the year following treatment. This study also found that approximately one-third of the study participants who were followed up either were still abstinent or were drinking without serious problems three years after the study ended. Other therapies that have been evaluated and found effective in reducing alcohol problems include brief intervention for alcohol abusers (individuals who are not dependent on alcohol) and behavioral marital therapy for married alcohol-dependent individuals.

- **Medications development:** NIAAA has made developing medications to treat alcoholism a high priority. We believe that a range of new medications will be developed based on the results of genetic and neuroscience research. In fact, neuroscience research has already led to studies of one medication—naltrexone

(ReVia)—as an anticraving medication. NIAAA-supported researchers found that this drug, in combination with behavioral therapy, was effective in treating alcoholism. Naltrexone, which targets the brain's reward circuits, is the first medication approved to help maintain sobriety after detoxification from alcohol since the approval of disulfiram (Antabuse) in 1949. Acamprosate, an anticraving medication, has been widely used in Europe and just recently was approved for use in the United States. Researchers believe that acamprosate works on different brain circuits to ease the physical discomfort that occurs when an alcoholic stops drinking. All of these new medications have their roots in neuroscience research, as do other drugs that are currently under investigation for the treatment of alcoholism.

- **Combined medications/behavioral therapies:** NIAAA-supported researchers have found that available medications work best with behavioral therapy. Thus, NIAAA has initiated a large-scale clinical trial to determine which of the currently available medications and which behavioral therapies work best together. Naltrexone and acamprosate will each be tested separately with different behavioral therapies. These medications will also be used together to determine if there is some interaction between the two that makes the combination more effective than the use of either one alone.

In addition to these efforts, NIAAA is sponsoring promising research in other vital areas, such as fetal alcohol syndrome, alcohol's effects on the brain and other organs, aspects of drinkers' environments that may contribute to alcohol abuse and alcoholism, strategies to reduce alcohol-related problems, and new treatment techniques. Together, these investigations will help prevent alcohol problems; identify alcohol abuse and alcoholism at earlier stages; and make available new, more effective treatment approaches for individuals and families.

Chapter 16

Commonly Abused Drugs and Their Health Effects

These days, drugs can be found everywhere, and it may seem like everyone's doing them. Many people are tempted by the excitement or escape that drugs seem to offer. But learning the facts about drugs can help you see the risks of chasing this excitement or escape. Read on to learn more.

The Deal on Substances

Thanks to medical and drug research, there are thousands of drugs that help people. Antibiotics and vaccines have revolutionized the treatment of infections. There are medicines to lower blood pressure, treat diabetes, and reduce the body's rejection of new organs. Medicines can cure, slow, or prevent disease, helping us to lead healthier and happier lives. But there are also lots of illegal, harmful drugs that people take to help them feel good or have a good time.

How do drugs work? Drugs are chemicals or substances that change the way our bodies work. When you put them into your body (often by swallowing, inhaling, or injecting them), drugs find their way into your bloodstream and are transported to parts of your body, such as your brain. In the brain, drugs may either intensify or dull your

Excerpted from "Drugs: What You Should Know." This information was provided by KidsHealth, one of the largest resources online for medically reviewed health information written for parents, kids, and teens. For more articles like this one, visit www.KidsHealth.org, or www.TeensHealth.org. © 2004 The Nemours Foundation.

senses, alter your sense of alertness, and sometimes decrease physical pain. A drug may be helpful or harmful. The effects of drugs can vary depending upon the kind of drug taken, how much is taken, how often it is used, how quickly it gets to the brain, and what other drugs, food, or substances are taken at the same time. Effects can also vary based on the differences in body size, shape, and chemistry.

Although substances can feel good at first, they can ultimately do a lot of harm to the body and brain. Drinking alcohol, smoking tobacco, taking illegal drugs, and sniffing glue can all cause serious damage to the human body. Some drugs severely impair a person's ability to make healthy choices and decisions. People who drink, for example, are more likely to get involved in dangerous situations, such as driving under the influence or having unprotected sex.

And just as there are many kinds of drugs available, there are as many reasons for trying drugs or starting to use drugs regularly. People take drugs just for the pleasure they believe they can bring. Often it's because someone tried to convince them that drugs would make them feel good or that they'd have a better time if they took them.

Some people believe drugs will help them think better, be more popular, stay more active, or become better athletes. Others are simply curious and figure one try won't hurt. Others want to fit in. A few use drugs to gain attention from others. Many people use drugs because they are depressed or think drugs will help them escape their problems. The truth is, drugs don't solve problems. Drugs simply hide feelings and problems. When a drug wears off, the feelings and problems remain— or become worse. Drugs can ruin every aspect of a person's life.

What are some of the more common drugs?

Alcohol

The oldest and most widely used drug in the world, alcohol is a depressant that alters perceptions, emotions, and senses.

How it's used: Alcohol is a liquid that is drunk.

Effects and Dangers

- Alcohol first acts as a stimulant, and then it makes people feel relaxed and a bit sleepy.

- High doses of alcohol seriously affect a person's judgment and coordination. Drinkers may have slurred speech, confusion, depression, short-term memory loss, and slow reaction times.

- Large volumes of alcohol drunk in a short period of time may cause alcohol poisoning.

Addictiveness: People who use alcohol can become psychologically dependent upon it to feel good, deal with life, or handle stress. In addition, their bodies may demand more and more to achieve the same kind of high experienced in the beginning. Some people are also at risk of becoming physically addicted to alcohol. Withdrawal from alcohol can be painful and even life threatening. Symptoms range from shaking, sweating, nausea, anxiety, and depression to hallucinations, fever, and convulsions.

Amphetamines

Amphetamines are stimulants that accelerate functions in the brain and body. They come in pills or tablets. Prescription diet pills also fall into this category of drugs.

Street names: Speed, uppers, dexies, bennies

How they're used: Amphetamines are swallowed, inhaled, or injected.

Effects and Dangers

- Swallowed or snorted, these drugs hit users with a fast high, making them feel powerful, alert, and energized.

- Uppers pump up heart rate, breathing, and blood pressure, and they can also cause sweating, shaking, headaches, sleeplessness, and blurred vision.

- Prolonged use may cause hallucinations and intense paranoia.

Addictiveness: Amphetamines are psychologically addictive. Users who stop report that they experience various mood problems, such as aggression and anxiety, and intense cravings for the drugs.

Cocaine and Crack

Cocaine is a white crystalline powder made from the dried leaves of the coca plant. Crack, named for its crackle when heated, is made from cocaine. It looks like white or tan pellets.

Street names for cocaine: Coke, snow, blow, nose candy, white, big C

Street names for crack: Freebase, rock

How they're used: Cocaine is inhaled through the nose or injected. Crack is smoked.

Effects and Dangers

- Cocaine is a stimulant that rocks the central nervous system, giving users a quick, intense feeling of power and energy. Snorting highs last between fifteen and thirty minutes; smoking highs last between five and ten minutes.

- Cocaine also elevates heart rate, breathing rate, blood pressure, and body temperature.

- Injecting cocaine can give you hepatitis or AIDS (acquired immunodeficiency syndrome) if you share needles with other users. Snorting can also put a hole inside the lining of your nose.

- First-time users of both cocaine and crack can stop breathing or have fatal heart attacks. Using either of these drugs even one time can kill you.

Addictiveness: These drugs are highly addictive, and as a result, the drug, not the user, calls the shots. Even after one use, cocaine and crack can create both physical and psychological cravings that make it very, very difficult for users to stop.

Cough and Cold Medicines (DXM)

Several over-the-counter cough and cold medicines contain the ingredient dextromethorphan (also called DXM). If taken in large quantities, these over-the-counter medicines can cause hallucinations, loss of motor control, and "out-of-body" (or dissociative) sensations.

Street names: Triple C, candy, C-C-C, dex, DM, drex, red devils, robo, rojo, skittles, tussin, velvet, vitamin D

How they're used: Cough and cold medicines, which come in tablets, capsules, gel caps, and lozenges as well as syrups, are swallowed. DXM is often extracted from cough and cold medicines, put into powder form, and snorted.

Effects and Dangers

- Small doses help suppress coughing, but larger doses can cause fever, confusion, impaired judgment, blurred vision, dizziness, paranoia, excessive sweating, slurred speech, nausea, vomiting, abdominal pain, irregular heartbeat, high blood pressure, head-ache, lethargy, numbness of fingers and toes, redness of face, dry and itchy skin, loss of consciousness, seizures, brain damage, and even death.

- Sometimes users mistakenly take cough syrups that contain other medications in addition to dextromethorphan. High doses of these other medications can cause serious injury or death.

Addictiveness: People who use cough and cold medicines and DXM regularly to get high can become psychologically dependent upon them (meaning they like the feeling so much they can't stop, even though they aren't physically addicted).

Depressants

Depressants, such as tranquilizers and barbiturates, calm nerves and relax muscles. Many are legally available by prescription (such as Valium and Xanax) and are bright-colored capsules or tablets.

Street names: Downers, goof balls, barbs, ludes

How they're used: Depressants are swallowed.

Effects and Dangers

- When used as prescribed by a doctor and taken at the correct dosage, depressants can help people feel calm and reduce angry feelings.

- Larger doses can cause confusion, slurred speech, lack of coordination, and tremors.

- Very large doses can cause a person to stop breathing and result in death.

- Depressants and alcohol should never be mixed—this combination greatly increases the risk of overdose and death.

Addictiveness: Depressants can cause both psychological and physical dependence.

Ecstasy (MDMA)

Ecstasy (methylenedioxymethamphetamine, or MDMA) is a designer drug created by underground chemists. It comes in powder, tablet, or capsule form. Ecstasy is a popular club drug because it is widely available at raves, dance clubs, and concerts.

Street names: XTC, X, Adam, E, Roll

How it's used: Ecstasy is swallowed or sometimes snorted.

Effects and Dangers

- This drug combines a hallucinogenic with a stimulant effect, making all emotions, both negative and positive, much more intense.

- Users feel a tingly skin sensation and an increased heart rate.

- Ecstasy can also cause dry mouth, cramps, blurred vision, chills, sweating, and nausea.

- Sometimes users clench their jaws while using. They may chew on something (like a pacifier) to relieve this symptom.

- Many users also experience depression, paranoia, anxiety, and confusion. There is some concern that these effects on the brain and emotion can become permanent with chronic use of ecstasy.

- Ecstasy also raises the temperature of the body. This increase can sometimes cause organ damage or even death.

Addictiveness: Although the physical addictiveness of Ecstasy is unknown, people who use it can become psychologically dependent upon it to feel good, deal with life, or handle stress.

GHB

GHB, which stands for gamma hydroxybutyrate, is often made in home basement labs, usually in the form of a liquid with no odor or color. It has gained popularity at dance clubs and raves and is a popular alternative to Ecstasy. The number of people brought to emergency departments because of GHB side effects is quickly rising in the United States. And according to the U.S. Drug Enforcement Agency (DEA), since 1995 GHB has killed more users than Ecstasy.

Street names: Liquid Ecstasy, G, Georgia Home Boy

How it's used: When in liquid or powder form (mixed in water), GHB is drunk; in tablet form it is swallowed.

Effects and Dangers

- GHB is a depressant drug that can cause both euphoric (high) and hallucinogenic effects.

- The drug has several dangerous side effects, including severe nausea, breathing problems, decreased heart rate, and seizures.

- GHB has been used for date rape because it is colorless and odorless and easy to slip into drinks.

- At high doses, users can lose consciousness within minutes. It's also easy to overdose. There is only a small difference between the dose used to get high and the amount that can cause an overdose.

- Overdosing GHB requires emergency care in a hospital right away. Within an hour GHB overdose can cause coma and stop someone's breathing, resulting in death.

- GHB (even at lower doses) mixed with alcohol is very dangerous—using it even once can kill you.

Addictiveness: When users come off GHB they may have withdrawal symptoms such as insomnia and anxiety. People may also become dependent upon it to feel good, deal with life, or handle stress.

Heroin

Heroin comes from the dried milk of the opium poppy, which is also used to create the class of painkillers called narcotics—medicines like codeine and morphine. Heroin can range from a white to dark brown powder to a sticky, tar-like substance.

Street names: Horse, smack, Big H, junk

How it's used: Heroin is injected, smoked, or inhaled (if it is pure).

211

Effects and Dangers

- Heroin gives you a burst of euphoric (high) feelings, especially if it's injected. This high is often followed by drowsiness, nausea, stomach cramps, and vomiting.

- Users feel the need to take more heroin as soon as possible just to feel good again.

- With long-term use, heroin ravages the body. It is associated with chronic constipation, dry skin, scarred veins, and breathing problems.

- Users who inject heroin often have collapsed veins and put themselves at risk of getting deadly infections such as HIV, hepatitis B or C, and bacterial endocarditis (inflammation of the lining of the heart) if they share needles with other users.

Addictiveness: Heroin is extremely addictive and easy to overdose on (which can cause death). Withdrawal is intense and symptoms include insomnia, vomiting, and muscle pain.

Inhalants

Inhalants are substances that are sniffed or "huffed" to give the user an immediate rush or high. They include household products like glues, paint thinners, dry cleaning fluids, gasoline, felt-tip marker fluid, correction fluid, hair spray, aerosol deodorants, and spray paint.

How it's used: Inhalants are breathed in directly from the original container (sniffing or snorting), from a plastic bag (bagging), or by holding an inhalant-soaked rag in the mouth (huffing).

Effects and Dangers

- Inhalants make you feel giddy and confused, as if you were drunk. Long-time users get headaches, nosebleeds, and may suffer loss of hearing and sense of smell.

- Inhalants are the most likely of abused substances to cause severe toxic reaction and death. Using inhalants, even one time, can kill you.

Addictiveness: Inhalants can be very addictive. People who use inhalants can become psychologically dependent upon them to feel good, deal with life, or handle stress.

Ketamine

Ketamine hydrochloride is a quick-acting anesthetic that is legally used in both humans (as a sedative for minor surgery) and animals (as a tranquilizer). At high doses, it causes intoxication and hallucinations similar to LSD (lysergic acid diethylamide).

Street names: K, Special K, vitamin K, bump, cat Valium

How it's used: Ketamine usually comes in powder that users snort. Users often do it along with other drugs such as Ecstasy (called kitty flipping) or cocaine or sprinkle it on marijuana blunts.

Effects and Dangers

- Users may become delirious, hallucinate, and lose their sense of time and reality. The trip—also called K-hole—that results from ketamine use lasts up to two hours.

- Users may become nauseated or vomit, become delirious, and have problems with thinking or memory.

- At higher doses, ketamine causes movement problems, body numbness, and slowed breathing.

- Overdosing on ketamine can stop you from breathing—and kill you.

Addictiveness: People who use it can become psychologically dependent upon it to feel good, deal with life, or handle stress.

LSD

LSD (which stands for lysergic acid diethylamide) is a lab-brewed hallucinogen and mood-changing chemical. LSD is odorless, colorless, and tasteless.

Street names: Acid, blotter, doses, microdots

How it's used: LSD is licked or sucked off small squares of blotting paper. Capsules and liquid forms are swallowed. Paper squares containing acid may be decorated with cute cartoon characters or colorful designs.

Effects and Dangers

- Hallucinations occur within thirty to ninety minutes of dropping acid. People say their senses are intensified and distorted—they see colors or hear sounds with other delusions such as melting walls and a loss of any sense of time. But effects are unpredictable, depending on how much LSD is taken and the user.

- Once you go on an acid trip, you can't get off until the drug is finished with you—at times up to about twelve hours or even longer!

- Bad trips may cause panic attacks, confusion, depression, and frightening delusions.

- Physical risks include sleeplessness, mangled speech, convulsions, increased heart rate, and coma.

- Users often have flashbacks in which they feel some of the effects of LSD at a later time without having used the drug again.

Addictiveness: People who use it can become psychologically dependent upon it to feel good, deal with life, or handle stress.

Marijuana

The most widely used illegal drug in the United States, marijuana resembles green, brown, or gray dried parsley with stems or seeds. A stronger form of marijuana called hashish (hash) looks like brown or black cakes or balls. Marijuana is often called a gateway drug because frequent use often leads to the use of stronger drugs.

Street names: Pot, weed, blunts, chronic, grass, reefer, herb, ganja

How it's used: Marijuana is typically smoked in cigarettes (joints), hollowed-out cigars (blunts), pipes (bowls), or water pipes (bongs). Some people mix it into foods or brew it as a tea.

Effects and Dangers

- Marijuana can affect mood and coordination. Users may experience mood swings that range from stimulated or happy to drowsy or depressed.

- Marijuana also elevates heart rate and blood pressure. Some people get red eyes and feel very sleepy or hungry. The drug can also make some people paranoid or cause them to hallucinate.

- Marijuana is as tough on the lungs as cigarettes—steady smokers suffer coughs, wheezing, and frequent colds.

Addictiveness: People who use marijuana can become psychologically dependent upon it to feel good, deal with life, or handle stress. In addition, their bodies may demand more and more marijuana to achieve the same kind of high experienced in the beginning.

Methamphetamine

Methamphetamine is a powerful stimulant.

Street names: Crank, meth, speed, crystal, chalk, fire, glass, crypto, ice

How it's used: It can be swallowed, snorted, injected, or smoked.

Effects and Dangers

- Users feel a euphoric rush from methamphetamine, particularly if it is smoked or shot up. But they can develop tolerance quickly—and will use more meth for longer periods of time, resulting in sleeplessness, paranoia, and hallucinations.

- Users sometimes have intense delusions such as believing that there are insects crawling under their skin.

- Prolonged use may result in violent, aggressive behavior, psychosis, and brain damage.

- The chemicals used to make methamphetamine can also be dangerous to both people and the environment.

Addictiveness: Methamphetamine is highly addictive.

Nicotine

Nicotine is a highly addictive stimulant found in tobacco. This drug is quickly absorbed into the bloodstream when smoked.

How it's used: Nicotine is typically smoked in cigarettes or cigars. Some people put a pinch of tobacco (called chewing or smokeless tobacco) into their mouths and absorb nicotine through the lining of their mouths.

Effects and Dangers

- Physical effects include rapid heartbeat, increased blood pressure, shortness of breath, and a greater likelihood of colds and flu.

- Nicotine users have an increased risk for lung and heart disease and stroke. Smokers also have bad breath and yellowed teeth. Chewing tobacco users may suffer from cancers of the mouth and neck.

- Withdrawal symptoms include anxiety, anger, restlessness, and insomnia.

Addictiveness: Nicotine is as addictive as heroin or cocaine, which makes it extremely difficult to quit. Those who start smoking before the age of twenty-one have the hardest time breaking the habit.

Rohypnol

Rohypnol (pronounced: ro-hip-nol) is a low-cost, increasingly popular drug. Because it often comes in presealed bubble packs, many people think that the drug is safe.

Street names: Roofies, roach, forget-me pill, date rape drug

How it's used: This drug is swallowed, sometimes with alcohol or other drugs.

Effects and Dangers

- Rohypnol is a prescription anti-anxiety medication that is ten times more powerful than Valium.

- It can cause the blood pressure to drop, as well as cause memory loss, drowsiness, dizziness, and an upset stomach.

- Though it's part of the depressant family of drugs, it causes some people to be overly excited or aggressive.

- Rohypnol has received a lot of attention because of its association with date rape. Many women report having been raped after having Rohypnol slipped into their drinks. The drug also causes "anterograde amnesia." This means it's hard to remember what happened while on the drug, like a blackout. Because of this it can be hard to give important details if a young woman wants to report the rape.

Addictiveness: Users can become physically addicted to Rohypnol, so it can cause extreme withdrawal symptoms when users stop.

Chapter 17

Getting Help for Addiction

What Are Substance Abuse and Addiction?

The difference between substance abuse and addiction is very slight. Addiction begins as abuse, or using a substance like marijuana or cocaine. You can abuse a drug (or alcohol) without having an addiction. For example, just because someone has smoked weed a few times doesn't mean that he or she has an addiction, but it does mean that he or she is abusing a drug—and that could lead to an addiction.

People can get addicted to all sorts of substances. When we think of addiction, we usually think of alcohol or illegal drugs. But people become addicted to medications, cigarettes, even glue! And some substances are more addictive than others: Drugs like crack or heroin are so addictive that they may be used only once or twice before the user loses control.

Addiction means a person has no control over whether he or she uses a drug or drinks. A person who's addicted to cocaine has grown so used to the drug that he or she has to have it. Addiction can be physical, psychological, or both.

Physical addiction is when a person's body actually becomes dependent on a particular substance (even smoking is physically addictive). It also means that a person builds tolerance to that substance,

Reprinted from "Dealing with Addiction." This information was provided by KidsHealth, one of the largest resources online for medically reviewed health information written for parents, kids, and teens. For more articles like this one, visit www.KidsHealth.org or www.TeensHealth.org. © 2004 The Nemours Foundation.

so that person needs a larger dose than ever before to get the same effects. When a person who is physically addicted stops using a substance like drugs, alcohol, or cigarettes, he or she may experience withdrawal symptoms. Withdrawal can be like having the flu—common symptoms are diarrhea, shaking, and generally feeling awful.

Psychological addiction happens when the cravings for a drug are psychological or emotional. People who are psychologically addicted feel overcome by the desire to have a drug. They may lie or steal to get it.

A person crosses the line between abuse and addiction when he or she is no longer trying the drug to have fun or get high, but because he or she has come to depend on it. His or her whole life centers around the need for the drug. An addicted person—whether it's a physical or psychological addiction or both—no longer has a choice in taking a substance.

Signs of Addiction

The most obvious sign of an addiction is the need to have a particular drug or substance. However, there are many other signs that can suggest a possible addiction, such as changes in mood or weight loss or gain. (These are also signs of other conditions, too, though, such as depression or eating disorders.)

Signs that you or someone you know may have a drug or alcohol addiction include both psychological and physical signals.

Psychological Signals

- Use of drugs or alcohol as a way to forget problems or to relax

- Withdrawal or keeping secrets from family and friends

- Loss of interest in activities that used to be important

- Problems with schoolwork, such as slipping grades or absences

- Changes in friendships, such as hanging out only with friends who use drugs

- Spending a lot of time figuring out how to get drugs

- Stealing or selling belongings to be able to afford drugs

- Failed attempts to stop taking drugs or drinking

- Anxiety, anger, or depression

- Mood swings

Physical Signals

- Changes in sleeping habits

- Feeling shaky or sick when trying to stop

- Needing to take more of the substance to get the same effect

- Changes in eating habits, including weight loss or gain

Getting Help

If you think you are addicted to drugs or alcohol, recognizing that you have a problem is the first step in getting help.

A lot of people think they can kick the problem on their own, but that doesn't work for most people. Find someone you trust to talk to.

Unfortunately, overcoming addiction is not easy. Quitting drugs or drinking is probably going to be the hardest thing you've ever done. It's not a sign of weakness if you need professional help from a trained drug counselor or therapist. Most people who try to kick a drug or alcohol program need professional assistance or treatment programs to do so.

Once you start a treatment program, try these tips to make the road to recovery less bumpy:

- Tell your friends about your decision to stop using drugs. Your true friends will respect your decision. This may mean that you need to find a new group of friends who will be 100 percent supportive. Unless everyone decides to kick their drug habit at once, you probably won't be able to hang out with the friends you did drugs with before.

- Ask your friends or family to be available when you need them. You may need to call someone in the middle of the night just to talk. If you're going through a tough time, don't try to handle things on your own—accept the help your family and friends offer.

- Accept invitations to events only that you know won't involve drugs or alcohol. Going to the movies is probably safe, but you may want to skip a Friday night party until you're feeling more secure. Plan activities that don't involve drugs. Go to the movies, try bowling, or take an art class with a friend.

- Have a plan about what you'll do if you find yourself in a place with drugs or alcohol. The temptation will be there sometimes, but if you know how you're going to handle it, you'll be OK.

- Remind yourself that having an addiction doesn't make you bad or weak. If you backslide a bit, talk to your treatment advisor as soon as possible. There's nothing to be ashamed about, but it's important to get help soon so that all of the hard work you put into your recovery is not lost.

If you're worried about a friend who has an addiction, use these tips to help him or her, too. For example, let your friend know that you are available to talk or offer your support. If you notice a friend backsliding, talk about it openly and ask what you can do to help.

Above all, offer a friend who's battling an addiction lots of encouragement and praise. It may seem corny, but hearing that you care is just the kind of motivation your friend needs.

Staying Clean

Recovering from a drug or alcohol addiction doesn't end with a six-week treatment program. It's a lifelong process. Many people find that joining a support group can help them stay clean. You'll meet people who have gone through the same experiences you have, and you'll be able to participate in real-life discussions about drugs that you won't hear anywhere else.

Many people find that helping others is also the best way to help themselves. Your understanding of how difficult the recovery process can be will help you to support others who are battling an addiction.

If you do have a relapse, recognizing the problem as soon as possible is critical. Get help right away so that you don't undo all the hard work you put into your initial recovery. And don't ever be afraid to ask for help!

Chapter 18

Other Behaviors That Can Affect Your Health

Chapter Contents

Section 18.1

Unsafe Sex and How to Avoid It

Reprinted from " Safe Sex," © 2007 A.D.A.M., Inc.
Reprinted with permission.

Definition

Safe sex means taking precautions during sex that can keep you from getting a sexually transmitted disease (STD), or from giving an STD to your partner. These diseases include genital herpes, genital warts, human immunodeficiency virus (HIV), Chlamydia, gonorrhea, syphilis, hepatitis B and C, and others.

Information

A STD is a contagious disease that can be transferred to another person through sexual intercourse or other sexual contact. Many of the organisms that cause sexually transmitted diseases live on the penis, vagina, anus, mouth, and skin of surrounding areas.

Most of the diseases are transferred by direct contact with a sore on the genitals or mouth. However, some organisms can be transferred in body fluids without causing a visible sore. They can be transferred to another person during oral, vaginal, or anal intercourse.

Some STDs can also be transferred by nonsexual contact with infected tissues or fluids, such as infected blood. For example, sharing needles when using intravenous (IV) drugs is a major cause of HIV and hepatitis B transmission. An STD can also be transmitted through contaminated blood transfusions and blood products, through the placenta from the mother to the fetus, and sometimes through breast-feeding.

The following factors increase your risk of getting a sexually transmitted disease (STD):

- Not knowing whether a partner has an STD

- Having a partner with a past history of any STD

- Having sex without a male or female condom

- Using drugs or alcohol in a situation where sex might occur

- If your partner is an IV drug user

- Having anal intercourse

Drinking alcohol or using drugs increase the likelihood that you will participate in high-risk sex. In addition, some diseases can be transferred through the sharing of used needles or other drug paraphernalia.

Abstinence is an absolute answer to preventing STDs. However, abstinence is not always a practical or desirable option.

Next to abstinence, the least risky approach is to have a monogamous sexual relationship with someone that you know is free of any STD. Ideally, before having sex with a new partner, each of you should get screened for STDs, especially HIV and hepatitis B, and share the test results with one another.

Use condoms to avoid contact with semen, vaginal fluids, or blood. Both male and female condoms dramatically reduce the chance you will get or spread an STD. However, condoms must be used properly:

- The condom should be in place from the beginning to end of sexual activity and should be used every time you have sex.

- Lubricants may help reduce the chance a condom will break. Use only water-based lubricants, because oil-based or petroleum-type lubricants can cause latex to weaken and tear. Do *not* use condoms with nonoxynol-9—these help prevent pregnancy, but may increase the chance of HIV transmission.

- Use latex condoms for vaginal, anal, and oral intercourse.

- Keep in mind that STDs can still be spread, even if you use a condom, because a condom does not cover surrounding skin areas. But a condom definitely reduces your risk.

Here are additional safe-sex steps:

- Know your partner. Before having sex, first establish a committed relationship that allows trust and open communication. You should be able to discuss past sexual histories, any previous STDs or IV drug use. You should not feel coerced or forced into having sex.

- Stay sober. Alcohol and drugs impair your judgment, communication abilities, and ability to properly use condoms or lubricants.

223

- Be responsible. If you have an STD, like HIV or herpes, advise any prospective sexual partner. Allow him or her to decide what to do. If you mutually agree on engaging in sexual activity, use latex condoms and other measures to protect the partner.

- If pregnant, take precautions. If you have an STD, learn about the risk to the infant before becoming pregnant. Ask your provider how to prevent the fetus from becoming infected. HIV-positive women should not breast-feed their infant.

In summary, safe sex requires prior planning and good communication between partners. Given that, couples can enjoy the pleasures of a sexual relationship while reducing the potential risks involved.

Section 18.2

The Dangers of Indoor Tanning

From "The Truth about Indoor Tanning," © American Osteopathic Association (www.osteopathic.org). Reprinted with permission. The text of this document is available online at http://www.osteopathic.org/index.cfm?PageID =you_indoortan; accessed February 5, 2007.

As the temperatures rise and shorts replace pants, pale winter skin may sway some to consider the speedy effects of indoor tanning to achieve a bronze summer glow. However, indoor tanning is even more dangerous than outdoor sun exposure.

"The myth of health associated with a suntan is simply that—a myth," explains Craig Wax, D.O., an osteopathic family physician practicing in Mullica Hill, New Jersey. "Some people expose themselves to the sun for the vitamin D. The amount of vitamin D made available is minimal compared with the risk of skin cancer with prolonged exposure."

He further explains that tanning is the body's way of protecting itself against ultraviolet (UV) ray exposure. The brown pigment melanin produced by skin is spread throughout the exposed areas. This pigment only minimally protects the skin against further damage from UV radiation.

Despite this information, the use of indoor tanning devices that emit ultraviolet light, both in tanning salons and at home, has never been more popular. The industry serves twenty-eight million people; generates $5 billion a year; and is represented by thirty thousand tanning facilities across the country, according to the Skin Cancer Foundation.

"Many patients consider indoor tanning to be a safer alternative to sun tanning," he explains. "But it is just the opposite: tanning beds emit up to twice as much skin-damaging radiation."

Dr. Wax explains that overexposure to UV rays can cause eye injury, premature wrinkling and aging of the skin, light-induced skin rashes, and increased chances of developing skin cancer.

"Young women are prone to use tanning salons," explains Dr. Wax, "because while the aging effects and skin cancer might take years to surface, the perceived social value of a tan is immediate." He warns that the dangers of tanning are serious and increase the potential for skin cancer, including:

- **Malignant melanoma:** The deadliest form of skin cancer, often surfacing as a flat or slightly raised discolored patch that has irregular borders. This is the result of intense exposure in childhood, resulting in multiple sunburns.

- **Basal cell carcinoma (BCC):** The most common form of skin cancer, BCC can be identified by an open sore, a red patch of skin, a shiny bump, a pink growth or scar-like area. This type of skin cancer follows a similar pattern to melanoma and is best identified by a physician.

Dr. Wax further explains that the health risks associated with UV radiation are even more likely with smoking, the use of birth control pills, anti-depressants, acne medication, ingredients found in antidandruff shampoos, lime oil, and some cosmetics.

"If you or someone you know is using an indoor tanning device, it is important to educate them on the hazards of tanning," explains Dr. Wax.

Further, he explains that if skin shows signs of possible cancer, it is important to consult a physician immediately.

Section 18.3

Tattoos and Permanent Makeup

Reprinted from the U.S. Food and Drug Administration
(www.fda.gov), August 2005.

Before getting a tattoo or permanent makeup, here is what you
should know. A tattoo is a mark or design on the skin. A permanent
tattoo is meant to last forever. It is made with a needle and colored
ink. The needle puts the ink into the skin.

Many colors used in tattoo inks are not approved by the U.S. Food
and Drug Administration (FDA) to be used on the skin. Some of these
colors are meant for printing or painting cars.

What types of tattoos are there?

There are many different kinds of tattoos:

- **Permanent tattoos:** A needle is used to insert colored ink into
  the skin.

- **Permanent makeup:** Permanent tattoos use a needle to insert
  colored ink into the skin. It makes it look like makeup, such as
  eyebrow pencil, lip liner, eyeliner, or blush.

- **Henna (mehndi) tattoos:** A natural plant dye called henna or
  mehndi is used to stain the skin. This kind of tattoo does not use
  needles. The color lasts two to three weeks. Use of henna in tattoos is illegal. Henna is approved only for use as a hair dye. It
  should not be put on the skin.

- **"Sticker" type temporary tattoos:** The tattoo design is on a
  piece of coated paper. It is put on the skin with water. Temporary
  tattoos last only a few days. Don't use tattoos from other countries.
  The FDA might not approve the colors. You might be allergic to
  them.

Why would someone want a tattoo?

- To restore a natural look to the face or breast, especially after
  surgery.

- They have trouble putting on makeup as a result of a medical condition.

- They have lost their eyebrows.

What are the risks?

Infection: Dirty needles can pass infections from one person to another person. These can be serious, like hepatitis and human immunodeficiency virus (HIV). Make sure that the needles are clean and germ-free.

You might be allergic to something used in your tattoo. This is rare, but can cause serious problems.

Lumps or bumps may form around the tattoo color.

People may have swelling or burning in the tattoo when they have magnetic resonance imaging (MRI). This happens rarely and does not last very long.

You may not like your tattoo even if it was done well. Not liking the tattoo is the most common reason people give for having one removed.

If you decide you want to get rid of a tattoo, it usually takes many treatments and costs a lot of money.

Scars may form when getting or removing a tattoo.

Think very carefully before getting a tattoo. Most tattoos are permanent. Removing tattoos and permanent makeup can be hard and can cost a lot of money. Sometimes, it cannot be done. It often means surgery and scarring.

How can I get rid of a tattoo?

Tattoo removal should be done by a doctor or clinic and not by a tattoo parlor. There are several ways to try to remove a tattoo, but they don't always work. It can cost a lot of money and you may need a lot of treatment. Here are some choices:

- **Laser treatment:** This is the most common way to remove a tattoo. Light from the laser breaks up the tattoo ink. The body itself gets rid of the treated areas over the next few weeks. Most tattoos need more than one laser treatment to be fully removed. Some inks cannot be removed by lasers.

- **Dermabrasion:** Sanding down to lower layers of skin is another way to remove a tattoo. The area to be sanded is numbed first to lessen pain. It may leave a scar.

- **Salabrasion:** A salt solution is used to remove the color. This is called salabrasion and is sometimes used with dermabrasion. Salabrasion is not used often.

- **Scarification:** This process removes the tattoo with acid and leaves a scar in its place.

- **Surgical removal:** You can have surgery to get rid of the tattoo.

- **Cover up:** New colors can be put into the skin to cover up the old tattoo.

Does the FDA control tattoos?

FDA does not control the tattoo parlors. Each state has its own laws for this.

How should I report a bad reaction or report a complaint?

They can be reported by contacting your FDA district office, or by contacting FDA's Center for Food Safety and Applied Nutrition Adverse Events Reporting System.

Section 18.4

Aggressive Driving

"Aggressive Driving," © 2007 American College of Emergency Physicians. All rights reserved. Reprinted with permission.

Main Points

Emergency physicians see the tragic consequences of aggressive driving every day and are dedicated to preventing injuries, including those involving motor vehicles.

Aggressive driving has been identified by the public as the number one problem on the nation's roadways.

The National Highway Traffic Safety Administration has estimated that aggressive drivers cause two-thirds of all fatal crashes and are responsible for nearly 35 percent of all crashes.

What is aggressive driving?

The National Highway Traffic Safety Administration (NHTSA) defines aggressive driving as operation of a motor vehicle that endangers or is likely to endanger people or property. It is a progression of unlawful driving actions that includes:

• **Speeding:** Exceeding the posted limit or driving too fast for conditions;

• **Improper or excessive lane changing:** Failing to signal intent or failing to see that movement can be made safely; or

• **Improper passing:** Failing to signal intent, using an emergency lane to pass, or passing on the shoulder.

Aggressive driving is a traffic offense. The exact number of motor vehicle crashes caused by aggressive drivers is unknown, but NHTSA estimates about 66 percent of all traffic fatalities annually are caused by aggressive driving behaviors, such as passing on the right, running red lights, and tailgating.

A nationwide study by NHTSA of fatal crashes at traffic signals in 1999 and 2000 estimated that 20 percent of the vehicles involved failed to obey the signals. In 2004, more than 900 people were killed and an estimated 168,000 were injured in crashes that involved red light running. About half of the deaths in red light running crashes are pedestrians and occupants in other vehicles who are hit by the red light runners.

According to the Insurance Institute for Highway Safety, disregarding red lights and other traffic control devices is the leading cause of urban crashes, representing 22 percent of the total number of crashes. The economic impact is estimated at $7 billion each year in medical costs, time off work, insurance rate increases, and property damage.

What is road rage?

NHTSA defines road rage as an "assault with a motor vehicle or other dangerous weapon by the operator or passenger(s) of another motor vehicle or an assault precipitated by an incident that occurred on a roadway. Road rage is a criminal offense."

What factors are linked to aggressive driving?

Some of the factors linked to aggressive driving include:

• Crowded roads;

• Being in a hurry;

- Roadwork;
- Stress from other areas of life;
- Dangerous driving attitudes;
- Selfishness.

What should you do when confronted by an aggressive driver?

You should:

- Make every attempt to get out of the way.
- Put your pride in the back seat. Do not challenge him or her by speeding up or attempting to "hold your own" in your travel lane.
- Wear your seat belt. It will hold you in your seat and behind the wheel in case you need to make an abrupt driving maneuver, and it will protect you in a crash.
- Avoid eye contact.
- Ignore gestures and refuse to return them.

Report aggressive drivers (once you are safe) to appropriate authorities; provide a vehicle description, license number, location, and if possible, direction of travel. If you have a cell phone, and can do it safely, call the police—many have special numbers (e.g., 9-1-1 or #77). If an aggressive driver is involved in a crash farther down the road, stop a safe distance from the crash scene, wait for police to arrive, and report the driving behavior you witnessed.

What preventive steps can be taken to avoid becoming the victim of an aggressive driver?

You should:

- Always merge with plenty of room. Never "cut" people off.
- If you are in the left lane and someone wants to pass, let him— even if you are going the speed limit.
- Never use obscene gestures.
- Drive defensively.

Part Three

Disease Prevention:
What Adults Should Know

Chapter 19

Preventing Cancer

Doctors often cannot explain why one person develops cancer and another does not. But research shows that certain risk factors increase the chance that a person will develop cancer. These are the most common risk factors for cancer:

- Growing older
- Tobacco
- Sunlight
- Ionizing radiation
- Certain chemicals and other substances
- Some viruses and bacteria
- Certain hormones
- Family history of cancer
- Alcohol
- Poor diet, lack of physical activity, or being overweight

Many of these risk factors can be avoided. Others, such as family history, cannot be avoided. People can help protect themselves by staying away from known risk factors whenever possible.

Excerpted from "What You Need to Know about Cancer—An Overview: Risk Factors," National Cancer Institute, October 4, 2006.

Tobacco

Tobacco use is the most preventable cause of death. Each year, more than 180,000 Americans die from cancer that is related to tobacco use.

Using tobacco products or regularly being around tobacco smoke (environmental or secondhand smoke) increases the risk of cancer.

Smokers are more likely than nonsmokers to develop cancer of the lung, larynx (voice box), mouth, esophagus, bladder, kidney, throat, stomach, pancreas, or cervix. They also are more likely to develop acute myeloid leukemia (cancer that starts in blood cells).

People who use smokeless tobacco (snuff or chewing tobacco) are at increased risk of cancer of the mouth.

Quitting is important for anyone who uses tobacco—even people who have used it for many years. The risk of cancer for people who quit is lower than the risk for people who continue to use tobacco. (But the risk of cancer is generally lowest among those who never used tobacco.)

Also, for people who have already had cancer, quitting may reduce the chance of getting another cancer.

Sunlight

Ultraviolet (UV) radiation comes from the sun, sunlamps, and tanning booths. It causes early aging of the skin and skin damage that can lead to skin cancer.

Doctors encourage people of all ages to limit their time in the sun and to avoid other sources of UV radiation:

- It is best to avoid the midday sun (from midmorning to late afternoon) whenever possible. You also should protect yourself from UV radiation reflected by sand, water, snow, and ice. UV radiation can penetrate light clothing, windshields, and windows.

- Wear long sleeves, long pants, a hat with a wide brim, and sunglasses with lenses that absorb UV.

- Use sunscreen. Sunscreen may help prevent skin cancer, especially sunscreen with a sun protection factor (SPF) of at least 15. But sunscreens cannot replace avoiding the sun and wearing clothing to protect the skin.

- Stay away from sunlamps and tanning booths. They are no safer than sunlight.

Ionizing Radiation

Ionizing radiation can cause cell damage that leads to cancer. This kind of radiation comes from rays that enter the earth's atmosphere from outer space, radioactive fallout, radon gas, x-rays, and other sources.

Radioactive fallout can come from accidents at nuclear power plants or from the production, testing, or use of atomic weapons. People exposed to fallout may have an increased risk of cancer, especially leukemia and cancers of the thyroid, breast, lung, and stomach.

Radon is a radioactive gas that you cannot see, smell, or taste. It forms in soil and rocks. People who work in mines may be exposed to radon. In some parts of the country, radon is found in houses. People exposed to radon are at increased risk of lung cancer.

Medical procedures are a common source of radiation:

- Doctors use radiation (low-dose x-rays) to take pictures of the inside of the body. These pictures help to diagnose broken bones and other problems.

- Doctors use radiation therapy (high-dose radiation from large machines or from radioactive substances) to treat cancer.

The risk of cancer from low-dose x-rays is extremely small. The risk from radiation therapy is slightly higher. For both, the benefit nearly always outweighs the small risk.

You should talk with your doctor if you are concerned that you may be at risk for cancer due to radiation.

If you live in a part of the country that has radon, you may wish to test your home for high levels of the gas. The home radon test is easy to use and inexpensive. Most hardware stores sell the test kit.

Certain Chemicals and Other Substances

People who have certain jobs (such as painters, construction workers, and those in the chemical industry) have an increased risk of cancer. Many studies have shown that exposure to asbestos, benzene, benzidine, cadmium, nickel, or vinyl chloride in the workplace can cause cancer.

Follow instructions and safety tips to avoid or reduce contact with harmful substances both at work and at home. Although the risk is highest for workers with years of exposure, it makes sense to be careful at home when handling pesticides, used engine oil, paint, solvents, and other chemicals.

Some Viruses and Bacteria

Being infected with certain viruses or bacteria may increase the risk of developing cancer:

- **Human papillomaviruses (HPVs):** HPV infection is the main cause of cervical cancer. It also may be a risk factor for other types of cancer.

- **Hepatitis B and hepatitis C viruses:** Liver cancer can develop after many years of infection with hepatitis B or hepatitis C.

- **Human T-cell leukemia/lymphoma virus (HTLV-1):** Infection with HTLV-1 increases a person's risk of lymphoma and leukemia.

- **Human immunodeficiency virus (HIV):** HIV is the virus that causes AIDS. People who have HIV infection are at greater risk of cancer, such as lymphoma and a rare cancer called Kaposi sarcoma.

- **Epstein-Barr virus (EBV):** Infection with EBV has been linked to an increased risk of lymphoma.

- **Human herpesvirus 8 (HHV8):** This virus is a risk factor for Kaposi sarcoma.

- *Helicobacter pylori*: This bacterium can cause stomach ulcers. It also can cause stomach cancer and lymphoma in the stomach lining.

Do not have unprotected sex or share needles. You can get an HPV infection by having sex with someone who is infected. You can get hepatitis B, hepatitis C, or HIV infection from having unprotected sex or sharing needles with someone who is infected.

You may want to consider getting the vaccine that prevents hepatitis B infection. Healthcare workers and others who come into contact with other people's blood should ask their doctor about this vaccine.

If you think you may be at risk for HIV or hepatitis infection, ask your doctor about being tested. These infections may not cause symptoms, but blood tests can show whether the virus is present. If so, the doctor may suggest treatment. Also, the doctor can tell you how to avoid infecting other people.

If you have stomach problems, see a doctor. Infection with *H. pylori* can be detected and treated.

Certain Hormones

Doctors may recommend hormones (estrogen alone or estrogen along with progestin) to help control problems (such as hot flashes, vaginal dryness, and thinning bones) that may occur during menopause. However, studies show that menopausal hormone therapy can cause serious side effects. Hormones may increase the risk of breast cancer, heart attack, stroke, or blood clots.

A woman considering menopausal hormone therapy should discuss the possible risks and benefits with her doctor.

Alcohol

Having more than two drinks each day for many years may increase the chance of developing cancers of the mouth, throat, esophagus, larynx, liver, and breast. The risk increases with the amount of alcohol that a person drinks. For most of these cancers, the risk is higher for a drinker who uses tobacco.

Doctors advise people who drink to do so in moderation. Drinking in moderation means no more than one drink per day for women and no more than two drinks per day for men.

Poor Diet, Lack of Physical Activity, or Being Overweight

People who have a poor diet, do not have enough physical activity, or are overweight may be at increased risk of several types of cancer. For example, studies suggest that people whose diet is high in fat have an increased risk of cancers of the colon, uterus, and prostate. Lack of physical activity and being overweight are risk factors for cancers of the breast, colon, esophagus, kidney, and uterus.

Having a healthy diet, being physically active, and maintaining a healthy weight may help reduce cancer risk. Doctors suggest the following:

- **Eat well:** A healthy diet includes plenty of foods that are high in fiber, vitamins, and minerals. This includes whole-grain breads and cereals and five to nine servings of fruits and vegetables every day. Also, a healthy diet means limiting foods high in fat (such as butter, whole milk, fried foods, and red meat).

- **Be active and maintain a healthy weight:** Physical activity can help control your weight and reduce body fat. Most scientists agree that it is a good idea for an adult to have moderate physical activity (such as brisk walking) for at least thirty minutes on five or more days each week.

Chapter 20

Preventing Disorders of the Heart and Blood Vessels

Chapter Contents

Section 20.1

Controlling Your Blood Cholesterol

Excerpted from "Your Guide to Lowering Your Cholesterol with TLC,"
National Heart, Lung, and Blood Institute, National Institutes of
Health, NIH Publication No. 06-5235, December 2005.

Cholesterol is a waxy, fat-like substance found in the walls of cells
in all parts of the body. The body uses cholesterol to make hormones,
bile acids, vitamin D, and other substances. The body makes all the
cholesterol it needs.

Cholesterol circulates in the bloodstream but cannot travel by itself.
As with oil and water, cholesterol (which is fatty) and blood (which is
watery) do not mix. So cholesterol travels in packages called lipoproteins, which have fat (lipid) inside and protein outside. Two main kinds
of lipoproteins carry cholesterol in the blood:

- Low density lipoprotein, or LDL, which also is called the "bad"
  cholesterol because it carries cholesterol to tissues, including the
  arteries. Most of the cholesterol in the blood is the LDL form. The
  higher the level of LDL cholesterol in the blood, the greater
  your risk for heart disease.

- High density lipoprotein, or HDL, which also is called the "good"
  cholesterol because it takes cholesterol from tissues to the liver,
  which removes it from the body. A low level of HDL cholesterol
  increases your risk for heart disease.

If there is too much cholesterol in the blood, some of the excess can
become trapped in artery walls. Over time, this builds up and is called
plaque. The plaque can narrow vessels and make them less flexible,
a condition called atherosclerosis or "hardening of the arteries."

This process can happen to blood vessels anywhere in the body,
including those of the heart, which are called the coronary arteries.
If the coronary arteries become partly blocked by plaque, then the
blood may not be able to bring enough oxygen and nutrients to the
heart muscle. This can cause chest pain, or angina. Some cholesterol-
rich plaques are unstable—they have a thin covering and can burst,

releasing cholesterol and fat into the bloodstream. The release can cause a blood clot to form over the plaque, blocking blood flow through the artery—and causing a heart attack.

What Affects Cholesterol Levels?

Various factors can cause unhealthy cholesterol levels. Some of the factors cannot be changed but most can be modified.

Factors you cannot change:

- **Heredity:** The amount of LDL cholesterol your body makes and how fast it is removed from your body is determined partly by genes. High blood cholesterol can run in families. However, very few people are stuck with a high cholesterol just by heredity— and everyone can take action to lower their cholesterol. Furthermore, even if high cholesterol does not run in your family, you can still develop it.

- **Age and sex:** Blood cholesterol begins to rise around age 20 and continues to go up until about age 60 or 65. Before age 50, men's total cholesterol levels tend to be higher than those of women of the same age—after age 50, the opposite happens.

Factors under your control:

- **Diet:** Three nutrients in your diet make LDL levels rise: saturated fat, a type of fat found mostly in foods that come from animals; trans fat, found mostly in foods made with hydrogenated oils and fats such as stick margarine, crackers, and French fries; and cholesterol, which comes only from animal products. Saturated fat raises your LDL cholesterol level more than anything else in your diet. Diets with too much saturated fat, trans fat, and cholesterol are the main cause for high levels of blood cholesterol—a leading contributor to the high rate of heart attacks among Americans.

- **Overweight:** Excess weight tends to increase your LDL level. Also, it typically raises triglycerides, a fatty substance in the blood and in food, and lowers HDL. Losing the extra pounds may help lower your LDL and triglycerides, while raising your HDL.

- **Physical inactivity:** Being physically inactive contributes to being overweight and can raise LDL and lower HDL. Regular physical activity can raise HDL and lower triglycerides, and can help you lose weight and, in that way, help lower your LDL.

Knowing Your Cholesterol Level

Most of the 65 million Americans with high cholesterol have no symptoms. So it's important to have your blood cholesterol levels checked. All adults age 20 and older should have their cholesterol levels checked at least once every 5 years. If you have an elevated cholesterol, you'll need to have it tested more often.

The recommended cholesterol test is called a "lipoprotein profile." It measures the levels of total cholesterol (which includes the cholesterol in all lipoproteins), LDL, HDL, and triglycerides. The lipoprotein profile is done after a 9- to 12-hour fast. A small sample of blood is taken from your finger or arm. The levels are measured as milligrams of cholesterol per deciliter of blood, or mg/dL.

Table 20.1. Cholesterol Classifications

Total Cholesterol

Less than 200 mg/dL	Desirable
200–239 mg/dL	Borderline high
240 mg/dL and above	High

LDL Cholesterol

Less than 100 mg/dL	Optimal (ideal)
100–129 mg/dL	Near optimal/above optimal
130–159 mg/dL	Borderline high
160–189 mg/dL	High
190 mg/dL and above	Very high

HDL Cholesterol

Less than 40 mg/dL	Major heart disease risk factor
60 mg/dL and above	Gives some protection against heart disease

Setting Your Goal

The main goal in treating high cholesterol is to lower your LDL level. The level to which your LDL must be lowered depends on the risk for developing heart disease or having a heart attack that you are found to have at the start of treatment. The higher your risk, the lower your goal LDL level. If the LDL level is in the "high" category and fewer than two other risk factors for heart disease are present, the goal is an LDL level lower than 160 mg/dL. If two or more risk factors are present, the goal is less than 130 mg/dL. If a patient already has heart disease, LDL levels should be 100 mg/dL or less.

Studies have proven that lowering LDL can prevent heart attacks and reduce deaths from heart disease in both men and women. It can slow, stop, or even reverse the buildup of plaque. It also can lower the cholesterol content in unstable plaques, making them more stable and less likely to burst and cause a heart attack. Lowering LDL is especially important for those who already have heart disease or have had a heart attack—it will reduce the risk of another heart attack.

Section 20.2

Coronary Heart Disease: Reducing Your Risk

"Preventing Heart Disease," © Pat and Jim Calhoun Cardiology Center, University of Connecticut Health Center (http://heart.uchc.edu.) Reprinted with permission. The text of this document is available online at http://heart.uchc.edu/patientcare/prevention/index.html; accessed March 6, 2007.

Given the prevalence of cardiovascular disease, there are many good reasons to take prevention to heart!

Certain risk factors increase the likelihood that you will develop cardiovascular disease. The three big risk factors are smoking, high blood pressure, and high cholesterol.

Smoking

Quitting smoking is important. And today, there's a lot of support available to patients, from counseling to medications, which can help people overcome addictions to nicotine. Cardiologists urge patients to speak to medical professionals if they need help breaking the habit.

High Cholesterol

Reducing saturated fat and cholesterol in your diet, shedding excess weight, and exercising can help you lower your cholesterol. If no improvement in cholesterol is seen after these modifications are made, your physician may recommend cholesterol-lowering medications. These days, there are many options to help patients get their cholesterol under control. For example, a class of anticholesterol drugs known as statins has been available since 1985 and has very few side effects.

High Blood Pressure

Blood pressure should normally be less than 140/90 mm Hg. Blood pressure that stays above this level is considered high. Diet, exercise, and medication can help to improve blood pressure. Also, note that blood pressure is highest in the morning, so you need to check it several times during the day to get an accurate reading.

Other Risk Factors for Heart Disease

Obesity: This can be treated through proper diet and exercise. Your doctor can help you develop a plan that works for you.

Diet: The U.S. Department of Agricultural guidelines recommend two to three servings of fruits and three to five servings of vegetables each day. Also, watch dietary cholesterol intake. The new cholesterol management guidelines from the National Heart, Lung and Blood Institute (NHLBI) include daily intakes of less than 7 percent of calories from saturated fat and less than 200 mg of dietary cholesterol. It is important to read food labels carefully.

Red meat has much more cholesterol than fish or skinless chicken. Aim to decrease your consumption of red meat. There is increasing evidence that fish may be your healthiest option. Certain fish contain a polyunsaturated fatty acid, called omega-3. The fatty acids may help reduce episodes of arrhythmia (or irregular heartbeat), which are a major cause of death from coronary heart disease. According to American Heart Association guidelines, you should have a minimum of two servings each week of the types of fish that may benefit heart health. These include mackerel, lake trout, herring, sardines, albacore tuna, and salmon.

Inactivity: Physical inactivity and a sedentary lifestyle are risk factors for heart disease. The surgeon general recommends every adult participate in moderate-intensity activity on most to all days of the week. The NHLBI suggests most people try to get 150 minutes of physical activity each week. Check with your doctor to assess risk factors for heart attack that may have gone undetected before starting any type of physical program. A cardiologist can give you a thorough check-up, including, if necessary, an exercise stress test, to make sure you're in good shape. Once you get your doctor's go-ahead, you're good to go. University of Connecticut cardiologists recommend that the elderly and those with arthritis pursue exercises that don't put a lot of wear and tear on the joints. Swimming and using a stationary bike are good examples.

Family history: Anyone with a family history of heart disease needs to have a thorough cardiology exam so a personalized heart disease prevention program can be implemented.

Diabetes: A complication of diabetes is heart disease. Studies show that long-term control of blood sugar can reduce the risk of cardiovascular problems down the road. Patients with diabetes are urged to talk to their physician about cardiovascular disease.

Hormones: Women rarely experience heart attacks before menopause. Researchers believe that estrogen offers some protection against the blood vessel blockage that causes heart attacks and strokes. But new research suggests that estrogen replacement therapy is not as protective as once thought. Certainly, hormone replacement isn't for everyone—women need to discuss the benefits and risks with their physician.

Section 20.3

Preventing High Blood Pressure

Excerpted from "Protect Your Heart! Prevent High Blood Pressure," National Heart, Lung, and Blood Institute, National Institutes of Health, NIH Publication No. 97-4062, September 1997. Revised by David A. Cooke, M.D., May 2007.

Anyone can develop high blood pressure, also called hypertension. The good news is that high blood pressure can be controlled, and better yet, it can be prevented!

What Is Blood Pressure?

Blood pressure is the force of blood pushing against your blood vessels. Your blood pressure is at its greatest when your heart contracts and is pumping blood. This is systolic blood pressure. When your heart rests between beats, your blood pressure falls. This is called diastolic blood pressure. Blood pressure is always given as these two numbers: the systolic and diastolic pressures. The numbers are usually written one above or before the other, with systolic first, for example, 120/80.

Is High Blood Pressure Really a Big Deal?

Yes! When your blood pressure is high, your heart has to work harder than it should to pump blood to all parts of the body. If it is not treated, high blood pressure can cause any of the following: stroke; heart attack; kidney problems; eye problems; and death.

Know Your Number

Have your blood pressure checked. It is easy, quick, and painless. Your blood pressure should be checked by your healthcare provider at least once each year. If you have prehypertension or high blood pressure, it should be checked more often. Check Table 20.2 to see where you fit in.

People whose blood pressure falls consistently in the prehypertensive range are at high risk for eventually developing high blood pressure. Risk of complications of high blood pressure rises sharply with higher readings. Strive for an optimal blood pressure of less than 120/80.

Table 20.2. Blood Pressure Categories (Adults Age 18 and Over)

Category		Systolic (mm/Hg)	Diastolic (mm/Hg)
Normal		Less than 120	Less than 80
Prehypertension		120–139	80–89
Hypertension			
	Stage 1	140–59	90–99
	Stage 2	160 or higher	100 or higher

Prevent High Blood Pressure

If your blood pressure is not high now, take steps to prevent it from becoming high. Here are some preventative steps you can take.

Aim for a Healthy Weight

- Choose foods lower in fat and calories.
- Eat smaller portions.
- Try not to gain extra weight. Lose weight if you are overweight.
- Be physically active every day.

Eat Less Salt and Sodium

- Read the food label. Choose foods with less salt and sodium.
- Prepare lower-sodium meals from scratch instead of using convenience foods that are high in sodium.
- Use spices, herbs, and salt-free seasoning blends instead of salt.
- Use only small amounts of cured or smoked meats for flavor.
- Use less salt when cooking.

Add Spice to Your Life

When you cook, try adding herbs and spices instead of salt. Following are some spicing suggestions:

- **Poultry:** Ginger, rosemary, thyme, curry powder, dill, sage, tarragon, oregano, cloves, orange rind
- **Fish:** Curry powder, pepper, lemon juice, ginger, marjoram, onion, paprika
- **Pork:** Garlic, onion, sage, ginger, curry, cloves, bay leaf, oregano
- **Greens:** Thyme, ginger, onion, dill, garlic
- **Potatoes:** Garlic, pepper, paprika, thyme, onion, sage
- **Beans:** Thyme, onion, dill, cumin, oregano, garlic, tarragon, rosemary
- **Okra:** Garlic, pepper, thyme, onion

Eat More Fruits and Vegetables

- Eat more fruits and vegetables in meals and as snacks.
- Add more vegetables to stews and casseroles.
- Serve fruit as a dessert more often.

Be Active Every Day

- Walk a little further each day or walk to the bus stop.
- Dance, skip, jump, run—take every opportunity to move your body.
- Use the stairs instead of the elevator.

Cut Back on Alcoholic Beverages

Alcohol raises blood pressure. Alcohol also adds calories and may make it harder to lose weight. Men who drink should have no more than two drinks a day. Women who drink should have no more than one drink a day.

Lower Your High Blood Pressure

If you have high blood pressure, you may be able to lower or keep your high blood pressure down. Practice these steps:

- Maintain a healthy weight.
- Be more active every day.
- Eat fewer foods high in salt and sodium.
- Cut back on alcoholic beverages.

You may also need medicine to lower your high blood pressure. Tell your doctor about any medicine you are already taking.
Follow these tips if you take medicine:

- Take your medicine the way your doctor tells you. To help you remember, plan to take your medicine at the same time every day.

- Tell the doctor right away if the medicine makes you feel strange or sick. The doctor may make changes in your medicine.

- Make sure you don't miss any days. Refill your prescription before you use up your medicine.

- Have your blood pressure checked often to be sure your medicine is working the way you and your doctor planned.

- Don't stop taking your medicine if your blood pressure is okay—that means the medicine is working.

Section 20.4

Stroke Prevention

Excerpted from "Stroke," U.S. Food and Drug Administration, 2007.

A stroke happens when the brain does not get enough blood. This kills brain cells. Many adults die from strokes.

Strokes can change the way a person thinks, speaks, sees, and moves. After a stroke, it may be harder to care for yourself or to have a job.

The good news is that many people who have had a stroke can get back some or all of their skills. Speech and physical therapy can help.

There are two major causes of stroke:

- A blood clot from another part of the body blocks a blood vessel or artery in the brain.

- An artery bleeds in or around the brain.

Who has strokes?

Adults over the age of forty are most likely to have strokes. Younger adults and kids can also have them. About the same number of men and women have strokes. People with heart disease may have a bigger risk of stroke. Certain kinds of heart disease can cause blood clots.

How can you lower your risk of stroke?

Control your blood pressure: Having high blood pressure adds to the chances of having a stroke. One out of three people with high blood pressure does not know it. Get your blood pressure checked often.

Control your diabetes: Diabetes can damage the blood vessels in the brain and increase the chance of having a stroke. Follow your doctor's advice to control your diabetes.

Stop smoking: Smoking can cause blood clots. It can also make blood pressure higher. Ask your doctor, pharmacist, or nurse about ways to quit.

Exercise daily: Exercise makes the heart stronger and blood flow better. It can also help you control your weight. Being heavy increases the chance of diseases.

Don't ignore the signs of a stroke. Even if you feel better in a few minutes or hours, you may have had a "mini-stroke." Mini-strokes may put you at risk for a full-blown stroke later. Call 911 if you have any of these warning signs (or have someone else call right away):

- Your face feels numb.
- Your arm or leg gets weak or numb.
- You lose part or all of your sight in one or both eyes.
- You have a hard time talking or understanding other people.
- You get a very bad headache for no reason.
- You get dizzy or fall all of a sudden.

FDA has approved a few drugs to prevent and treat stroke. Ask your doctor for more information.

Chapter 21

Minimizing the Risk of Chronic Obstructive Pulmonary Disease

Did You Know?

Chronic obstructive pulmonary disease (COPD) is the fourth-leading cause of death in the United States. The disease kills more than 120,000 Americans each year—that's one death every four minutes— and causes serious, long-term disability. The number of people with COPD is increasing. More than twelve million people have been diagnosed with COPD and an additional twelve million likely have the disease and don't even know it.

What is COPD?

COPD is a serious lung disease that over time makes it hard to breathe. You may have heard COPD called other names, like emphysema or chronic bronchitis.

In people who have COPD, the airways—tubes that carry air in and out of your lungs—are partly blocked, which makes it hard to get air in and out.

What Are the Symptoms?

Many people with COPD avoid activities that they used to enjoy because they become short of breath more easily.

Reprinted from "COPD: Are You at Risk?" National Heart, Lung, and Blood Institute, National Institutes of Health, September 2006.

Symptoms of COPD include the following:

- Constant coughing, sometimes called "smoker's cough"
- Shortness of breath while doing activities you used to be able to do
- Excess sputum production
- Feeling like you can't breathe
- Not being able to take a deep breath
- Wheezing

When COPD is severe, shortness of breath and other symptoms can get in the way of doing even the most basic tasks, such as doing light housework, taking a walk, and even bathing and getting dressed.

COPD develops slowly, and can worsen over time, so be sure to report any symptoms you might have to your doctor as soon as possible, no matter how mild they may seem.

Are You at Risk?

Most people who are at risk for getting COPD have never even heard of it and, in many cases, don't even realize that the condition has a name. There are several things that put you at risk for COPD.

Smoking: COPD most often occurs in people age forty and over with a history of smoking (either current or former smokers), although as many as one out of six people with COPD never smoked. Smoking is the most common cause of COPD—it accounts for as many as nine out of ten COPD-related deaths.

Environmental exposure: COPD can also occur in people who have had long-term exposure to things that can irritate your lungs, like certain chemicals, dust, or fumes in the workplace. Heavy or long-term exposure to secondhand smoke or other air pollutants may also contribute to COPD.

Genetic factors: In some people, COPD is caused by a genetic condition known as alpha-1 antitrypsin, or AAT, deficiency. While very few people know they have AAT deficiency, it is estimated that as many as 100,000 Americans have it. People with AAT deficiency can get COPD even if they have never smoked or had long-term exposure to harmful pollutants.

Getting Tested

Everyone at risk for COPD who has a cough, sputum production, or shortness of breath should be tested for the disease. The test for COPD is called spirometry.

Spirometry

Spirometry can detect COPD before symptoms become severe. It is a simple, noninvasive breathing test that measures the amount of air a person can blow out of the lungs (volume) and how fast he or she can blow it out (flow). Based on this test, your doctor can tell if you have COPD, and if so, how severe it is. The spirometry reading can help your doctor determine the best course of treatment.

How Spirometry Works

Spirometry is one of the best and most common lung function tests. The test is done with a spirometer, a machine that measures how well your lungs function, records the results, and displays them on a graph for your doctor. You will be asked to take a deep breath, then blow out as hard and as fast as you can using a mouthpiece connected to the machine with tubing. The spirometer then measures the total amount of air exhaled, called the forced vital capacity or FVC, and how much you exhaled in the first second, called the forced expiratory volume in 1 second or FEV1. Your doctor will use the results to assess how well your lungs are working and whether or not you have COPD.

Taking Action

There are many things people at risk for COPD can do.

Quit smoking: If you smoke, the best thing you can do to prevent more damage to your lungs is to quit. To help you quit, there are many online resources and several new aids available from your doctor.

Avoid exposure to pollutants: Try to stay away from other things that could irritate your lungs, like dust and strong fumes. Stay indoors when the outside air quality is poor. You could also stay away from places where there might be cigarette smoke.

Visit your doctor on a regular basis: See your doctor regularly even if you are feeling fine. Make a list of your breathing symptoms and think about any activities that you can no longer do because of shortness of breath. Be sure to bring a list of all the medicines you are taking to each doctor's visit.

Take precautions against the flu: Do your best to avoid crowds during flu season. It is also a good idea to get a flu shot every year, since the flu can cause serious problems for people with COPD. You should also ask your doctor about the pneumonia vaccine.

Learn More, Breathe Better

If you think you might be at risk for COPD, get a simple breathing test. Talk with your doctor about treatment options. You can take steps to make breathing easier and live a longer and more active life.

Chapter 22

Preventing Diabetes and Kidney Disease

Chapter Contents

Section 22.1

Preventing Diabetes and Diabetes Complications

"Preventing Diabetes" is reprinted from "Frequently Asked Questions: Preventing Diabetes," Centers for Disease Control and Prevention, June 2006. "Preventing Diabetes Complications" is excerpted from "National Diabetes Fact Sheet," Centers for Disease Control and Prevention, January 2005.

Preventing Diabetes

What are the most important things to do to prevent diabetes?

The Diabetes Prevention Program (DPP), a major federally funded study of 3,234 people at high risk for diabetes, showed that people can delay and possibly prevent the disease by losing a small amount of weight (5 to 7 percent of total body weight) through thirty minutes of physical activity five days a week and healthier eating.

When should I be tested for diabetes?

Anyone aged forty-five years or older should consider getting tested for diabetes, especially if you are overweight. If you are younger than forty-five, but are overweight and have one or more additional risk factors (see following), you should consider testing.

What are the risk factors that increase the likelihood of developing diabetes?

- Being overweight or obese

- A parent, brother, or sister with diabetes

- African American, American Indian, Asian American, Pacific Islander, or Hispanic American/Latino heritage

- Prior history of gestational diabetes or birth of at least one baby weighing more than nine pounds

- High blood pressure measuring 140/90 or higher

- Abnormal cholesterol with high density lipoprotein (HDL, or "good") cholesterol of 35 or lower, or triglyceride level of 250 or higher

- Physical inactivity—exercising fewer than three times a week

How does body weight affect the likelihood of developing diabetes?

Being overweight or obese is a leading risk factor for type 2 diabetes. Being overweight can keep your body from making and using insulin properly, and can also cause high blood pressure. The Diabetes Prevention Program (DPP), a major federally funded study of 3,234 people at high risk for diabetes, showed that moderate diet and exercise of about 30 minutes or more, five or more days per week, or of 150 or more minutes per week resulting in a 5 percent to 7 percent weight loss can delay and possibly prevent type 2 diabetes.

What is pre-diabetes?

People with blood glucose levels that are higher than normal but not yet in the diabetic range have "pre-diabetes." Doctors sometimes call this condition impaired fasting glucose (IFG) or impaired glucose tolerance (IGT), depending on the test used to diagnose it. Insulin resistance and pre-diabetes usually have no symptoms. You may have one or both conditions for several years without noticing anything.

If you have pre-diabetes, you have a higher risk of developing type 2 diabetes. Studies have shown that most people with pre-diabetes go on to develop type 2 diabetes within ten years, unless they lose weight through modest changes in diet and physical activity. People with pre-diabetes also have a higher risk of heart disease.

Can vaccines cause diabetes?

No. Carefully performed scientific studies show that vaccines do not cause diabetes or increase a person's risk of developing diabetes. In 2002, the Institute of Medicine reviewed the existing studies and released a report concluding that the scientific evidence favors rejection of the theory that immunizations cause diabetes. The only evidence suggesting a relationship between vaccination and diabetes comes from Dr. John B. Classen, who has suggested that certain vaccines if given at birth may decrease the occurrence of diabetes, whereas if initial vaccination is performed after two months of age the occurrence of diabetes increases. Dr. Classen's studies have a number of limitations and have not been verified by other researchers.

Preventing Diabetes Complications

Diabetes can affect many parts of the body and can lead to serious complications such as blindness, kidney damage, and lower-limb amputations. Working together, people with diabetes and their healthcare providers can reduce the occurrence of these and other diabetes complications by controlling the levels of blood glucose, blood pressure, and blood lipids and by receiving other preventive care practices in a timely manner.

Glucose Control

Research studies in the United States and abroad have found that improved glycemic control benefits people with either type 1 or type 2 diabetes. In general, for every 1 percent reduction in results of A1C blood tests (e.g., from 8.0 percent to 7.0 percent), the risk of developing microvascular diabetic complications (eye, kidney, and nerve disease) is reduced by 40 percent.

Blood Pressure Control

Blood pressure control can reduce cardiovascular disease (heart disease and stroke) by approximately 33 to 50 percent and can reduce microvascular disease (eye, kidney, and nerve disease) by approximately 33 percent.

In general, for every 10 millimeters of mercury (mm Hg) reduction in systolic blood pressure, the risk for any complication related to diabetes is reduced by 12 percent.

Control of Blood Lipids

Improved control of cholesterol or blood lipids can reduce cardiovascular complications by 20 to 50 percent.

Preventive Care Practices for Eyes, Kidneys, and Feet

Detecting and treating diabetic eye disease with laser therapy can reduce the development of severe vision loss by an estimated 50 to 60 percent.

Comprehensive foot care programs can reduce amputation rates by 45 to 85 percent.

Detecting and treating early diabetic kidney disease by lowering blood pressure can reduce the decline in kidney function by 30 to 70 percent. Treatment with angiotensin converting enzyme (ACE) inhibitors and angiotensin receptor blockers (ARBs) is more effective in reducing the decline in kidney function than other blood pressure–lowering drugs.

Section 22.2

Preventing Kidney Disease

Excerpted from "You Have the Power to Prevent Kidney Disease,"
National Kidney Disease Education Program, National Institutes of
Health, 2005.

Learn the Risks

Kidney disease is a growing problem in the United States. It is a problem that affects adults of all ages and races. People with diabetes, high blood pressure, or a family member with kidney failure are more likely to develop kidney disease. African Americans with any of these risk factors have an even greater chance of developing this disease.

Healthy kidneys filter your blood. They remove waste and extra water. They help control the amount of certain chemicals in your blood like sodium, phosphorus, and potassium. The right balance of these chemicals helps your body work well. Healthy kidneys help keep this balance.

When kidneys are diseased they slowly stop doing these jobs. If not treated, kidney disease can lead to kidney failure. When that happens, dialysis or a kidney transplant are the only options for keeping a person alive.

Stop a Disease That Comes without Warning

Early kidney disease is a silent problem, like high blood pressure. Kidney disease can become kidney failure with little or no warning, and is usually discovered right before the kidneys fail. If you have diabetes, high blood pressure, or a family member with kidney failure, a doctor or healthcare professional should test your blood and urine for early signs of kidney disease. You can take steps to keep your kidneys working if the tests show kidney disease.

Steps to Protect Your Kidneys

- Control your blood pressure and diabetes.

- Ask your doctor or healthcare professional to test your blood and urine for kidney disease.

- If these tests show kidney disease, special medicines called angiotensin converting enzyme (ACE) Inhibitors or angiotensin receptor blockers (ARBs) can help. Talk to your doctor about these medications.

What to Ask Your Doctor or Healthcare Professional

- Based on my medical and family history, am I at risk for kidney disease?

- Would lowering my blood pressure help reduce my risk of developing kidney disease?

- Do my blood and urine tests show signs of kidney disease?

- How can I prevent or control kidney disease?

Are You at Risk for Kidney Disease?

- Do you have diabetes?

- Do you have high blood pressure?

- Did your mother, father, sister, or brother ever have kidney disease or failure?

- Has a doctor ever told you that you had protein in your urine?

If you answered "yes" to any of these questions, you are at risk for kidney disease. Now is the time to talk to your doctor or healthcare professional about getting tested. It could save your life.

Tips for Talking with Your Doctor or Healthcare Professional

- Know as much as you can about your family's medical history.

- Take this book with you so you don't forget what to ask.

- Write down the answers you get and ask more questions if you need to.

- Bring someone else with you for support and to help you remember what you learn.

Do You Have Diabetes?

Diabetes is the most common cause of kidney failure. Your kidneys keep you healthy by maintaining the chemicals in your blood. Diabetes damages small blood vessels in your body. When the blood vessels in your kidneys are hurt, your kidneys are not able to do this job well. Both type 1 and type 2 diabetes can lead to kidney disease. The longer you have diabetes, the greater your risk for kidney disease.

But, kidney failure can be prevented. One way to help prevent kidney disease is to control your diabetes. Medication can also help prevent or slow kidney disease. Kidney disease has no early symptoms so it's important that people with diabetes get tested for kidney disease every year.

If you have diabetes, please read this chapter and ask your healthcare provider to test your blood and urine for early signs of kidney disease.

Do You Have High Blood Pressure?

High blood pressure is the second leading cause of kidney failure. Your kidneys play a key role in keeping your blood pressure in a healthy range. And blood pressure, in turn, can affect the health of your kidneys. High blood pressure makes your heart work harder, and over time can damage blood vessels throughout your body, including those in your kidneys.

But, kidney failure can be prevented. One way to help prevent kidney disease is to control your blood pressure. Medication can also help prevent or slow kidney disease. Kidney disease has no early symptoms so it's important that people with high blood pressure get tested for kidney disease.

If you have high blood pressure, please read this chapter and ask your healthcare provider to test your blood and urine for early signs of kidney disease.

You have the power to prevent kidney disease.

Chapter 23

Caring for Your Liver and Preventing Hepatitis

Caring for Your Liver

Basic Liver Care

Your liver depends on you to take care of it . . . so it can take care of you. It serves as your body's engine, pantry, refinery, food processor, garbage disposal, and "guardian angel." The trouble is, your liver is a silent partner; when something's wrong it does not complain until the damage is far advanced. So it needs your help every day to keep it healthy and hepatitis-free. To do that, you need to eat a healthy diet, exercise, get lots of fresh air, and avoid things that can cause liver damage.

What Does My Liver Do?

Sadly, people generally have little knowledge of the complexities and importance of the thousands of vital functions their livers perform nonstop.

The liver is about the size of a football—the largest organ in your body. It plays a vital role in regulating life processes. Before you were born, it served as the main organ of blood formation. Now, its primary functions are to refine and detoxify everything you eat, breathe, and absorb through your skin. It is your body's internal chemical power plant, converting nutrients in the food you eat into muscles, energy, hormones, clotting factors, and immune factors.

It stores certain vitamins, minerals (including iron) and sugars, regulates fat stores, and controls the production and excretion of cholesterol. The bile, produced by liver cells, helps you to digest your food and absorb important nutrients. It neutralizes and destroys poisonous substances and metabolizes alcohol. It helps you resist infection and removes bacteria from the bloodstream, helping you to stay healthy. Arguably, your liver isn't just your silent partner—it's your best friend.

Three Things to Avoid for Liver Health

Avoid excessive alcohol: Most people know that the liver acts as a filter and can be badly damaged by drinking too much alcohol. Liver specialists suggest that more than two drinks a day for men—and more than one drink a day for women—may even be too much for some people.

One of the most remarkable accomplishments of this miraculous organ is its ability to regenerate. (Three quarters of the liver can be removed and it will grow back in the same shape and form within a few weeks!) However, overworking your liver by heavy alcohol consumption can cause liver cells (the "employees" in the power plant) to become permanently damaged or scarred. This is called cirrhosis.

Avoid drugs and medicines taken with alcohol: Medicines—especially the seemingly harmless acetaminophen (the active ingredient in Tylenol and other over-the-counter medications)—should never be taken with alcoholic beverages. Many prescribed and over-the-counter drugs and medicines (including herbal medications) are made up of chemicals that could be potentially hazardous to your precious liver cells, especially if taken with alcohol.

If you are ill with a virus or metabolic disorder, liver damage may result from the medications you take. In such cases, you should ask your physician about possible liver cell damage.

Avoid environmental pollutants: Fumes from paint thinners, bug sprays, and other aerosol sprays are picked up by the tiny blood vessels in your lungs and carried to your liver, where they are detoxified and discharged in your bile. The amount and concentration of those chemicals should be controlled to prevent liver damage. Make certain you have good ventilation, use a mask, cover your skin, and wash off any chemicals you get on your skin with soap and water as soon as possible.

Diet and Your Liver

Overview: Poor nutrition is rarely a cause of liver disease, but good nutrition in the form of a balanced diet, may help liver cells damaged by hepatitis viruses to regenerate, forming new liver cells. Nutrition can be an essential part of treatment. Many chronic liver diseases are associated with malnutrition.

Watch the protein: To quickly determine your daily protein in grams, divide your weight in pounds by 2. Too much daily protein may cause hepatic encephalopathy (mental confusion). This occurs when the amount of dietary protein is greater than the liver's ability to use the protein. This causes a buildup of toxins that can interfere with brain function. Protein is restricted in patients with clinical evidence of encephalopathy. However, controversy exists regarding the type of protein a diet should contain. Vegetable and dairy protein may be tolerated better than meat protein. Medications, such as lactulose and neomycin, may be used to help control hepatitis-related encephalopathy. Due to the body's need for proteins, protein restriction should be undertaken only with a doctor's advice.

Watch the calories: Excess calories in the form of carbohydrates can add to liver dysfunction and can cause fat deposits in the liver. No more than 30 percent of a person's total calories should come from fat because of the danger to the cardiovascular system. To figure out your daily calorie needs, you'll need a minimum of 15 calories a day for each pound you weigh.

Watch the salt: Good nutrition also helps to maintain the normal fluid and electrolyte balances in the body. Patients with fluid retention and swelling of the abdomen (ascites) or the legs (peripheral edema) may need diets low in salt to avoid sodium retention that contributes to fluid retention. Avoiding foods such as canned soups and vegetables, cold cuts, dairy products, and condiments such as mayonnaise and ketchup can reduce sodium intake. Read food labels carefully, as many prepared foods contain large amounts of salt. The best-tasting salt substitute is lemon juice.

Watch vitamins A and D: Excessive amounts of some vitamins may be an additional source of stress to the liver that must act as a filter for the body. Mega-vitamin supplements, particularly if they contain vitamins A and D, may be harmful. Excess vitamin A is very toxic to the liver.

Beware of alcohol: You'll need to stop drinking completely to give your liver a break—a chance to heal, a chance to rebuild, a chance for new liver cells to grow. This means avoiding beer, wine, cocktails, champagne, and liquor in any other form. If you continue to drink, your liver will pay the price, and if your doctor is checking your liver function tests, it may be hard to determine if a change in a test means there has been damage to your liver due to the disease itself or because of the alcohol.

Beware of alcohol and acetaminophen: Acetaminophen is an ingredient in some over-the-counter pain relievers, and is contained in many over-the-counter drugs used for colds or coughs. Taken with alcohol, these products can cause a condition called sudden and severe hepatitis, which could cause fatal liver failure. Clearly, you should never combine these two substances. If you have any doubt about what medicines to take simultaneously, ask your doctor.

Beware of "nutritional therapies": Herbal treatments and alternative liver medicines need to undergo rigorous scientific study before they can be recommended. "Natural" or diet treatments and herbal remedies can be quite dangerous. Plants of the Senecio, Crotalaria and Heliotropium families, plus chaparral, germander, comfrey, mistletoe, skullcap, margosa oil, mate tea, Gordolobo yerba tea, pennyroyal, and Jin Bu Huan are all toxic to the liver.

Preventing Hepatitis

This infectious virus is complex—it comes in three primary forms in the United States (A, B, and C) and two more less prevalent forms (D and E). Yet there is much you can do to help prevent hepatitis. Safe and effective vaccines exist to prevent hepatitis A and B. Although hepatitis C does not have a vaccine yet, there are ways to reduce the risk of contracting it. Today, about four million people in the United States have been infected with hepatitis C.

Here's what you can do to prevent or reduce your chances of getting hepatitis.

Preventing Hepatitis A (HAV)

Vaccinate: Immunization of children (one to eighteen years of age) consists of two or three doses of the vaccine. Adults need a booster dose six to twelve months following the initial dose of vaccine. The vaccine is thought to be effective for fifteen to twenty years or more. Vaccines to prevent HAV infection prior to exposure provide protection against the virus as early as two to four weeks after vaccination. Other people who should be vaccinated include the following:

- Users of illegal injected drugs

- Restaurant workers and food handlers

- Young people living in dorms or in close contact with others

- Children living in communities that have high rates of hepatitis

- Children and workers in daycare centers

- People engaging in anal or oral sex

- People with chronic liver disease

- Laboratory workers who handle live hepatitis A virus.

If you eat raw shellfish frequently, ask your physician about being vaccinated.

Common sense hygiene: Hands should be washed with soap and water following bowel movements and before food preparation.

Traveler precautions: People who travel to developing countries where sanitary conditions are poor should be vaccinated two months prior to departure. For those exposed to HAV, immune globulin (IG) should be given as soon as possible and no later than two weeks after initial exposure.

Preventing Hepatitis B (HBV)

Vaccinate: Safe and effective vaccines can prevent HBV. Vaccines provide protection against hepatitis B for fifteen years and possibly much longer. Currently, the Center for Disease Control and Prevention recommends that all newborns and individuals up to eighteen years of age and adults participating in activities putting them at risk of infection be vaccinated. Three injections over a six- to twelve-month period are required to provide full protection.

Newborns exposed to HBV at birth by an infected mother should receive Hepatitis B immune globulin plus the first dose of hepatitis B vaccine within twelve hours of birth and two additional doses of vaccine at one and six to twelve months of age.

All children and adolescents should be vaccinated, since most cases of HBV occur in sexually active young adults. Those who engage in high-risk behaviors should be vaccinated as well.

Everyone who handles blood or blood products in his or her daily work should be vaccinated.

Practice safer sex (use latex condoms): If you have hepatitis, or if you have more than one sex partner within a six-month period, you should consider vaccination. Unvaccinated individuals who have been exposed to HBV-infected persons through unprotected sex or contact with infected blood or body fluids should receive an intramuscular injection of hepatitis B immune globulin (HBIG) within fourteen days of exposure plus the hepatitis B vaccine.

Don't share: If you are a user of injected drugs, never share drug needles, cocaine straws, or any drug paraphernalia. No one should share anything that could have an infected person's blood on it (e.g., toothbrush, razor, nail clipper, body piercing instruments, etc.).

Handle blood spills correctly: If there is blood spill, even a small one, clean it up with a 10 percent solution of household bleach (believed to kill the virus). Wear protective gloves.

Preventing Hepatitis C (HCV)

There is *no* vaccine to prevent HCV. Vaccines for hepatitis A and B do not provide immunity against hepatitis C (although those who are HCV infected should receive both hepatitis A and hepatitis B vaccination). The source of HCV infection remains a mystery in about 10 percent of the cases. That means preventive measures are your first line of defense against HCV.

Preventive actions for HCV are the same as for hepatitis B.

Hepatitis Vaccinations

Hepatitis A Vaccination

Is the hepatitis A vaccine safe and effective? The HAV vaccine, made from inactive hepatitis A virus (synthetic), is highly effective in preventing the hepatitis A infection when given prior to exposure. However, its safety when given during pregnancy has not been determined. Currently, the hepatitis A vaccine is *not* licensed for children less than one year of age in the United States.

Who should be vaccinated against hepatitis A? Just about anyone is a candidate to get hepatitis A; however, those at higher risk for hepatitis A include: users of illegal drugs; individuals who have chronic liver disease or blood clotting disorders (e.g., hemophilia); those who have close physical contact with people who live in areas with poor sanitary conditions; men who have sex with men; those who travel or work in developing countries; and children in populations that have repeated epidemics of hepatitis A (e.g., Alaska natives, American Indians, and certain closed religious communities).

What is the dosage regimen? Recommended dosages and schedules vary with the patient's age and which specific vaccine is used. Whether you are a child over one or an adult, more than one shot is needed for long-term protection. Check with your doctor or nurse to determine how many shots are needed and when to return for the next dose. The vaccine provides protection about four weeks after the first injection; a second injection protects you longer, possibly up to twenty years. Twinrix, a combined hepatitis A and B vaccine may be given to those over eighteen years of age.

Hepatitis B Vaccination

Is the hepatitis B vaccine safe and effective? Yes. The hepatitis B vaccine has been available since 1982. Use of hepatitis B vaccine and other vaccines is strongly endorsed by the medical, scientific, and public health communities as a safe and effective way to prevent disease and death. Hepatitis B vaccines have been shown to be very safe when given to infants, children, and adults.

Could vaccinations eradicate hepatitis B? Eradication of hepatitis B is possible through a comprehensive vaccination program. The way to do this is to make sure all newborns, children under nineteen, and adults at risk are vaccinated against HBV.

Who should be vaccinated? All newborns and children up to the age of nineteen, especially adoptees; all individuals living in the same household with a chronically infected individual; those who are in positions where they are exposed to blood at work or through drug use, or who have multiple sex partners; and individuals with hepatitis C and other chronic liver diseases should be vaccinated for hepatitis B.

Why is it so important to vaccinate children against hepatitis B? Parents and guardians are encouraged to have their children vaccinated at an early age to prevent the serious complications that can occur when youngsters under the age of five are infected. HBV, a sexually transmitted disease, is one hundred times more infectious than human immunodeficiency virus (the virus that causes AIDS).

What is the Vaccines for Children program? The Vaccines for Children Program provides free hepatitis B vaccines to young people under the age of nineteen years who are on Medicaid, who have no insurance, or whose insurance does not cover immunizations.

Can the babies of infected mothers be vaccinated? Yes. All newborns, especially those whose mothers are HBV infected, should get three vaccination shots for hepatitis B—the first within twelve hours of birth, the second at one to two months, and the third at six months. In addition, babies born to infected mothers should receive a shot called HBIG (hepatitis B immune globulin) within twelve hours of delivery. All women should be screened for hepatitis B surface antigen during pregnancy to determine if they are a carrier (chronically infected) of HBV. Without the above intervention, 90 percent of babies born to infected mothers will become chronically infected, reducing their life expectancy. It is safe to vaccinate pregnant women.

What is the dosage regimen? HBV vaccines require three injections to obtain long-lasting immunity. Hepatitis B vaccine is given as an intramuscular injection, and can be given to children at the same time as other vaccinations. It can be given in a number of schedules, each of which provides excellent protection. For infants, vaccination should begin at birth. A second dose at one month of age and the third dose at six months of age may be given.

Chapter 24

Preventing Disorders of the Teeth and Bones

Chapter Contents

Section 24.1

Oral Health for Adults

Reprinted from the National Center for Chronic Disease Prevention and Health Promotion, Centers for Disease Control and Prevention, December 21, 2006.

The baby boomer generation will be the first where the majority will maintain their natural teeth over their entire lifetime, having benefited from water fluoridation and fluoride toothpastes.

Over the past ten years, the number of adults missing all their natural teeth has declined from 31 percent to 25 percent for those aged sixty years and older, and from 9 percent to 5 percent for those adults between forty and fifty-nine years. However, 5 percent means a surprising one out of twenty middle-aged adults are missing all their teeth.

Over 40 percent of poor adults (twenty years and older) have at least one untreated decayed tooth compared to 16 percent of non-poor adults.

Toothaches are the most common pain of the mouth or face reported by adults. This pain can interfere with vital functions such as eating, swallowing, and talking. Almost one of every four adults reported some form of facial pain in the past six months.

Most adults show signs of gum disease. Severe gum disease affects about 14 percent of adults aged forty-five to fifty-four years.

Signs and symptoms of soft tissue diseases such as cold sores are common in adults and affect about 19 percent of those aged twenty-five to forty-four years.

Chronic disabling diseases such as jaw joint diseases, diabetes, and osteoporosis affect millions of Americans and compromise oral health and functioning.

Women report certain painful mouth and facial conditions (temporomandibular [TMD] disorders, migraine headaches, and burning mouth syndrome) more often than men.

Every year more than four hundred thousand cancer patients undergoing chemotherapy suffer from oral problems such as painful mouth ulcers, impaired taste, and dry mouth.

Patients with weakened immune systems, such as those infected with human immunodeficiency virus (HIV) and other medical conditions (including organ transplants) and who use some medications (e.g., steroids), are at higher risk for some oral problems.

Employed adults lose more than 164 million hours of work each year due to oral health problems or dental visits. Customer service industry employees lose two to four times more work hours than executives or professional workers.

For every adult nineteen years or older without medical insurance, there are three without dental insurance.

Seventy percent of adults reported visiting a dentist in the past twelve months. Those with incomes at or above the poverty level are much more likely to report a visit to a dentist in the past twelve months than those with lower incomes.

What You Can Do to Maintain Good Oral Health

Drink fluoridated water and use a fluoride toothpaste. Fluoride's protection against tooth decay works at all ages.

Take care of your teeth and gums. Thorough tooth brushing and flossing to reduce dental plaque can prevent gingivitis—the mildest form of gum disease.

Avoid tobacco. In addition to the general health risks posed by tobacco, smokers have four times the risk of developing gum disease compared to nonsmokers. Tobacco use in any form—cigarette, pipes, and smokeless (spit) tobacco—increases the risk for gum disease, oral and throat cancers, and oral fungal infection (candidiasis). Spit tobacco containing sugar increases the risk of tooth decay.

Limit alcohol. Heavy use of alcohol is also a risk factor for oral and throat cancers. When used alone, alcohol and tobacco are risk factors for oral cancers, but when used in combination the effects of alcohol and tobacco are even greater.

Eat wisely. Adults should avoid snacks full of sugars and starches. Limit the number of snacks eaten throughout the day. The recommended five-a-day helping of fiber-rich fruits and vegetables stimulates salivary flow to aid remineralization of tooth surfaces with early stages of tooth decay.

Visit the dentist regularly. Check-ups can detect early signs of oral health problems and can lead to treatments that will prevent further damage, and in some cases, reverse the problem. Professional tooth cleaning (prophylaxis) also is important for preventing oral problems, especially when self-care is difficult.

Diabetic patients should work to maintain control of their disease. This will help prevent the complications of diabetes, including an increased risk of gum disease.

If medications produce a dry mouth, ask your doctor if there are other drugs that can be substituted. If dry mouth cannot be avoided, drink plenty of water, chew sugarless gum, and avoid tobacco and alcohol.

Have an oral health check-up before beginning cancer treatment. Radiation to the head or neck and/or chemotherapy may cause problems for your teeth and gums. Treating existing oral health problems before cancer therapy may help prevent or limit oral complications or tissue damage.

Section 24.2

Osteoporosis Prevention

Reprinted with permission from the National Osteoporosis Foundation website, http://www.nof.org/prevention/index.htm, July 2007. © 2007 National Osteoporosis Foundation, Washington, D.C. All rights reserved.

Osteoporosis is largely preventable for most people. Prevention of this disease is very important because, while there are treatments for osteoporosis, there is currently no cure. There are five steps to prevent osteoporosis. No one step alone is enough to prevent osteoporosis but all five may.

National Osteoporosis Foundation's Five Steps to Bone Health and Osteoporosis Prevention (© 2002 NOF):

- Get your daily recommended amounts of calcium and vitamin D.

- Engage in regular weight-bearing exercise.

- Avoid smoking and excessive alcohol.

- Talk to your healthcare provider about bone health.

- When appropriate, have a bone density test and take medication.

Calcium

Calcium is needed for the heart, muscles, and nerves to function properly and for blood to clot. Inadequate calcium is thought to contribute to the development of osteoporosis. National nutrition surveys have shown that many women and young girls consume less than half the amount of calcium recommended to maintain healthy bones.

According to National Osteoporosis Foundation (NOF) recommendations, adults under age fifty need 1,000 mg of calcium daily, and adults age fifty and over need 1,200 mg of calcium daily. If you have difficulty getting enough calcium from the foods you eat, you may take a calcium supplement to make up the difference.

Vitamin D

Vitamin D is needed for the body to absorb calcium. Without enough vitamin D, you will be unable to absorb calcium from the foods you eat, and your body will have to take calcium from your bones. Vitamin D comes from two sources: through the skin following direct exposure to sunlight and from the diet. According to NOF recommendations, adults under age fifty need 400–800 international units (IU) of vitamin D_3 daily, and adults age fifty and over need 800–1,000 IU of vitamin D_3 daily. Vitamin D_3 is the form of vitamin D that best supports bone health. It is also called cholecalciferol. Vitamin D can also be obtained from fortified milk, egg yolks, saltwater fish, liver, and supplements.

Exercise

If you exercise regularly in childhood and adolescence, you are more likely to reach your peak bone density than those who are inactive. The best exercise for your bones is weight-bearing exercise such as walking, dancing, jogging, stair-climbing, racquet sports, and hiking. If you have been sedentary most of your adult life, be sure to check with your healthcare provider before beginning any exercise program.

Medications for Prevention and Treatment

Although there is no cure for osteoporosis, currently bisphosphonates (alendronate, ibandronate, and risedronate), calcitonin, estrogens, parathyroid hormone, and raloxifene are approved by the U.S. Food and Drug Administration (FDA) for the prevention and treatment of osteoporosis.

Bone Mineral Density Tests

Since osteoporosis can develop undetected for decades until a fracture occurs, early diagnosis is important.

A bone mineral density test (BMD) measures the density of your bones and is necessary to determine whether you need medication to help maintain your bone mass, prevent further bone loss, and reduce fracture risk. This test is accurate, painless, and noninvasive.

Part Four

Screening for Common Diseases and Disorders

Chapter 25

Stay Healthy at Any Age: Screening Tests for Men and Women

Women: Stay Healthy at Any Age

What can you do to stay healthy and prevent disease? You can get certain screening tests, take preventive medicine if you need it, and practice healthy behaviors.

Top health experts from the U.S. Preventive Services Task Force suggest that when you go for your next checkup, talk to your doctor or nurse about how you can stay healthy no matter what your age.

Screening Tests for Women: What You Need and When

Here are the most important things you can do to stay healthy:

- Get recommended screening tests.

- Be tobacco free.

- Be physically active.

- Eat a healthy diet.

- Stay at a healthy weight.

- Take preventive medicines if you need them.

Reprinted from "Women: Stay Healthy at Any Age," Agency for Healthcare Research and Quality, AHRQ Publication No. 07-IP005-A, February 2007, and "Men: Stay Healthy at Any Age," Agency for Healthcare Research and Quality, AHRQ Publication No. 07-IP006-A. February 2007.

Screening tests can find diseases early when they are easier to treat. Health experts from the U.S. Preventive Services Task Force have made recommendations, based on scientific evidence, about testing for the following conditions. Talk to your doctor about which ones apply to you and when and how often you should be tested.

Obesity: Have your body mass index (BMI) calculated to screen for obesity. (BMI is a measure of body fat based on height and weight.) [You can also find your own BMI with the BMI calculator in Chapter 12 of this book.]

Breast cancer: Have a mammogram every one to two years starting at age forty.

Cervical cancer: Have a Pap smear every one to three years if you:

• Have ever been sexually active;

• Are between the ages of twenty-one and sixty-five.

High cholesterol: Have your cholesterol checked regularly starting at age forty-five. If you are younger than forty-five, talk to your doctor about whether to have your cholesterol checked if:

• You have diabetes;

• You have high blood pressure;

• Heart disease runs in your family;

• You smoke.

High blood pressure: Have your blood pressure checked at least every two years. High blood pressure is 140/90 or higher.

Colorectal cancer: Have a test for colorectal cancer starting at age fifty. Your doctor can help you decide which test is right for you. If you have a family history of colorectal cancer, you may need to be screened earlier.

Diabetes: Have a test for diabetes if you have high blood pressure or high cholesterol.

Depression: Your emotional health is as important as your physical health. If you have felt "down," sad, or hopeless over the last two weeks or have felt little interest or pleasure in doing things, you may be depressed. Talk to your doctor about being screened for depression.

Osteoporosis (thinning of the bones): Have a bone density test beginning at age sixty-five to screen for osteoporosis. If you are between the ages of sixty and sixty-four and weigh 154 lbs. or less, talk to your doctor about being tested.

Chlamydia and other sexually transmitted infections: Have a test for chlamydia if you are twenty-five or younger and sexually active. If you are older, talk to your doctor about being tested. Also ask whether you should be tested for other sexually transmitted diseases.

Human immunodeficiency virus (HIV): Have a test to screen for HIV infection if you:

- Have had unprotected sex with multiple partners;
- Are pregnant;
- Have used or now use injection drugs;
- Exchange sex for money or drugs or have sex partners who do;
- Have past or present sex partners who are HIV-infected, are bisexual, or use injection drugs;
- Are being treated for sexually transmitted diseases;
- Had a blood transfusion between 1978 and 1985.

Daily Steps to Health

Don't smoke: If you do smoke, talk to your doctor about quitting. If you are pregnant and smoke, quitting now will help you and your baby. Your doctor or nurse can help you.

Be physically active: Walking briskly, mowing the lawn, dancing, swimming, and bicycling are just a few examples of moderate physical activity. If you are not already physically active, start small and work up to thirty minutes or more of moderate physical activity most days of the week.

Eat a healthy diet: Emphasize fruits, vegetables, whole grains, and fat-free or low-fat milk and milk products; include lean meats, poultry, fish, beans, eggs, and nuts; and eat foods low in saturated fats, trans fats, cholesterol, salt (sodium), and added sugars.

Stay at a healthy weight: Balance calories from foods and beverages with calories you burn off by your activities. To prevent gradual weight gain over time, make small decreases in food and beverage calories and increase physical activity.

Drink alcohol only in moderation: If you drink alcohol, have no more than one drink a day. (A standard drink is one 12-ounce bottle of beer or wine cooler, one 5-ounce glass of wine, or 1.5 ounces of 80-proof distilled spirits.) If you are pregnant, avoid alcohol.

Should You Take Medicines to Prevent Disease?

Hormones: Do not take hormones to prevent disease. Talk to your doctor if you need relief from the symptoms of menopause.

Breast cancer drugs: If your mother, sister, or daughter has had breast cancer, talk to your doctor about the risks and benefits of taking medicines to prevent breast cancer.

Aspirin: Ask your doctor about taking aspirin to prevent heart disease if you are older than forty-five or younger than forty-five and:

- Have high blood pressure;
- Have high cholesterol;
- Have diabetes;
- Smoke.

Immunizations: Stay up-to-date with your immunizations:

- Have a flu shot every year starting at age fifty. If you are younger than fifty, ask your doctor whether you need a flu shot.
- Have a pneumonia shot once after you turn sixty-five. If you are younger, ask your doctor whether you need a pneumonia shot.

Men: Stay Healthy at Any Age

What can you do to stay healthy and prevent disease? You can get certain screening tests, take preventive medicine if you need it, and practice healthy behaviors.

Top health experts from the U.S. Preventive Services Task Force suggest that when you go for your next checkup, you should talk to your doctor or nurse about how you can stay healthy no matter what your age.

Here are the most important things you can do to stay healthy:

- Get recommended screening tests.
- Be tobacco free.
- Be physically active.
- Eat a healthy diet.
- Stay at a healthy weight.
- Take preventive medicines if you need them.

Screening Tests for Men: What You Need and When

Screening tests can find diseases early when they are easier to treat. Health experts from the U.S. Preventive Services Task Force have made recommendations, based on scientific evidence, about testing for the following conditions. Talk to your doctor about which ones apply to you and when and how often you should be tested.

Obesity: Have your body mass index (BMI) calculated to screen for obesity. (BMI is a measure of body fat based on height and weight.) [You can also find your own BMI with the BMI calculator in Chapter 12 of this book.]

High cholesterol: Have your cholesterol checked regularly starting at age thirty-five. If you are younger than thirty-five, talk to your doctor about whether to have your cholesterol checked if:

- You have diabetes;
- You have high blood pressure;
- Heart disease runs in your family;
- You smoke.

High blood pressure: Have your blood pressure checked at least every two years. High blood pressure is 140/90 or higher.

Colorectal cancer: Have a test for colorectal cancer starting at age fifty. Your doctor can help you decide which test is right for you. If you have a family history of colorectal cancer, you may need to be screened earlier.

Diabetes: Have a test for diabetes if you have high blood pressure or high cholesterol.

Depression: Your emotional health is as important as your physical health. If you have felt "down," sad, or hopeless over the last two weeks or have felt little interest or pleasure in doing things, you may be depressed. Talk to your doctor about being screened for depression.

Sexually transmitted infections: Talk to your doctor to see whether you should be tested for gonorrhea, syphilis, Chlamydia, or other sexually transmitted infections.

Human immunodeficiency virus (HIV): Talk to your doctor about HIV screening if you:

- Have had sex with men since 1975;
- Have had unprotected sex with multiple partners;
- Have used or now use injection drugs;
- Exchange sex for money or drugs or have sex partners who do;
- Have past or present sex partners who are HIV-infected, are bisexual, or use injection drugs;
- Are being treated for sexually transmitted diseases;
- Had a blood transfusion between 1978 and 1985.

Abdominal aortic aneurysm: If you are between the ages of sixty-five and seventy-five and have ever smoked (one hundred or more cigarettes during your lifetime), you need to be screened once for abdominal aortic aneurysm, which is an abnormally large or swollen blood vessel in your abdomen.

Daily Steps to Health

Don't smoke: If you do smoke, talk to your doctor about quitting. Your doctor or nurse can help you.

Be physically active: Walking briskly, mowing the lawn, dancing, swimming, and bicycling are just a few examples of moderate physical activity. If you are not already physically active, start small and work up to thirty minutes or more of moderate physical activity most days of the week.

Eat a healthy diet: Emphasize fruits, vegetables, whole grains, and fat-free or low-fat milk and milk products; include lean meats, poultry, fish, beans, eggs, and nuts; and eat foods low in saturated fats, trans fats, cholesterol, salt (sodium), and added sugars.

Stay at a healthy weight: Balance calories from foods and beverages with calories you burn off by your activities. To prevent gradual weight gain over time, make small decreases in food and beverage calories and increase physical activity.

Drink alcohol only in moderation: If you drink alcohol, have no more than two drinks a day. (A standard drink is one 12-ounce bottle of beer or wine cooler, one 5-ounce glass of wine, or 1.5 ounces of 80-proof distilled spirits.)

Should You Take Medicines to Prevent Disease?

Aspirin: Ask your doctor about taking aspirin to prevent heart disease if you are older than forty-five or younger than forty-five and:

- Have high blood pressure;
- Have high cholesterol;
- Have diabetes;
- Smoke.

Immunizations: Stay up-to-date with your immunizations:

- Have a flu shot every year starting at age fifty. If you are younger than fifty, ask your doctor whether you need a flu shot.
- Have a pneumonia shot once after you turn sixty-five. If you are younger, ask your doctor whether you need a pneumonia shot.

Chapter 26

Self-Examinations Can Lead to Early Cancer Detection

Chapter Contents

Section 26.1

How to Do a Breast Self-Examination

This information is excerpted with permission from the American Institute for Cancer Research brochure "Questions and Answers about Breast Health and Breast Cancer." © 2005 American Institute for Cancer Research. Figures 26.1–6 are from the National Cancer Institute (NCI)'s Visuals Online at http://visualsonline.cancer.gov.

Breast Self-Examination

Breast self-examination (BSE) should be done once a month so you become familiar with the usual appearance and feel of your breasts. Familiarity makes it easier to notice any changes. Early discovery of a change from what is normal for you is the main purpose of BSE.

The best time to do BSE is one week after your period ends, when your breasts are least likely to be tender and swollen. After menopause, or if you have had a hysterectomy, perform your BSE on the first day of each month.

How to Do a Breast Self-Examination

1. Stand before a mirror with your arms at your sides. Look at both breasts for anything unusual, such as puckering, dimpling, scaling of the skin, or fluid leaking from the nipples.

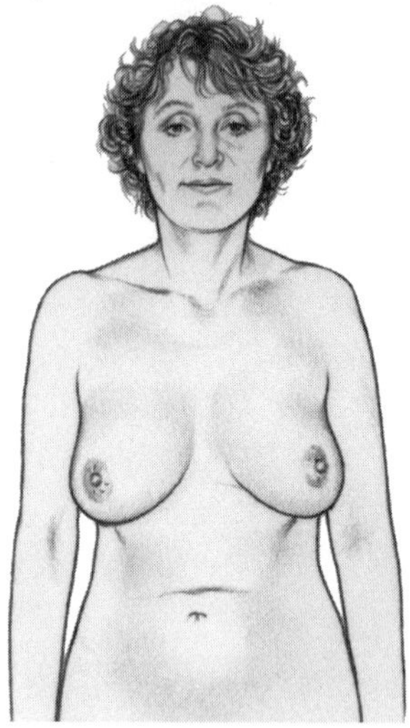

The next two steps are designed to emphasize any change in the shape or contour of your breasts. As you do them you should be able to feel your chest muscles tighten.

Figure 26.1. Breast self-exam: Step one (Source: NCI).

2. Clasp your hands behind your head and press your hands forward. Look closely at your breasts in the mirror.

3. Press your hands firmly on your hips and bow slightly toward the mirror as you pull your shoulders and elbows forward. Once again, look closely at your breasts in the mirror.

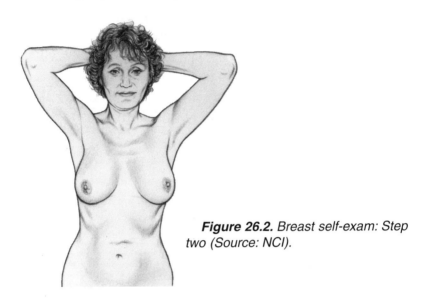

Figure 26.2. Breast self-exam: Step two (Source: NCI).

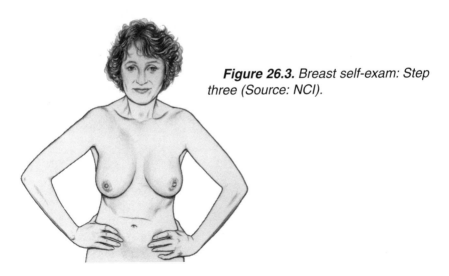

Figure 26.3. Breast self-exam: Step three (Source: NCI).

Some women do the next part of the exam in the shower. Fingers glide over soapy skin, making it easy to concentrate on the texture underneath.

4. Raise your left arm. Use three or four fingers of your right hand to explore your left breast carefully. Beginning at the outer edge, firmly press the flat part of your fingers in small circles, moving the circles slowly around the breast. Gradually work toward the nipple. Be sure to cover the entire breast. Pay special attention to the area between the breast and armpit, including the armpit itself. Feel for any unusual lumps or masses under the skin.

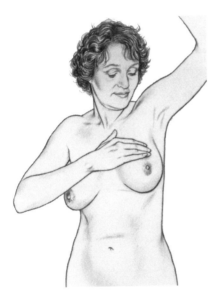

Figure 26.4. Breast self-exam: Step four (Source: NCI).

5. Gently squeeze the nipple and look for any fluid discharge. Repeat steps 4 and 5 on your right breast. The last part of the exam should be done while lying down.

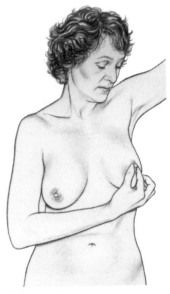

Figure 26.5. Breast self-exam: Step five (Source: NCI).

6. Lie flat on your back with your left arm over your head and a
    pillow or folded towel under your left shoulder. This position
    flattens the breast and makes it easier to examine. Using the
    same motions described in steps 4 and 5, examine your left
    breast, underarm area, and nipple. Repeat on your right side.

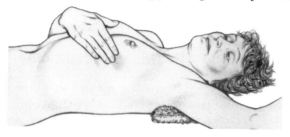

Figure 26.6. Breast self-exam: Step six (Source: NCI).

Section 26.2

Skin Cancer Self-Examination:
How to Spot Skin Cancer

Reprinted from "Self-Examination" and "Warning Signs: The ABCDEs
of Melanoma," © 2007 Skin Cancer Foundation (www.skincancer.org).
Reprinted with permission.

Self-Examination

Coupled with a yearly skin exam by a doctor, self-examination of
your skin once a month is the best way to detect the early warning
signs of basal cell carcinoma, squamous cell carcinoma, and melanoma, the three main types of skin cancer. Look for a new growth or
any skin change.

What you'll need: a bright light; a full-length mirror; a hand mirror; two chairs or stools; a blow dryer.

Examine head and face, using one or both mirrors. Use blow dryer
to inspect scalp.

Check hands, including nails. In full-length mirror, examine elbows,
arms, underarms.

Focus on neck, chest, torso. Women: Check under breasts.

With back to the mirror, use hand mirror to inspect back of neck, shoulders, upper arms, back, buttocks, legs.

Sitting down, check legs and feet, including soles, heels, and nails. Use hand mirror to examine genitals.

Melanoma, the deadliest form of skin cancer, is especially hard to stop once it has spread (metastasized) to other parts of the body. But it can be readily treated in its earliest stages.

Warning Signs: The ABCDEs of Melanoma

Moles, brown spots, and growths on the skin are usually harmless—but not always. Anyone who has more than one hundred moles is at greater risk for melanoma. The first signs can appear in one or more of these moles. That's why it's so important to get to know your skin very well, so you can recognize any changes in the moles on your body. Look for the ABCDEs of melanoma, and if you see one or more, make an appointment with a dermatologist immediately.

Asymmetry: If you draw a line through the mole, the two halves will not match, meaning it is asymmetrical, a warning sign for melanoma.

Border: The borders of an early melanoma tend to be uneven. The edges may be scalloped or notched.

Color: Having a variety of colors is another warning signal. A number of different shades of brown, tan, or black could appear. A melanoma may also become red, white, or blue.

Diameter: Melanomas usually are larger in diameter than the size of the eraser on your pencil (¼ inch or 6 mm), but they may sometimes be smaller when first detected.

Evolving: Any change—in size, shape, color, elevation, or another trait, or any new symptom such as bleeding, itching, or crusting—points to danger.

Prompt action is your best protection. Common moles and melanomas do not look alike.

Table 26.1. Characteristics of Benign and Malignant Skin Growths

Benign	Malignant
Symmetrical	Asymmetrical
Borders are even	Borders are uneven
One shade	Two or more shades
Smaller than ¼ inch	Larger than ¼ inch

Section 26.3

How to Do a Testicular Self-Examination

Reprinted from "How to Perform a Testicular Self-Examination." This information was provided by TeensHealth, one of the largest resources online for medically reviewed health information written for parents, kids, and teens. For more articles like this one, visit www.TeensHealth.org, or www.KidsHealth.org. © 2005 The Nemours Foundation.

The testicular self-examination (TSE) is an easy way for guys to check their own testicles to make sure there aren't any unusual lumps or bumps—which can be the first sign of testicular cancer.

Although testicular cancer is rare in teenage guys, overall it is the most common cancer in males between the ages of fifteen and thirty-five. It's important to try to do a TSE every month so you can become familiar with the normal size and shape of your testicles, making it easier to tell if something feels different or abnormal in the future.

Here's what to do:

- It's best to do a TSE during or right after a hot shower or bath. The scrotum (skin that covers the testicles) is most relaxed then, which makes it easier to examine the testicles.

- Examine one testicle at a time. Use both hands to gently roll each testicle (with slight pressure) between your fingers. Place your thumbs over the top of your testicle, with the index and middle fingers of each hand behind the testicle, and then roll it between your fingers.

- You should be able to feel the epididymis (the sperm-carrying tube), which feels soft, rope-like, and slightly tender to pressure, and is located at the top of the back part of each testicle. This is a normal lump.

- Remember that one testicle (usually the right one) is slightly larger than the other for most guys—this is also normal.

- When examining each testicle, feel for any lumps or bumps along the front or sides. Lumps may be as small as a piece of rice or a pea.

- If you notice any swelling, lumps, or changes in the size or color of a testicle, or if you have any pain or achy areas in your groin, let your doctor know right away.

Lumps or swelling may not be cancer, but they should be checked by your doctor as soon as possible. Testicular cancer is almost always curable if it is caught and treated early.

Chapter 27

Cancer Screening Tests

Chapter Contents

Section 27.1

Breast Cancer Screening: Mammograms

Reprinted from "Mammograms," National Women's Health
Information Center, April 2006.

What is the best method of detecting breast cancer?

A mammogram, or x-ray of the breast, along with a clinical breast
exam (an exam done by your doctor) is the most effective way to detect breast cancer early. Mammograms have both benefits and limitations. For example, some cancers can't be detected by a
mammogram, but may be detectable by breast exam.

Checking your own breasts for lumps or other changes is called a
breast self-exam (BSE). Studies so far have not shown that BSE alone
reduces the numbers of deaths from breast cancer. BSE should not
take the place of a clinical breast exam and a mammogram.

What is a mammogram?

A mammogram is a safe test used to look for any problems with a
woman's breasts. The test uses a special, low-dose x-ray machine to
take pictures of both breasts. The results are recorded on x-ray film
or directly onto a computer for a radiologist to examine.

Mammograms allow the doctor to have a closer look for breast
lumps and changes in breast tissue. They can show small lumps or
growths that a doctor or woman may not be able to feel when doing a
clinical breast exam. "Mammography" is the best screening tool that
doctors have for finding breast cancer.

If a lump is found, your doctor may order other tests, such as ultrasound or a biopsy—a test where a small amount of tissue is taken
from the lump and area around the lump. The tissue is sent to a lab
to look for cancer or changes that may mean cancer is likely to develop. Breast lumps or growths can be benign (not cancer) or malignant (cancer). Finding breast cancer early means that a woman has
a better chance of surviving the disease. There are also more choices
for treatment when breast cancer is found early.

Are there different types of mammograms?

Screening mammograms: These are done for women who have no symptoms of breast cancer. When you reach age forty, you should have a mammogram every one to two years.

Diagnostic mammograms: These are done when a woman has symptoms of breast cancer or a breast lump. This mammogram takes longer than screening mammograms because more pictures of the breast are taken.

Digital mammograms: These take an electronic image of the breast and store it directly in a computer. Current research has not shown that digital images are better at finding cancer than x-ray film images.

How is a mammogram done?

You stand in front of a special x-ray machine. The person who takes the x-rays, called a radiologic technologist, places your breasts (one at a time) between two plastic plates. The plates press your breast to make it flat. You will feel pressure on your breast for a few seconds. It may cause you some discomfort; you might feel squeezed or pinched. But, the flatter your breast, the better the picture. Most often, two pictures are taken of each breast—one from the side and one from above. A screening mammogram takes about fifteen minutes from start to finish.

What if I have breast implants?

If you have breast implants, be sure to tell your mammography facility that you have them when you make your appointment. You will need an x-ray radiologic technologist who is trained in x-raying patients with implants. This is important because breast implants can hide some breast tissue, which could make if difficult for the radiologist to see breast cancer when looking at your mammograms. For this reason, to take a mammogram of a breast with an implant, the x-ray technician might gently lift the breast tissue slightly away from the implant.

How often should I get a mammogram?

Women forty years and older should get a mammogram every one to two years.

Women who have had breast cancer or other breast problems or who have a family history of breast cancer might need to start getting mammograms before age forty or they might need to get them more often. Talk to your doctor about when to start and how often you should have a mammogram.

Where can I get a mammogram?

Be sure to get a mammogram from a facility certified by the U.S. Food and Drug Administration (FDA). These places must meet high standards for their x-ray machines and staff. Check out the FDA's website on the internet for a list of FDA-certified mammography facilities. Some of these facilities also offer digital mammograms.

Your doctor, local medical clinic, or local or state health department can tell you where to get no-cost or low-cost mammograms.

How do I get ready for my mammogram?

First, check with the place you are having the mammogram for any special instructions you may need to follow before you go. Here are some general guidelines to follow:

- Make your mammogram appointment for one week after your period. Your breasts hurt less after your period.

- If you have breast implants, be sure to tell your mammography facility that you have them when you make your appointment.

- Wear a shirt with shorts, pants, or a skirt. This way, you can undress from the waist up and leave your shorts, pants, or skirt on when you get your mammogram.

- Don't wear any deodorant, perfume, lotion, or powder under your arms or on your breasts on the day of your mammogram appointment. These things can make shadows show up on your mammogram.

Are there any problems with mammograms?

As with any medical test, mammograms have limits. These limits include:

- They are only part of a complete breast exam. Your doctor also should do a clinical breast exam. If your mammogram finds something abnormal, your doctor will order other tests.

- "False negatives" can happen. This means everything may look normal, but cancer is actually present. False negatives don't happen often. Younger women are more likely to have a false negative mammogram than are older women. This is because the breast tissue is denser, making cancer harder to spot.

• "False positives" can happen. This is when the mammogram results look like cancer is present, even though it is not. False positives are more common in younger women than older women.

Section 27.2

Screening for Cervical Cancer: Pap Tests

Reprinted from "Pap Test," National Women's Health Information Center, March 2006.

What is a Pap test?

The Pap test, also called a Pap smear, checks for changes in the cells of your cervix. The cervix is the lower part of the uterus (womb) that opens into the vagina (birth canal). The Pap test can tell if you have an infection, abnormal (unhealthy) cervical cells, or cervical cancer.

Why do I need a Pap test?

A Pap test can save your life. It can find the earliest signs of cervical cancer—a common cancer in women. If caught early, the chance of curing cervical cancer is very high. Pap tests also can find infections and abnormal cervical cells that can turn into cancer cells. Treatment can prevent most cases of cervical cancer from developing.

Getting regular Pap tests is the best thing you can do to prevent cervical cancer. About 13,000 women in America will find out they have cervical cancer this year. In 2004, 3,500 women died from cervical cancer in the United States.

Do all women need Pap tests?

It is important for all women to have Pap tests, along with pelvic exams, as part of their routine health care. You need a Pap test if you are:

- Twenty-one years or older;

- Under twenty-one years old and have been sexually active for three years or more.

There is no age limit for the Pap test. Even women who have gone through menopause (when a woman's periods stop) need regular Pap tests.

How often do I need to get a Pap test?

It depends on your age and health history. Talk with your doctor about what is best for you. The American College of Obstetricians and Gynecologists recommends the following:

- If you are younger than thirty years old, you should get a Pap test every year.

- If you are age thirty or older and have had three normal Pap tests for three years in a row, talk to your doctor about spacing out Pap tests to every two or three years.

- If you are ages sixty-five to seventy and have had at least three normal Pap tests and no abnormal Pap tests in the last ten years, ask your doctor if you can stop having Pap tests.

You should have a Pap test every year no matter how old you are if any of the following are true:

- You have a weakened immune system because of organ transplant, chemotherapy, or steroid use.

- Your mother was exposed to diethylstilbestrol (DES) while pregnant.

- You are human immunodeficiency virus (HIV)–positive.

Women who are living with HIV, the virus that causes AIDS, are at a higher risk of cervical cancer and other cervical diseases. The U.S. Centers for Disease Control and Prevention recommends that all HIV-positive women get an initial Pap test, and get re-tested six months later. If both Pap tests are normal, then these women can get yearly Pap tests in the future.

Who does not need regular Pap tests?

The only women who do not need regular Pap tests are the following:

- Women over age sixty-five who have had a number of normal Pap tests and have been told by their doctors that they don't need to be tested anymore.

- Women who do not have a cervix and are at low risk for cervical cancer. These women should speak to their doctor before stopping regular Pap tests.

If had a hysterectomy do I still need Pap tests?

It depends on the type of hysterectomy (surgery to remove the uterus) you had and your health history. Women who have had a hysterectomy should talk with their doctor about whether they need routine Pap tests.

Usually during a hysterectomy, the cervix is removed with the uterus. This is called a total hysterectomy. Women who have had a total hysterectomy for reasons other than cancer may not need regular Pap tests. Women who have had a total hysterectomy because of abnormal cells or cancer should be tested yearly for vaginal cancer until they have three normal test results. Women who have had only their uterus removed but still have a cervix need regular Pap tests. Even women who have had hysterectomies should see their doctors yearly for pelvic exams.

How can I reduce my chances of getting cervical cancer?

Aside from getting Pap tests, the best way to avoid cervical cancer is by steering clear of the human papilloma virus (HPV). HPV is a major cause of cervical cancer. HPV infection is also one of the most common sexually transmitted diseases (STD). So, a woman boosts her chances of getting cervical cancer if she:

- Starts having sex before age eighteen;
- Has many sex partners;
- Has sex partners who have other sex partners;
- Has or has had a sexually transmitted disease (STD).

What should I know about human papilloma viruses (HPV)?

Human papilloma viruses are a group of more than one hundred different viruses. About forty types of HPV are spread during sex. Some types of HPVs can cause cervical cancer when not treated. HPV infection is one of the most common sexually transmitted diseases. About 75 percent of sexually active people will get HPV sometime in their life. Most women with untreated HPV do not get cervical cancer. Some HPVs cause genital warts but these HPVs do not cause cervical cancer. Since HPV rarely causes symptoms, most people don't know they have the infection.

How would I know if I had human papilloma virus (HPV)?

Most women never know they have HPV. It usually stays hidden and doesn't cause symptoms like warts. When HPV doesn't go away on its own, it can cause changes in the cells of the cervix. Pap tests usually find these changes.

How do I prepare for a Pap test?

Many things can cause wrong test results by washing away or hiding abnormal cells of the cervix. So, doctors suggest that for two days before the test you avoid the following:

- Douching
- Using tampons
- Using vaginal creams, suppositories, and medicines
- Using vaginal deodorant sprays or powders
- Having sex

Should I get a Pap test when I have my period?

No. Doctors suggest you schedule a Pap test when you do not have your period. The best time to be tested is ten to twenty days after the first day of your last period.

How is a Pap test done?

Your doctor can do a Pap test during a pelvic exam. It is a simple and quick test. While you lie on an exam table, the doctor puts an instrument called a speculum into your vagina, opening it to see the cervix. He or she will then use a special stick or brush to take a few cells from inside and around the cervix. The cells are placed on a glass slide and sent to a lab for examination. While usually painless, a Pap test is uncomfortable for some women.

When will I get the results of my Pap test?

Usually it takes three weeks to get Pap test results. Most of the time, test results are normal. If the test shows that something might be wrong, your doctor will contact you to schedule more tests. There are many reasons for abnormal Pap test results. It usually does not mean you have cancer.

What do abnormal Pap test results mean?

It is scary to hear that your Pap test results are "abnormal." But abnormal Pap test results usually do not mean you have cancer. Most often there is a small problem with the cervix.

Some abnormal cells will turn into cancer. But most of the time, these unhealthy cells will go away on their own. By treating these unhealthy cells, almost all cases of cervical cancer can be prevented. If you have abnormal results, to talk with your doctor about what they mean.

My Pap test was "abnormal"—what happens now?

There are many reasons for "abnormal" Pap test results. If results of the Pap test are unclear or show a small change in the cells of the cervix, your doctor will probably repeat the Pap test.

If the test finds more serious changes in the cells of the cervix, the doctor will suggest more powerful tests. Results of these tests will help your doctor decide on the best treatment. These include the following:

- **Colposcopy:** The doctor uses a tool called a colposcope to see the cells of the vagina and cervix in detail.

- **Endocervical curettage:** The doctor takes a sample of cells from the endocervical canal with a small spoon-shaped tool called a curette.

- **Biopsy:** The doctor removes a small sample of cervical tissue. The sample is sent to a lab to be studied under a microscope.

The U.S. Food and Drug Administration (FDA) recently approved the LUMA® Cervical Imaging System. The doctor uses this device right after a colposcopy. This system can help doctors see areas on the cervix that are likely to contain precancerous cells. The device shines a light on the cervix and looks at how different areas of the cervix respond to this light. It gives a score to tiny areas of the cervix. It then makes a color map that helps the doctor decide where to further test the tissue with a biopsy. The colors and patterns on the map help the doctor tell the difference between healthy tissue and tissue that might be diseased.

My Pap test result was a "false positive." What does this mean?

Pap tests are not always 100 percent correct. False positive and false negative results can happen. This can be upsetting and confusing. A false positive Pap test is when a woman is told she has abnormal cervical cells, but the cells are really normal. If your doctor says your Pap results were a false positive, there is no problem.

A false negative Pap test is when a woman is told her cells are normal, but in fact there is a problem with the cervical cells that was missed. False negatives delay the discovery and treatment of unhealthy cells of the cervix. But having regular Pap tests boosts your chances of finding any problems. If abnormal cells are missed at one time, they will probably be found on your next Pap test.

I don't have health insurance; how can I get a free or low-cost Pap test?

Programs funded by the National Breast and Cervical Cancer Early Detection Program (NBCCEDP) offer free or low-cost Pap tests to women in need. These and other programs are available throughout the United States. Also, your state or local health department can direct you to places that offer free or low-cost Pap tests.

Section 27.3

Colorectal Cancer Screening

Reprinted from "Colorectal Cancer: Basic Facts on Screening," U.S. Centers for Disease Control and Prevention, January 2006.

What Is Colorectal Cancer?

Colorectal cancer is cancer that occurs in the colon or rectum. Sometimes it is called colon cancer, for short. The colon is the large intestine or large bowel. The rectum is the passageway that connects the colon to the anus.

It's the Second Leading Cancer Killer

Colorectal cancer is the second leading cancer killer in the United States, but it doesn't have to be. If everybody age fifty or older had regular screening tests, at least one-third of deaths from this cancer could be avoided. So if you are fifty or older, start screening now.

Who Gets Colorectal Cancer?

- Both men and women can get colorectal cancer.
- Colorectal cancer is most often found in people fifty and older.
- The risk for getting colorectal cancer increases with age.

Are You at High Risk?

Your risk for colorectal cancer may be higher than average if any of the following are true:

- You or a close relative have had colorectal polyps or colorectal cancer.
- You have inflammatory bowel disease.

People at high risk for colorectal cancer may need earlier or more frequent tests than other people. Talk to your doctor about when you should begin screening and how often you should be tested.

Screening Saves Lives

If you're fifty or older, getting a screening test for colorectal cancer could save your life. Here's how:

- Colorectal cancer usually starts from polyps in the colon or rectum. A polyp is a growth that shouldn't be there.

- Over time, some polyps can turn into cancer.

- Screening tests can find polyps, so they can be removed before they turn into cancer.

- Screening tests can also find colorectal cancer early. When it is found early, the chance of being cured is good.

Colorectal Cancer Can Start with No Symptoms

People who have polyps or colorectal cancer sometimes don't have symptoms, especially at first. This means that someone could have polyps or colorectal cancer and not know it. That is why having a screening test is so important.

What Are the Symptoms?

Some people with colorectal polyps or colorectal cancer do have symptoms. They may include the following:

- Blood in or on your stool (bowel movement)

- Pain, aches, or cramps in your stomach that happen a lot and you don't know why

- A change in bowel habits, such as having stools that are narrower than usual

- Losing weight and you don't know why

If you have any of these symptoms, talk to your doctor. These symptoms may also be caused by something other than cancer. However, the only way to know what is causing them is to see your doctor.

Types of Screening Tests

There are several different screening tests that can be used to find polyps or colorectal cancer. Each one can be used alone. Sometimes they are used in combination with each other. Talk to your doctor about which test or tests are right for you and how often you should be tested.

- **Fecal Occult Blood Test or Stool Test:** For this test, you receive a test kit from your doctor or healthcare provider. At home, you put a small piece of stool on a test card. You do this for three bowel movements in a row. Then you return the test cards to the doctor or a lab. The stool samples are checked for blood. This test should be done every year.

- **Flexible sigmoidoscopy:** For this test, the doctor puts a short, thin, flexible, lighted tube into your rectum. The doctor checks for polyps or cancer inside the rectum and lower third of the colon. This test should be done every five years.

- **Fecal occult blood test plus flexible sigmoidoscopy:** Your doctor may ask you to have both tests. Some experts believe that by using both tests, there is a better chance of finding polyps or colorectal cancer.

- **Colonoscopy:** This test is similar to flexible sigmoidoscopy, except the doctor uses a longer, thin, flexible, lighted tube to check for polyps or cancer inside the rectum and the entire colon. During the test, the doctor can find and remove most polyps and some cancers. This test should be done every ten years. Colonoscopy may also be used as a follow-up test if anything unusual is found during one of the other screening tests.

- **Double contrast barium enema:** This test is an x-ray of your colon. You are given an enema with a liquid called barium. Then the doctor takes an x-ray. The barium makes it easy for the doctor to see the outline of your colon on the x-ray to check for polyps or other abnormalities. This test should be done every five years.

Will Insurance or Medicare Pay for Screening Tests?

Many insurance plans and Medicare help pay for colorectal cancer screening tests. Check with your plan to find out which tests are covered for you.

The Bottom Line

If you're fifty or older, talk with your doctor about getting screened.

Section 27.4

Prostate Cancer Screening: A Decision Guide

Currently, digital rectal examination (DRE) and prostate specific antigen (PSA) are used for prostate cancer detection. The age at which time screening for prostate cancer should begin is not known with certainty. However, most experts agree that healthy men over the age of fifty should consider prostate cancer screening with a DRE and PSA test. Screening should occur earlier, at age forty, in those who are at a higher risk of prostate cancer such as African-American men or those with a family history of prostate cancer. Men who are concerned about their future risk of prostate cancer should be screened to assess their baseline risk for developing the disease.

Digital rectal exam (DRE): The DRE is performed with the man either bending over, lying on his side, or with his knees drawn up to his chest on the examining table. The physician inserts a gloved finger into the rectum and examines the prostate gland, noting any abnormalities in size, contour, or consistency. DRE is inexpensive, easy to perform, and allows the physician to note other abnormalities such as blood in the stool or rectal masses, which may allow for the early detection of rectal or colon cancer. However, DRE is not the most effective way to detect an early cancer, so it should be combined with a PSA test.

Prostate specific antigen test: The PSA test is usually performed in addition to DRE and increases the likelihood of prostate cancer detection. The test measures the level of PSA, a substance produced only by the prostate, in the bloodstream. The PSA should be less than 1.0 ng/ml The median for men in their forties is 0.7 ng/ml. If the PSA is higher than the age-specific median, the risk of developing prostate cancer and the risk of having an aggressive form of the disease are increased. Accordingly, the patient might be well advised to have more frequent screening to detect a rise in the PSA level over time.

This blood test can be performed in a clinical laboratory, hospital, or physician's office and requires no special preparation on the part of the patient. Ideally, the test should be taken before a digital rectal examination is performed or any catheterization or instrumentation of the urinary tract. Furthermore, because ejaculation can transiently elevate the PSA level for twenty-four to forty-eight hours, men should abstain from sexual activity for two days prior to having a PSA test. A tourniquet or rubber strap is tied around the upper arm to mildly restrict the flow of blood and keep blood in the vein. Then, a needle with a tube-like container attached is inserted into a vein, usually in the bend of the elbow or the top of the hand. After a sufficient sample of blood is obtained, the needle is withdrawn, a bandage is placed on the puncture site, and firm pressure is held until the bleeding stops. The entire test takes less than five minutes and produces only mild discomfort. Afterward, the patient may experience slight bruising at the puncture site.

Very little PSA escapes from a healthy prostate into the bloodstream, but certain prostatic conditions can cause larger amounts of PSA to leak into the blood. One possible cause of a high PSA level is benign (noncancerous) enlargement of the prostate, otherwise known as benign prostatic hyperplasia (BPH). Inflammation of the prostate, called prostatitis, is another common cause of PSA elevation, as is recent ejaculation. Prostate cancer is the most serious possible cause of an elevated PSA level. The frequency of PSA testing remains a matter of some debate. The American Urological Association (AUA) encourages men to have annual PSA testing starting at age fifty. The AUA also recommends annual PSA testing for men over the age of forty who are African-American or have a family history of the disease (for example, a father or brother who was diagnosed with prostate cancer), or for those who are interested in an early risk assessment. Some experts have suggested that men with an initial normal DRE and PSA level of less than 2.5 ng/ml can have PSA testing performed every two years. However, a disadvantage of infrequent testing is that it limits the ability to detect a rapidly rising PSA level that can signal aggressive prostate cancer. Recently, several refinements have been made in the PSA blood test in an attempt to determine more accurately who has prostate cancer and who has false-positive PSA elevations caused by other conditions like BPH. These refinements include PSA density, PSA velocity, PSA age-specific reference ranges, and use of free-to-total PSA ratios. Such refinements may increase the ability to detect cancer and these should be discussed with your physician.

Currently, it is recommended that both a DRE and a PSA test be used for the early detection of prostate cancer. It is important to realize that in most cases an abnormality in either test is not due to cancer but to benign conditions, the most common being BPH or prostatitis. For instance, it has been shown that only 18 to 30 percent of men with serum PSA values between 4 and 10 ng/ml have prostate cancer. This number rises to approximately 42 to 70 percent for those men whose PSA values exceed 10 ng/ml.

Chapter 28

Screening for High Cholesterol

High cholesterol is a leading risk factor for heart disease. Cholesterol, together with other substances, can build up inside the walls of the arteries that feed the heart and brain, forming a thick, hard deposit that can clog those arteries. When the blood flow is blocked, or partially blocked, to the heart muscle, the heart starves for oxygen and a heart attack may result. If a clot blocks blood flow to part of the brain, a stroke may occur.

Cholesterol is produced by the liver, circulated by the bloodstream, and found in all of the body's cells. It helps form cell membranes, certain hormones, Vitamin D, and tissue, and helps process dietary fats.

The body manufactures all the cholesterol it needs. The rest of the cholesterol in the bloodstream is derived from an individual's diet, with saturated fat being the main dietary cause of high blood cholesterol. The American Heart Association (AHA) recommends that you limit saturated fat intake to less than 7 percent of total calories each day to maintain healthy levels of cholesterol.

A cholesterol reading is the sum of low-density lipoprotein, or LDL (often referred to as "bad" cholesterol), high-density lipoprotein, or HDL (often referred to as "good" cholesterol), and other lipoproteins, such as triglycerides, measured in milligrams per deciliter (mg/dL).

According to the AHA, a desirable level of total cholesterol is 200 mg/dL or less. Borderline high-risk level is between 200 and 239 mg/dL, and high risk is 240 mg/dL or greater. An even more accurate

From "Cholesterol Testing Information," © 2007 College of American Pathologists (www.cap.org). All rights reserved. Reprinted with permission.

indicator than total cholesterol level is the level of LDL in the bloodstream. The lower the level of LDL cholesterol, the better.

In general, people who have a total cholesterol level greater than 240 have twice the risk of heart attack as those who have a cholesterol level of 200. This means that if your total cholesterol is less than 200 mg/dL, your heart attack risk is relatively low, unless you have other risk factors or an elevated LDL cholesterol level. No matter what your cholesterol level is, it is always better to eat foods low in saturated fat and cholesterol. Being physically active also helps reduce cholesterol levels.

How Often Should I Have My Cholesterol Checked?

The College of American Pathologists (CAP) recommends that all people twenty years or older have their cholesterol checked at least every five years, or more frequently if recommended by their doctor. Men over the age of forty-five and women older than fifty-five should be tested more frequently, according to their physicians' advice. This check-up should measure total cholesterol, LDL cholesterol, HDL cholesterol, and triglycerides.

Management and Treatment: Lowering Cholesterol Reduces Your Risk of Heart Disease

Have your blood cholesterol checked regularly. If the LDL level is high, follow your physician's recommendations to lower it.

If you are in the high-normal to borderline-high cholesterol range, diet and lifestyle changes can often improve your cholesterol levels:

- Eat foods low in saturated fat, cholesterol, and sodium.

- Maintain a healthy weight and lose weight if needed. Exercise for a half hour to an hour each day, if possible.

- Don't smoke, and avoid exposure to tobacco smoke.

- Reduce your alcohol consumption.

- Have your blood pressure checked regularly and take steps to reduce it if it is high.

If dietary changes and exercise do not produce results, your physician may prescribe a drug to lower your cholesterol.

In extreme cases in which there is a severe genetic cholesterol disorder, a blood-cleansing procedure called LDL apheresis may be considered. In this procedure, blood is removed from the body over a period of several hours and is chemically cleansed of LDL cholesterol before being returned to the body. Treatments every two to three weeks can reduce average LDL cholesterol by 50 to 80 percent, but are costly and time consuming.

Why Is LDL Cholesterol Considered "Bad"?

LDL is thought to carry cholesterol to tissues throughout the body. An LDL level of 130 mg/dL or greater increases the risk of heart disease because at that level, LDL begins causing plaque buildup in the arteries feeding the heart and brain. Most cholesterol-lowering treatments target reduction of LDL cholesterol.

Optimal LDL: Less than 100 mg/dL
Near optimal LDL: 100–129 mg/dL
Borderline high LDL: 130–159 mg/dL
High LDL: 160–189 mg/dL
Very high LDL: 190 mg/dL and higher

Why Is HDL Cholesterol Considered "Good"?

HDL cholesterol carries excess cholesterol to the liver for elimination from the body, and may actually protect against heart disease. An HDL level of 60 mg/dL or above helps protect against heart disease, while an HDL cholesterol level of less than 40 mg/dL may result in a greater risk for heart disease.

What Are Triglycerides?

Triglycerides are naturally occurring compounds that are the main component of fat, both in food and in the body. Calories consumed that are not used immediately are converted into triglycerides and transported to fat cells to be stored. Hormones regulate the release of triglycerides from fat tissue so they meet the body's needs for energy between meals.

What Happens in a Cholesterol Screening Test? Must a Doctor Perform It?

A simple blood test can assess your cholesterol levels. You may be asked to fast, and you may be told not to take certain drugs before the test. Your healthcare provider will take a small blood sample. Your arm will be cleaned with antiseptic and an elastic band briefly tightened around it to make the veins stand out. A needle will be inserted into a vein, and the blood will be collected in a sterile container. The band will be removed once the needle is inserted. When a small quantity of blood has been drawn, the needle will be removed and the puncture site will be covered. The blood will then sent to a laboratory for analysis.

The test does not necessarily have to be performed in a doctor's office. Cholesterol testing is often offered at public and private health fairs. If you participate in one of these public screenings, make sure that a reputable company does the screening and that you share the results with your regular healthcare professional afterward.

It is important to have a doctor interpret the results of the test. Only your doctor can correctly interpret your cholesterol numbers based on risk factors such as age, family history, smoking, and high blood pressure.

Make sure the test measures LDL cholesterol and triglyceride levels in addition to total cholesterol and HDL cholesterol levels. Although knowing your total cholesterol can provide a general idea of your risk for heart disease, it is more beneficial in assessing your risk and treatment options to obtain a "lipid profile" that includes your levels of HDL cholesterol, LDL cholesterol, and triglycerides, as well as your total cholesterol.

Measuring only your total cholesterol can be misleading because some people have low levels of HDL cholesterol and high levels of triglycerides, but normal or even high levels of LDL cholesterol. In these cases, a total cholesterol measurement might appear normal. Even with a "desirable" total cholesterol level, if you have high LDL or low HDL levels, you may be at increased risk for heart disease.

Chapter 29

Screening for Diabetes

Diagnosing Diabetes

In diagnosing diabetes, physicians primarily depend upon the results of specific glucose tests. However, test results are just part of the information that goes into the diagnosis of diabetes. Doctors also take into account your physical exam, presence or absence of symptoms, and medical history. Some people who are significantly ill will have transient problems with elevated blood sugars which will then return to normal after the illness has resolved. Also, some medications may alter your blood glucose levels (most commonly steroids and certain diuretics [water pills]). The two main tests used to measure the presence of blood sugar problems are (1) the direct measurement of glucose levels in the blood during an overnight fast, and (2) measurement of the body's ability to appropriately handle the excess sugar presented after drinking a high glucose drink.

1. **Fasting blood glucose (blood sugar) level:** The "gold standard" for diagnosing diabetes is an elevated blood sugar level after an overnight fast (not eating anything after midnight). A value above 140 mg/dl on at least two occasions typically means a person has diabetes. Normal people have fasting sugar levels that generally run between 70 and 110 mg/dl.

2. **The oral glucose tolerance test:** An oral glucose tolerance test is one that can be performed in a doctor's office or a lab. The person being tested starts the test in a fasting state (having no food or drink except water for at least ten hours but not greater than sixteen hours). An initial blood sugar is drawn and then the person is given a "Glucola" bottle with a high amount of sugar in it (75 grams of glucose, or 100 grams for pregnant women). The person then has his or her blood tested again thirty minutes, one hour, two hours, and three hours after drinking the high-glucose drink.

For the test to give reliable results, you must be in good health (not have any other illnesses, not even a cold). Also, you should be normally active (for example, not lying down or confined to a bed like a patient in a hospital) and taking no medicines that could affect your blood glucose. The morning of the test, you should not smoke or drink coffee. During the test, you need to lie or sit quietly.

The oral glucose tolerance test is conducted by measuring blood glucose levels five times over a period of three hours. In a person without diabetes, the glucose levels in the blood rise following drinking the glucose drink, but then fall quickly back to normal (because insulin is produced in response to the glucose, and the insulin has a normal effect of lowing blood glucose.) In a diabetic, glucose levels rise higher than normal after drinking the glucose drink and come down to normal levels much slower (insulin is either not produced, or it is produced but the cells of the body do not respond to it).

As with fasting or random blood glucose tests, a markedly abnormal oral glucose tolerance test is diagnostic of diabetes. However, blood glucose measurements during the oral glucose tolerance test can vary somewhat. For this reason, if the test shows that you have mildly elevated blood glucose levels, the doctor may run the test again to make sure the diagnosis is correct.

Glucose tolerance tests may lead to one of the following diagnoses:

- **Normal response:** A person is said to have a normal response when the two-hour glucose level is less than or equal to 110 mg/dl.

- **Impaired fasting glucose:** When a person has a fasting glucose equal to or greater than 110 and less than 126 mg/dl, he or she is said to have impaired fasting glucose. This is considered a risk factor for future diabetes, and will likely trigger another test in the future, but by itself, does not make the diagnosis of diabetes.

- **Impaired glucose tolerance:** A person is said to have impaired glucose tolerance when the two-hour glucose results from the oral glucose tolerance test are greater than or equal to 140 but less than 200 mg/dl. This is also considered a risk factor for future diabetes. There has recently been discussion about lowering the upper value to 180 mg/dl to diagnose more mild diabetes to allow earlier intervention and hopefully prevention of diabetic complications.

- **Diabetes:** A person has diabetes when oral glucose tolerance tests show that the blood glucose level at two hours is equal to or more than 200 mg/dl. This must be confirmed by a second test (any of the three) on another day. There has recently been discussion about lowering the upper value to 180 mg/dl to diagnose more people with mild diabetes to allow earlier intervention and hopefully prevention of diabetic complications.

- **Gestational diabetes:** A woman has gestational diabetes when she is pregnant and has any two of the following: a fasting plasma glucose of more than 105 mg/dl, a one-hour glucose level of more than 190 mg/dl, a two-hour glucose level of more than 165 mg/dl, or a three-hour glucose level of more than 145 mg/dl.

Chapter 30

Hearing and Vision Screening

Chapter Contents

Section 30.1

Hearing Screening

Excerpted from "Audiology," © 2007 A.D.A.M., Inc.
Reprinted with permission.

An audiology exam tests your ability to hear sounds. Sounds vary according to the intensity (volume or loudness) and the tone (the speed of sound wave vibrations).

Hearing occurs when sound waves move to the nerves of the inner ear and then the brain.

Intensity of sound is measured in decibels (dB):

- A whisper is about 20 dB.

- Loud music (some concerts) is around 80 to 120 dB.

- A jet engine is about 140 to 180 dB

Usually, sounds greater than 85 dB can cause hearing loss in a few hours. Louder sounds can cause immediate pain, and hearing loss can develop in a very short time.

Tone of sound is measured in cycles per second (cps) or Hertz (Hz):

- Low bass tones range around 50 to 60 Hz.

- Shrill, high-pitched tones range around 10,000 Hz or higher.

The normal range of human hearing is about 20 Hz to 20,000 Hz, and some animals can hear up to about 50,000 Hz.

How the Test Is Performed

The first steps are used to estimate the need for an audiogram. The specific procedures may vary, but they generally involve blocking one ear at a time and checking for the ability to hear whispers, then spoken words or the sound of a ticking watch.

A tuning fork may be used. The tuning fork is tapped and held in the air on each side of the head to test the ability to hear by air conduction. It is tapped and placed against the mastoid bone behind each ear to test bone conduction.

Audiometry provides a more precise measurement of hearing. Air conduction is tested by having you wear earphones attached to the audiometer. Pure tones of controlled intensity are delivered, to one ear at a time. You are asked to raise a hand, press a button, or otherwise indicate when you hear a sound. The minimum intensity (volume) required to hear each tone is graphed. An attachment called a bone oscillator is placed against the bone behind each ear (mastoid bone) to test bone conduction.

How the Test Will Feel

There is no discomfort. The length of time varies. An initial screening may take about five to ten minutes. Detailed audiometry may take about one hour.

Why the Test Is Performed

This may be a screening test to detect a hearing loss at an early stage. It may also be used when there is difficulty in hearing from any cause.

Common causes of hearing loss include:

- Chronic ear infections;
- Ruptured eardrum;
- Acoustic trauma;
- Occupational hearing loss;
- Head injury;
- Inherited conditions;
- Diseases of the inner ear;
- Medications that can be toxic to the nerve of the inner ear, including certain antibiotics (such as neomycin), diuretics, and large doses of salicylates (such as aspirin).

Normal Values

- The ability to hear a whisper, normal speech, and a ticking watch is normal.
- The ability to hear a tuning fork through air and bone is normal.

- In detailed audiometry, hearing is normal if tones from 250 Hz through 8000 Hz can be heard at 25 dB or lower.

What Abnormal Results Mean

There are many different kinds and degrees of hearing loss. Some include only the loss of the ability to hear high or low tones, or the loss of only air or bone conduction. The inability to hear pure tones below 25 dB indicates some extent of hearing loss.

The following conditions may affect test results:

- Acoustic neuroma
- Acoustic trauma
- Age-related hearing loss
- Alport syndrome
- Labyrinthitis
- Ménière disease
- Occupational hearing loss
- Otosclerosis
- Ruptured or perforated eardrum

Special Considerations

There are many different hearing function tests. Simple screenings involve making a loud noise and watching to see if it startles the patient. Detailed screenings include brainstem auditory evoked response testing (BAER). This test uses electroencephalogram to detect brain wave activity when sounds are made.

A newer hearing test called otoacoustic emission testing (OAE) can be used in the very young (such as newborns) or when standard tests do not produce reliable results.

Section 30.2

Vision Screening

Excerpted from "Age-Related Eye Disease Doesn't Have to Steal Your Sight," *Word on Health*, National Institutes of Health, January 1999. Reviewed by David A. Cooke, M.D., May 2007.

According to the National Eye Institute, a comprehensive eye exam should include at least the following three tests:

- **Visual acuity test:** The familiar eye chart measures how well you see at various distances.

- **Pupil dilation:** An eye care professional places drops into the eye to widen the pupil. This reveals more of the retina and other signs of disease.

- **Tonometry:** A standard test that determines the fluid pressure inside the eye. There are many types of tonometry. One uses a purple light to measure pressure; another, an "air puff" test, which measures the resistance of the eye to a puff of air. Elevated pressure is a possible sign of glaucoma.

In addition, several special examinations may be recommended to detect other eye disorders, including signs of age-related eye diseases:

- **Visual field:** This test measures your side (peripheral) vision. It helps your eye care professional find out if you have lost side vision, a sign of glaucoma.

- **Amsler grid:** While conducting the examination, your eye care professional may ask you to look at an Amsler grid. It is a pattern that resembles a checkerboard. You will be asked to cover one eye and stare at a black dot in the center of the grid. While staring at the dot, if you notice that the straight lines in the pattern appear wavy, it may be a sign of wet age-related macular degeneration (AMD). If your eye care professional suspects you have wet AMD, you may need to have a test called fluorescein angiography. In this test, a special dye is injected into a vein in your arm. Pictures are then taken as the dye passes through the blood vessels in the retina. The photos help your eye care professional evaluate leaking blood vessels to determine whether they can be treated.

- **Ophthalmoscopy:** The eye care professional looks through a device with a special magnifying lens that provides a narrow view of the retina, or looks through a special magnifying glass and gains a wide view of the retina. Your eye care professional will look at your retina for early signs of retinal disease.

Chapter 31

Screening for Osteoporosis

Osteoporosis is a condition of low bone density that can progress silently over a long period of time. If diagnosed early, the fractures associated with the disease can often be prevented. Unfortunately, osteoporosis frequently remains undiagnosed until a fracture occurs.

An examination to diagnose osteoporosis can involve several steps that predict your chances of future fracture, diagnose osteoporosis, or both. It might include an initial physical exam; various x-rays that detect skeletal problems; laboratory tests that reveal important information about the metabolic process of bone breakdown and formation; and a bone density test to detect low bone density.

Before performing any tests, your doctor will record information about your medical history and lifestyle and will ask questions related to the following:

- Risk factors, including information about any fractures you have had
- Your family history of disease, including osteoporosis
- Medication history
- General intake of calcium and vitamin D
- Exercise pattern
- For women, menstrual history

Reprinted from "Osteoporosis: The Diagnosis," National Institute of Arthritis and Musculoskeletal and Skin Diseases, National Institutes of Health, November 2005.

In addition, the doctor will note medical problems and medications you may be taking that can contribute to bone loss (including glucocorticoids, such as cortisone). He or she will also check your height for changes and your posture to note any curvature of the spine from vertebral fractures, which is known as kyphosis.

Risk Factors

Risk factors for osteoporotic fracture include the following:

- Personal history of fracture as an adult
- History of fracture in a first-degree relative
- Caucasian or Asian race, although African Americans and Hispanic Americans are at significant risk as well
- Advanced age
- Being female
- Dementia
- Poor health, frailty, or both
- Current cigarette smoking
- Low body weight
- Anorexia nervosa
- Estrogen deficiency (past menopause, menopause before age forty-five, having both ovaries removed, or the absence of menstrual periods for a year or more prior to menopause)[1]
- Low testosterone levels in men
- Use of certain medications such as corticosteroids and anticonvulsants
- Lifelong low calcium intake
- Excessive alcohol intake
- Impaired eyesight despite adequate correction
- Recurrent falls
- Inadequate physical activity

X-ray Tests

If you have back pain, your doctor may order an x-ray of your spine to determine whether you have had a fracture. An x-ray also may be appropriate if you have experienced a loss of height or a change in posture. However, since an x-ray can detect bone loss only after 30 percent of the skeleton has been depleted, the presence of osteoporosis may be missed.

Bone Mineral Density Tests

A bone mineral density (BMD) test is the best way to determine your bone health. BMD tests can identify osteoporosis, determine your risk for fractures (broken bones), and measure your response to osteoporosis treatment. The most widely recognized bone mineral density test is called a dual-energy x-ray absorptiometry or DXA test. It is painless: a bit like having an x-ray, but with much less exposure to radiation. It can measure bone density at your hip and spine.

During a BMD test, an extremely low energy source is passed over part or all of the body. The information is evaluated by a computer program that allows the doctor to see how much bone mass you have. Since bone mass serves as an approximate measure of bone strength, this information also helps the doctor accurately detect low bone mass, make a definitive diagnosis of osteoporosis, and determine your risk of future fractures.

BMD tests provide doctors with a measurement called a T-score, a number value that results from comparing your bone density to optimal bone density. When a T-score appears as a negative number such as -1, -2 or -2.5, it indicates low bone mass. The more negative the number, the greater the risk of fracture.

Although no bone density test is 100 percent accurate, this type of test is the single most important predictor of whether a person will fracture in the future.

Bone Scans

For some people, a bone scan may be ordered. A bone scan is different from the BMD test just described, although the term "bone scan" often is used incorrectly to describe a bone density test. A bone scan can tell the doctor whether there are changes that may indicate cancer, bone lesions, inflammation, or new fractures. In a bone scan, the person being tested is injected with a dye that allows a scanner to identify differences in the conditions of various areas of bone tissue.

Laboratory Tests

A number of laboratory tests may be performed on blood and urine samples. The results of these tests can help your doctor identify conditions that may be contributing to your bone loss. The most common blood tests evaluate:

- Blood calcium levels;
- Blood vitamin D levels;
- Thyroid function;
- Parathyroid hormone levels;
- Estradiol levels to measure estrogen (in women);
- Follicle stimulating hormone (FSH) test to establish menopause status;
- Testosterone levels (in men);
- Osteocalcin levels to measure bone formation.

The most common urine tests are as follows:

- Twenty-four-hour urine collection to measure calcium metabolism
- Tests to measure the rate at which a person is breaking down or resorbing bone

Treatment

In addition to diagnosing osteoporosis, results from BMD tests assist the doctor in deciding whether to begin a prevention or treatment program. Once you and your doctor have definitive information based on your history, physical examination, and diagnostic tests, a specific treatment program can be developed for you.

Recommendations for optimizing bone health include a comprehensive program that consists of a well-balanced diet rich in calcium and vitamin D, physical activity, and a healthy lifestyle (including not smoking, avoiding excessive alcohol use, and recognizing that some prescription medications and chronic diseases can cause bone loss). If you already have experienced a fracture, your doctor may refer you to a specialist in physical therapy or rehabilitation medicine to help you with daily activities, safe movement, and exercises to improve your strength and balance.

Notes

1. Women lose bone rapidly in the first four to eight years following menopause, making them more susceptible to osteoporosis.

Part Five

Understanding How the Aging Process Affects Wellness

Chapter 32

The Aging Process

As we age, our bodies change in many ways that affect the function of both individual cells and organ systems. These changes occur little by little and progress inevitably over time. However, the rate of this progression can be very different from person to person. Research in aging is beginning to find out the reasons for these changes and the genetic and environmental factors that control them.

Genetic and Environmental Factors

The aging process depends on a combination of both genetic and environmental factors. Recognizing that every individual has his or her own unique genetic makeup and environment, which interact with each other, helps us understand why the aging process can occur at such different rates in different people. Overall, genetic factors seem to be more powerful than environmental factors in determining the large differences among people in aging and lifespan. There are even some specific genetic disorders that speed up the aging process, such as Hutchinson-Gilford, Werner, and Down syndromes. However, many environmental conditions, such as the

Used with permission from the American Geriatrics Society Foundation for Health in Aging, http://www.healthinaging.org/ from the Public Education Forums web page, http://www.healthinaging.org/public_education/pef and from the Aging in the Know website, http://www.healthinaging.org/agingintheknow/. For more information visit AGS online at www.americangeriatrics.org.

quality of health care that you receive, have a substantial effect on aging. A healthy lifestyle is an especially important factor in healthy aging and longevity. These environmental factors can significantly extend lifespan.

Behaviors of a Healthy Lifestyle

- Not smoking

- Drinking alcohol in moderation

- Exercising

- Getting adequate rest

- Eating a diet high in fruits and vegetables

- Coping with stress

- Having a positive outlook

Cellular Changes Associated with Aging

Aging causes functional changes in cells. For example, the rate at which cells multiply tends to slow down as we age. Certain cells that are important for our immune system to work properly (called T-cell lymphocytes) also decrease with age. In addition, age causes changes in our responses to environmental stresses or exposures, such as ultraviolet light, heat, not enough oxygen, poor nutrition, and toxins (poisons), among others.

Age also interferes with an important process called apoptosis, which programs cells to self-destruct or die at appropriate times. This process is necessary for tissues to remain healthy, and it is especially important in slowing down immune responses once an infection has been cleared from the body.

Different diseases that are common in elderly people can affect this process in different ways. For example, cancer results in a loss of apoptosis. The cancer cells continue to multiply and invade or take over surrounding tissue, instead of dying as originally programmed. Other diseases may cause cells to die too early. In Alzheimer disease, a substance called amyloid builds up and causes the early death of brain cells, which results in a progressive loss of memory and other brain functions. Toxins produced as byproducts of nerve cell transmissions are also thought to be involved in the death of nerve cells in Parkinson disease.

Bodily Changes Associated with Aging

Our bodies normally change in appearance as we age.

Changes in Height

We all lose height as we age, although when the height loss begins and how quickly it progresses vary quite a bit among different people. Generally, our height increases until our late forties and then decreases about two inches by age eighty. The reasons for height loss include the following:

- Changes in posture
- Changes in the growth of vertebrae (the bones that make up the spine)
- A forward bending of the spine
- Compression of the discs between the vertebrae
- Increased curvature of the hips and knees
- Decreased joint space in the trunk and extremities
- Joint changes in the feet
- Flattening of the arches

The length of the bones in our legs does not change much.

Changes in Weight

In men, body weight generally increases until their mid-fifties; then it decreases, with weight being lost faster in their late sixties and seventies. In women, body weight increases until the late sixties and then decreases at a rate slower than that of men.

People that live in less technologically developed societies do not show this pattern of weight change. This suggests that reduced physical activity and changes in eating habits may be causes of the change in body weight rather than the aging process.

Changes in Body Composition

The proportion of the body that is made up of fat doubles between age twenty-five and age seventy-five. Exercise programs may prevent or reverse much of the proportional decrease in muscle mass and increase in total body fat. This change in body composition is important to consider in nutritional planning and level of activity. The change in body composition also has an important effect on how the body handles various drugs. For example, when our body fat increases, drugs that are dissolved in fatty tissues remain in the body much longer than when our body was younger and more muscular.

Other Changes with Aging

Normal aging in the absence of disease is a remarkably benign process. In other words, our body can remain healthy as we age. Although our organs may gradually lose some function, we may not even notice these changes except during periods of great exertion or stress. We may also experience slower reaction times.

Normal Aging and Disease

Aging and disease are related in subtle and complex ways. Several conditions that were once thought to be part of normal aging have now been shown to be due to disease processes that can be influenced by lifestyle. For example, heart and blood vessel diseases are more common in people who eat a lot of meat and fat. Similarly, cataract formation in the eye largely depends on the amount of exposure to direct sunlight.

We should remember that there is a range of individual response to aging. Biologic and chronologic ages are not the same. In addition, body systems do not age at the same rate within any individual. For example, you might have severe arthritis or loss of vision while the function of your heart or kidneys is excellent. Even those aging changes that are considered "usual" or "normal" are not inevitable consequences of aging.

Changes in the Regulation of Body Systems

The way our body regulates certain systems changes with age. Some examples are listed here:

- Progressive changes in the heart and blood vessels interfere with your body's ability to control blood pressure.

- Your body cannot regulate its temperature as it could when you were younger. This can result in dangerously low body temperature from prolonged exposure to the cold or in heat stroke if the outside temperature is too high.

- There may be aging-related changes in your body's ability to develop a fever in response to an infection.

- The regulation of the amount and makeup of body fluids is slowed down in healthy older persons. Usual (resting) levels of the hormones that control the amount of body fluids are unchanged, but problems in fluid regulation commonly develop during illness or other stress. Also, elderly people don't feel as thirsty after water deprivation as they did when younger.

What do these age-related changes in our body systems mean?

First, with advancing age, we become less like each other biologically, so our healthcare needs to be more individualized.

Body systems that can be minimally affected by age are often profoundly influenced by lifestyle behaviors such as cigarette smoking, physical activity, and nutritional intake, and by circumstances such as financial means.

Finally, it's helpful to consider ahead of time our possible choices in case certain situations arise. For example, if you become less physically able to take part in an athletic activity you did before, is there a different activity you might enjoy? Are there things you might like to do to keep your mind active? More serious situations to consider might include death of a spouse, or if you find your abilities becoming more and more limited. Have you discussed how you would like to handle such situations and your wishes with your family?

It is important to remember that the ability to learn and adjust continues throughout life and is strongly influenced by interests, activities, and motivation. With years of rich experience and reflection, we can rise above our own circumstances. Old age, despite the physical limitations, can be a time of variety, creativity, and fulfillment.

Chapter 33

Depression and Other Mental Health Issues Associated with Aging

Chapter Contents

Section 33.1

Psychological and Social Issues Related to Aging

Used with permission from the American Geriatrics Society Foundation for Health in Aging, http://www.healthinaging.org/ from the Public Education Forums web page, http://www.healthinaging.org/public_education/pef and from the Aging in the Know website, http://www.healthinaging.org/agingintheknow. For more information visit AGS online at www.americangeriatrics.org.

For young people, time seems to have no end. But, as time passes we suddenly realize that the number of remaining years is limited. The realization that we are growing old can be traumatic. Our ideas about and attitudes toward aging are very important in how well we cope with and enjoy the passing years.

Some psychological characteristics of aging get passed down from generation to generation through our genes. Others can result from real or perceived changes in our bodies as we age (e.g., mental or physical limitations). Social and cultural differences also affect how we deal with aging. Men and women think about aging differently, because of biological, social, and psychological differences between the sexes. For example, women tend to live longer than men, so they generally experience more losses of family members and friends. All these factors influence our overall well-being as we age.

How Our Minds Change as We Age

Losing mental function is perhaps the most feared aspect of aging. In fact, the fear itself often begins to wear down our quality of life. We begin to believe the stereotype that we are losing (or will lose) our mental function. This can lead to loss of self-esteem and withdrawal from others. However, mental function does not have to decrease with age. Our fears are usually groundless.

Learning

The ability to learn continues throughout life, although we may learn in different ways as we age. Older people often require more time and effort to absorb new information. We may need to read instructions more carefully to be able to organize and understand new information. As we get older, we tend to avoid learning things that are not meaningful or rewarding to us, or that cannot be linked to one of our other senses, such as sight or hearing. The reasons for these changes in learning are not known, but they may be partly caused by changes in our sight, hearing, and other senses that we use for memory.

Memory

Older people may have trouble remembering some things, but not others. Short-term memory (i.e., less than thirty minutes) worsens as we age. Although we often hear that long-term memory (weeks to months) also worsens as we age, this may depend more on getting information into our memory, rather than remembering it later. Very long-term memory (months to years) is basically permanent, collected through a lifetime of day-to-day education and experience. This type of memory increases from the age of twenty to about the age of fifty and then remains essentially the same until well after seventy.

Most of us learn to adapt to changes in learning and memory. We slow down and do things more carefully. We think about things a little longer to remember them. We may avoid new or strange environments. As a result, any memory losses may not even be noticed until we experience a major life change, such as moving or the death of a spouse.

Reaction Time

As we age, we tend to process information at a slower pace. This means it takes longer to figure out what is going on and what to do about it (if anything). Most of this "slow down" is caused by changes in the nervous system over time. We tend to slow down even further when doing tasks that require more thought or are more complicated. When an event is a surprise, we are particularly slow to respond. However, older people tend to make fewer mistakes in their responses than younger people.

Intelligence

Whether intelligence declines as we age is hotly debated. Although overall intelligence stays about the same throughout life, older people don't do as well as younger people on many standardized intelligence tests. In formal tests of performance, older people also slow down with age—but they make fewer mistakes. This is because we learn to value

339

correctness as we age. So although we may be slower to respond, our answers are more accurate. We tend to be more cautious and less willing than younger people to make a mistake in judgment, which is a valuable characteristic in many real-life situations.

Life Skills

You should keep in mind that most intelligence tests do not address things that we deal with in our daily lives. For example, older people tend to do better than younger people on tests that deal with practical activities, such as using a telephone directory. In fact, as we age, most of us get much better at being able to manage our daily affairs. It is usually only in times of stress or loss that we may be pushed beyond our limits, and having a support network to help us cope is very important. Older adults can continue to gain support, care, respect, status, and a sense of purpose by interacting with younger people. And younger people can learn from the experience, cultural meaning, stability, and continuity of older people.

Stresses

Older adults often must face a great number of stresses that can be caused by a broad range of events and situations. Stresses can be physical or social. They can be an ongoing part of day-to-day life, or caused by sudden traumatic events. Common stresses for older people include the following:

- Diseases or health conditions, possibly chronic (e.g., arthritis)

- Perceived loss of social status after retirement

- Death of a spouse

Stress often affects our physical health and can have an even stronger effect on our mental well-being. Too much stress can be associated with a number of psychological and physical conditions, such as anxiety, headaches, and ulcers.

Caregiving

Chronic diseases and conditions affect most older adults. Family members, especially spouses, are most often the caregivers. More than forty-four million Americans (mostly women) care for family members of all ages. Many older adults are also caregivers for another family member.

Although caregiving can be rewarding, it is also very stressful. Caregivers have twice the risk of others for mental and physical health problems (e.g., burnout, substance abuse, depression, etc.). They are also more than twice as likely to be taking medications to relieve anxiety or stress. Social isolation, family disagreements, and financial hardships are common problems associated with long-term caregiving.

Caregivers can benefit greatly from training, information, and support. Programs that provide education, counseling, and behavioral therapy can decrease the stress of caregiving. Support groups for individuals with specific diseases (e.g., Alzheimer support groups) often have information about support programs for caregivers.

Loss and Grief

As we get older, the death of friends and family becomes more common. Losing and grieving for a spouse is one of the most traumatic situations commonly faced by older adults. More than 1 million spouses (mostly women) were widowed in the United States in 2003. This number is estimated to increase to 1.5 million every year by 2030. Other losses that may also cause grief include loss of sight or hearing and losses in function caused by illnesses (e.g., trouble walking from arthritis). These and other negative life events place a heavy burden on older adults.

Most people grieve intensely for six to twelve months after a major loss. Generally, we feel depressed and withdraw from others. After about a year, we begin to accept the loss and start to interact more with friends and family. Going through the grieving process is an important part of emotional healing, and we shouldn't try to ignore it or pretend it isn't there. Getting treatment for depression can also help avoid the mental and physical health problems associated with a grieving process that goes on far longer than usual.

Changing Roles as We Age

People shift through many roles throughout their lives. We are children, parents, friends, workers, patients, students, sports enthusiasts, artists, etc. One of the most dramatic changes involves retirement. When older adults retire, they leave work and social roles that likely provided economic rewards as well as social status.

In addition, older people may find that there are changes in their personal relationships after retirement. For example, spouses may

341

find themselves spending much more time together than they ever did before. Older parents may add the role of grandparent or even great-grandparent, which brings both new rewards and new demands.

Losses in function may place older adults in the position of asking for help, rather than providing it. Similarly, another's losses may place someone in a caregiving role. These role changes can be stressful and affect mental and physical health.

Social Status

Many social factors affect how we think about ourselves and how others think about us. Our sex, race, and economic status all affect our real and perceived social status. These factors also can affect the resources that are available to us to help cope with aging and health. For example, it's difficult for poorer people to use support programs or community activities that cost money. Ethnic or cultural backgrounds may also have a major effect on our outlook and how we deal with situations. For example, women from some cultures do not feel comfortable exercising in public.

Many people are uncomfortable discussing some illnesses. Others may agree to only those treatments that are acceptable in their culture. Some cultures view hospice care as a wish to bring about the death of the person. Similarly, a procedure like autopsy may strongly violate certain cultural or religious beliefs.

Healthy Ways to Cope with Stress

Everyone must learn to manage both the stresses caused by major life events and the routine stresses of day-to-day life. Too much stress can greatly affect our physical health and ability to function, as well as our mental health and overall well-being. This includes enthusiasm for life and the ability to enjoy social interactions.

Problems caused by stress often relate to how we deal with the stressful situation. There are positive ways to deal with stress, even when the stress is beyond our control (e.g., the death of a loved one). Learning positive behaviors can improve how we understand and cope with stress. For example, we can learn how to take more control of a stressful situation. We can also become more aware of social services and programs that are available. Family counseling and therapy can also strengthen social relationships with family and friends.

Belief in Yourself

One of the best ways to cope with all kinds of stress is through a strong belief in yourself and your ability to deal with situations. Believing in yourself has many positive effects on health, both physical and mental. The way a person deals with a stressful situation has a big effect on what happens and how he or she feels about it. This is true for many kinds of stress, including those related to disease, loss in function, and changes in social roles. In fact, feelings of self-confidence and personal control can go a long way toward improving function and overall quality of life, even in the face of physical disability.

Benefits of Believing in Yourself and Your Ability to Control Situations

* Lessens the negative effects of stress

* Contributes to overall physical health and ability

* Helps maintain overall function

* Slows loss of function

* Contributes to being able to make good decisions and follow through

* Contributes to ability to get more done

More good news is that there are effective ways to strengthen your belief in yourself. Your sense of personal control and self-confidence increases when you succeed at something new or when you see others like yourself succeed. Encouragement and empathy also can increase self-confidence and a feeling of personal control. A number of training programs are available for improving performance in specific areas. Examples include programs to reduce the fear of falling or to stick with an exercise regimen after a heart attack.

Coping Strategies

Coping strategies are emotional and mental responses that help us deal with stress. They provide positive reinforcement and reinforce self-esteem. There are many coping strategies that we can try. For example, thinking confidently and optimistically in the face of bad news might help us meet the challenge and increase the likelihood of a good result.

Another coping strategy that people tend to adopt with age is to cut down on the number and kinds of things they do, but to keep doing those activities that they like the most and do well. In other words, people spend more time doing a few selected activities and getting the most enjoyment from them. Although performance and abilities may lessen over time, you can continue to do the things you like, but perhaps you might simplify them. For example, a person who enjoys preparing fancy dinners might choose a simpler main course that he or she has prepared many times, along with several simple side dishes.

Social Involvement

Participating in family and community activities is a major source of personal satisfaction. Being involved plays an important role in improving self-esteem and giving meaning to life. This is true for people of all ages, but is especially important for older adults.

Becoming more involved and finding ways to contribute to the broader world can improve overall well-being. There are many ways to get involved, including providing family assistance (e.g., baby-sitting), participating in group activities, volunteering, and even taking a job. Social involvement also helps to fight depression, which is more common among those who withdraw from their friends, family, and community. Social isolation is a strong risk factor for health problems and early death.

Social Networks

Social networks provide many benefits that improve our overall well-being. Social networks provide emotional and physical support in times of crisis. For example, family and friends can support older adults through the death of a spouse or close friend. They can also provide help if an older adult experiences functional losses. However, we shouldn't allow ourselves to rely completely on social networks. Older people, particularly men, who receive too much assistance may be less motivated to manage and overcome a disability. If a person receives too much help or isn't encouraged to care for him- or herself, permanent disability can result. So although the social network is very helpful, the person should also be encouraged to regain maximal function.

Benefits of Social Networks

- Less risk of early death
- Better physical and mental health

- Less risk of disability or decline in activities of daily living
- Better chance of recovering ability to perform activities of daily living
- Buffered impact of major life events
- Greater feeling of personal control

Having social relationships that are enjoyable and meaningful is more important than having a large number of social interactions. Close personal relationships, such as a happy marriage or close relationships with family or friends, seem to be the most important. However, close relationships that are filled with disagreements and conflict work in the opposite direction. Having a large social network can have both positive and negative effects. A large social network offers the opportunity for greater involvement and contribution. However, a large social network also means a greater number of losses (death or disability) within the network.

Spiritual or Religious Involvement

Religion plays an important part in the lives of many older adults, who are generally more actively involved than younger people in religious services and practices. More than 50 percent of all older adults report frequent attendance at religious events. This involvement generally has overall benefits. Religious activity contributes to social interaction and encourages involvement.

Healthy Behaviors

Healthy behaviors have positive effects on overall well-being at any age. Positive behaviors include the following:

- Being physically active
- Eating a healthy diet
- Not smoking
- Drinking alcohol only in moderation
- Practicing relaxation or stress-reduction techniques

Although these are physical behaviors, they are also important psychologically and socially. For example, older adults with strong feelings of personal control and self-esteem are more likely to practice healthy behaviors. Similarly, healthy behaviors are likely to promote self-esteem and feelings of accomplishment in older adults.

Strong social networks generally encourage healthy behaviors, making them easier and more enjoyable. Seeing friends and family gain health benefits from exercise encourages a person to increase his or her physical activity as well. For example, an older adult may be able to join a friend or family member on daily walks or tai chi classes.

Section 33.2

Depression and Aging

"Depression in Late Life: Not a Natural Part of Aging,"
© 2005 Geriatric Mental Health Foundation (www.gmhfonline.org).
Reprinted with permission.

Everyone Feels Sad or Blue Sometimes

It is a natural part of life. But when the sadness persists and interferes with everyday life, it may be depression. Depression is not a normal part of growing older. It is a treatable medical illness, much like heart disease or diabetes.

Depression is a serious illness affecting approximately fifteen out of every one hundred adults over age sixty-five in the United States. The disorder affects a much higher percentage of people in hospitals and nursing homes. When depression occurs in late life, it sometimes can be a relapse of an earlier depression. But when it occurs for the first time in older adults, it usually is brought on by another medical illness. When someone is already ill, depression can be both more difficult to recognize and more difficult to endure.

Depression Is Not a Passing Mood

Sadness associated with normal grief or everyday "blues" is different from depression. A sad or grieving person can continue to carry on with regular activities. The depressed person suffers from symptoms that interfere with his or her ability to function normally for a prolonged period of time.

Recognizing depression in the elderly is not always easy. It often is difficult for the depressed elder to describe how he or she is feeling. In addition, the current population of older Americans came of age at a time when depression was not understood to be a biological disorder and medical illness. Therefore, some elderly fear being labeled "crazy," or worry that their illness will be seen as a character weakness.

The depressed person or his or her family members may think that a change in mood or behavior is simply "a passing mood," and the person should just "snap out of it." But someone suffering from depression cannot just "get over it." Depression is a medical illness that must be diagnosed and treated by trained professionals. Untreated, depression may last months or even years.

Untreated depression can:

- Lead to disability;

- Worsen symptoms of other illnesses;

- Lead to premature death;

- Result in suicide.

When it is properly diagnosed and treated, more than 80 percent of those suffering from depression recover and return to their normal lives.

The most common symptoms of late-life depression include:

- Persistent sadness (lasting two weeks or more);

- Feeling slowed down;

- Excessive worries about finances and health problems;

- Frequent tearfulness;

- Feeling worthless or helpless;

- Weight changes;

- Pacing and fidgeting;

- Difficulty sleeping;

- Difficulty concentrating;

- Physical symptoms such as pain or gastrointestinal problems.

One important sign of depression is when people withdraw from their regular social activities. Rather than explaining their symptoms as a medical illness, often depressed persons will give different explanations such as: " It's too much trouble"; " I don't feel well enough"; or " I don't have the energy."

For the same reasons, they often neglect their personal appearance, or may begin cooking and eating less. Like many illnesses, there are varying levels and types of depression. A person may not feel "sad" about anything, but may exhibit symptoms such as difficulty sleeping, weight loss, or physical pain with no apparent explanation. This person still may be clinically depressed. Those same symptoms also may be a sign of another problem—only a doctor can make the correct diagnosis.

It Can Happen to Anyone

Sometimes depression will occur for no apparent reason. In other words, nothing necessarily needs to "happen" in one's life for depression to occur. This can be because the disease often is caused by biological changes in the brain. However, in older adults, there usually are understandable reasons for the depression. As the brain and body age, a number of natural biochemical changes begin to take place. Changes as the result of aging, medical illnesses, or genetics may put the older adult at a greater risk for developing depression.

Life Changes

Chronic or serious illness is the most common cause of depression in the elderly. But even when someone is struggling with a chronic illness such as arthritis, it is not natural to be depressed. Depression is defined as an illness if it lasts two weeks or more and if it affects one's ability to lead a normal life.

Many factors can contribute to the development of depression. Often people describe one specific event that triggered their depression, such as the death of a partner or loved one, or the loss of a job through layoff or retirement. What seems like a normal period of sadness or grief may lead to a prolonged, intense grief that requires medical attention.

The loss of a lifelong partner or a friend is a frequent occurrence in later life. It is normal to grieve after such a loss. But it may be depression rather than bereavement if the grief persists, or is accompanied by any of the following symptoms:

- Guilt unconnected with the loved one's death;

- Thoughts of one's own death;

- Persistent feelings of worthlessness;

- Inability to function at one's usual level;

- Difficulty sleeping;

- Weight loss.

If any of these symptoms are triggered by a loss, a physician should be consulted.

Changes in the older adult's sensory abilities or environment may contribute to the development of depression. Examples of such changes include:

- Changes in vision and hearing;

- Changes in mobility;

- Retirement;

- Moving from the family home;

- Neighborhood changes.

Other Illnesses

In the older population, medical illnesses are a common trigger for depression, and often depression will worsen the symptoms of other illnesses. The following illnesses are common causes of late-life depression:

- Cancer

- Parkinson disease

- Heart disease

- Stroke

- Alzheimer disease

In addition, certain medical illnesses may hide the symptoms of depression. When a depressed person is preoccupied with physical symptoms resulting from a stroke, gastrointestinal problems, heart disease, or arthritis, he or she may attribute the depressive symptoms to an existing physical illness, or may ignore the symptoms entirely. For this reason, he or she may not report the depressive symptoms to his or her doctor, creating a barrier to becoming well.

Depression Is Treatable

Most depressed elderly people can improve dramatically from treatment. In fact, there are highly effective treatments for depression in late life. Common treatments prescribed by physicians include the following:

- Psychotherapy
- Antidepressant medications
- Electroconvulsive therapy (ECT)

Psychotherapy can play an important role in the treatment of depression with, or without, medication. This type of treatment is most often used alone in mild to moderate depression. There are many forms of short-term therapy (ten to twenty weeks) that have proven to be effective. It is important that the depressed person find a therapist with whom he or she feels comfortable and who has experience with older patients.

Antidepressants work by increasing the level of neurotransmitters in the brain. Neurotransmitters are the brain's "messengers." Many feelings, including pain and pleasure, are a result of the neurotransmitters' function. When the supply of neurotransmitters is imbalanced, depression may result.

A frequent reason some people do not respond to antidepressant treatment is because they do not take the medication properly. Missing doses or taking more than the prescribed amount of the medication compromises the effect of the antidepressant. Similarly, stopping the medication too soon often results in a relapse of depression. In fact, most patients who stop taking their medication before four to six months after recovery will experience a relapse of depression.

Usually, antidepressant medication is taken for at least six months to a year. Typically, it takes four to twelve weeks to begin seeing results from antidepressant medication. If after this period of time the depression does not subside, the patient should consult his or her physician. Antidepressant drugs are not habit-forming or addictive. And because depression is often a recurrent illness, it usually is necessary to stay on the medication for six months after recovery to prevent new episodes of depression.

Electroconvulsive therapy (ECT) is a treatment that unnecessarily evokes fear in many people. In reality, ECT is one of the most safe, fast-acting, and effective treatments for severe depression. It can be life saving. ECT often is the best choice for the person who has a life-threatening depression that is not responding to antidepressant medication or for the person who cannot tolerate the medication.

After a thorough evaluation, a physician will determine the treatment best suited for a person's depression. The treatment of depression demands patience and perseverance for the patient and the physician. Sometimes several different treatments must be tried before full recovery. Each person has individual biological and psychological characteristics that require individualized care.

Suicide

Suicide is more common in older people than in any other age group. The population over age sixty-five accounts for more than 25 percent of the nation's suicides. In fact, white men over age eighty are six times more likely to commit suicide than the general population, constituting the largest risk group. Suicide attempts or severe thoughts or wishes by older adults must always be taken seriously.

It is appropriate and important to ask a depressed person the following questions:

- Do they feel as though life is no longer an option for them?
- Have they had thoughts about harming themselves?
- Are they planning to do it?
- Is there a collection of pills or guns in the house?
- Are they often alone?

Most depressed people welcome care, concern, and support, but they are frightened and may resist help. In the case of a potentially suicidal elder, caring friends or family members must be more than understanding. They must actively intervene by removing pills and weapons from the home and calling the family physician, mental health professional, or, if necessary, the police.

Caring for a Depressed Person

The first step in helping an elderly person who may be depressed is to make sure he or she gets a complete physical checkup. Depression may be a side effect of a preexisting medical condition or of a medication. If the depressed older adult is confused or withdrawn, it is helpful for a caring family member or friend to accompany the person to the doctor and provide important information.

The physician may refer the older adult to a psychiatrist with geriatric training or experience. If a person is reluctant to see a psychiatrist, he or she may need assurance that an evaluation is necessary to determine if treatment is needed to reduce symptoms, improve functioning, and enhance well-being.

It is important to remember that depression is a highly treatable medical condition and is not a normal part of growing older. Therefore, it is crucial to understand and recognize the symptoms of the illness. As with any medical condition, the primary care physician should be consulted if someone has symptoms that interfere with everyday life. An older person who is diagnosed with depression also should know that there are trained professionals who specialize in treating the elderly (called "geriatric psychiatrists") who may be able to help.

Section 33.3

Divorce: Coping with Stress and Change

"Divorce Matters: Coping with Stress and Change," © 1996
Iowa State University Extension, reviewed November 2003.
Reprinted with permission.

Marital separation and divorce can be two of the most difficult events in an adult's life. Much stress comes from three sources:

- The daily tasks and responsibilities that must be reorganized

- The loss of significant relationships and possessions

- The need to establish a new identity as an individual

Restructuring the Family

For most couples with children, a divorce does not mean the end of a family. Instead, it means the family must restructure the way it handles household chores, family finances, parenting roles, and relationships with extended family and friends. This reorganization can create much stress.

Household chores: Tasks such as cleaning, cooking, and shopping must be managed. Each parent may have to assume tasks formerly shared by two adults, a situation that may feel overwhelming.

Family finances: Financial arrangements often must be reworked, adding considerably more stress and tension between parents. Finances may become a leading source of anger.

Parenting roles: If one parent is the main wage earner and the other the main caretaker, each may have to cover both roles after a divorce. Parents must answer various childcare questions: Who will stay home with a sick child? Who will leave work early to take a child to the dentist?

Relationships with extended family and friends: Interaction with extended family and friends must be reconsidered. Family members may take sides, disrupting relationships and removing potential sources of guidance and comfort.

Losing Significant Relationships, Possessions, and Dreams

Everyone needs the love, security, closeness, and belonging that come from relationships with others. Marriage is one of the most significant relationships. Its loss causes much of the stress and emotional turmoil of divorce.

Not all individuals experience loss with the same intensity, in the same way, or at the same time. Some people experience loss of closeness when they realize the relationship is ending. For others, the idea of separation can be overwhelming, and they hang onto the hope that the relationship can be saved.

Other losses resulting from separation and divorce undermine a person's sense of security and well-being. Although they do not realize it, many people become attached to a way of life, a home and possessions, pets, and daily contact with children.

Changing Identity

Divorce is a crisis that affects a person's identity. Individuals no longer occupy the role of husband or wife. At the same time, they must rethink changes in their roles as parents, workers, and caretakers. People often are caught off guard by the need to reconsider questions such as "Who am I?" and "What do I want to do with my life?"

353

Detecting Personal Stress Symptoms

People develop patterns of thought, feeling, and behavior that signal stress. If you are not aware of these patterns, you might ignore their signals. On the list below, check the responses you make to stressful situations.

Behavioral Changes

- Crying
- Withdrawal from others
- Aggression
- Substance misuse (drugs, alcohol, tobacco, food)
- Agitation
- Exhaustion
- Restlessness
- Disrupted sleep
- Other emotional changes
- Sadness
- Guilt
- Depression
- Anxiety
- Tension
- Irritability
- Fear
- Fatigue
- Mood swings
- Other

Thoughts and Feelings Related to Stress

- Thinking you cannot cope
- Feeling frightened for an unknown reason
- Worrying about everything, large or small
- Feeling afraid that something bad will happen

- Feeling that you are about to fall apart
- Having the same worrisome thought over and over
- Having a negative view of yourself
- Having a negative view of the world
- Feeling bored with everything
- Being unable to concentrate
- Having nightmares
- Feeling helpless
- Feeling hopeless
- Feeling worthless
- Feeling unable to make decisions
- Feeling confused
- Blaming yourself
- Other

Taking Charge of Your Life

One way to reduce stress is to take charge of your life. Here are some suggestions for ways you can regain personal control.

Relax by:

- Sitting in a quiet place and thinking of nothing;
- Listening to music and floating with the melody; and
- Tensing and relaxing your muscles.

Control your environment by:

- Scheduling activities so you don't have to rush;
- Setting priorities and sticking to them;
- Taking on one task at a time;
- Taking drugs only when a doctor prescribes them;
- Saying no to a request; and
- Balancing work and play.

Slow down by:

- Eating slowly;
- Walking slowly;
- Talking slowly;
- Listening until others are finished speaking;
- Starting activities early; and
- Getting enough rest.

Control your anger by:

- Telling someone how you feel before you lose control;
- Walking away from a situation until you cool off;
- Doing something physical to work off pent-up energy;
- Respecting another person's right to have a different opinion; and
- Praising others more than criticizing them.

Schedule recreation by:

- Going somewhere you enjoy with a friend or relative;
- Playing your favorite sport;
- Working on your favorite hobby; and
- Engaging in a relaxing activity.

Understand yourself by:

- Talking over personal feelings and concerns with a trusted friend or relative;
- Listing your good points and posting the list where you and others can see it; and
- Building close relationships with people who make you feel important and appreciated.

Remember, if your negative emotions begin to interfere with your role as a parent or employee, it may be helpful to seek support from a professional counselor or therapist.

Adjusting to Divorce

Although individuals are different, most adults need two or three years to adapt to the changes separation and divorce bring. People who also encounter problems such as job loss or illness during this period need additional time for adjustment. For adults, this involves three basic tasks.

Task 1—Accepting the Divorce

Individuals must accept that the marriage is over and establish an identity that is not tied to their former spouse. For this to occur, the individual must be convinced that there is no use investing further in this relationship.

Former spouses must make peace with each other. This involves realizing that continued nastiness only creates more nastiness in return. Often this realization creates a more balanced view of the relationship. An individual able to forgive the former spouse for the marriage's end is able to appreciate what is good about that person.

Individuals also must recognize their part in the breakup. They must stop blaming their former spouses and examine honestly their own role in the relationship. Such self-examination includes:

- Remembering the reasons for originally choosing the mate and making necessary revisions in expectations for future mates;

- Accepting individual contributions to the destructive patterns of behavior within the marriage so that these patterns are not repeated in future relationships; and

- Exploring how individual experiences growing up may play a role in marital struggles.

Task 2—Balancing Being a Single Person and a Single Parent

Individuals must establish sources of support for each of these roles. They need to begin feeling competent as a single person and as a single parent.

Task 3—Establishing Future-Oriented Instead of Past-Oriented Goals

People who are adjusting well are ready to move on. They begin to have new hobbies or leisure activities, or enter into new dating relationships. In contrast, those not ready to move on may need more time to mourn the loss of a spouse. These individuals may not have exhausted their efforts to rekindle the relationship. They may not realize that the relationship is over.

A Final Note

Dealing with the stress and change from a separation or divorce is not easy. It helps to become familiar with your sources of stress and your style of coping. Take time to think about ways that you can take charge of your life by controlling your environment and your anger with positive coping skills.

Realize that adjusting to divorce takes time. Be sure to pat yourself on the back occasionally as you move forward in reestablishing your life. Baby steps toward adjustment can sometimes be as significant as giant steps. The important thing is to keep moving forward.

Section 33.4

When a Spouse Dies

"When a Spouse Dies," © Bereaved Families of Ontario-York Region. Reprinted with permission. This document is available online at http://www.bfoyr.com/spouse_dies.htm; accessed March 6, 2007.

Helping Yourself Heal

Your life has changed, and the emptiness may at times feel overwhelming. Your life journey has taken a new and unexpected direction, but you do have the strength to step along this path, which will lead to peace and healing.

Allow yourself to grieve. Accept the reality of your loss and acknowledge your thoughts and feelings. Healing cannot begin until you have given yourself permission to grieve.

Accept that your grief is unique. Everyone grieves differently, because each person and relationship is different. Don't compare this grief with others, or expect it to last a certain period of time. Try to take things one day at a time.

Expect to feel many different emotions. You may feel confusion, fear, guilt, anger, or other strong emotions. Don't let these feelings frighten you. They are normal, healthy expressions of grief. Try to understand and learn from them.

Share your thoughts and feelings. Expressing your grief openly doesn't mean that you are losing control. Talk about your spouse and share your memories with supportive friends and family.

Be compassionate with yourself. Some days will be more difficult than others. Holidays, birthdays, and special occasions are particularly emotional times. Do what feels right for you at these times.

Treasure your memories. Allow good memories to bring you comfort. Difficult memories can also bring healing, if you can express them openly. Whether they make you laugh or cry, memories are a lasting part of your relationship.

Some Things to Consider

- It's easy to ignore your own health. Try to get sufficient food, sleep, and exercise.

- Many people have physical symptoms such as heaviness in the chest or extreme fatigue. If you or others are concerned, see your doctor.

- Avoid addictive behavior. Your doctor may recommend medication for anxiety, or to help you sleep. Please be careful: drugs and alcohol will only mask the pain, not cure it.

- Try not to make major decisions during the first year. It's hard to know if you've made the right choices, when you still are unsure of your new status.

- Take time with your spouse's belongings. Don't force yourself to go through his or her things until you are ready.

- Recognize that you may not be able to do everything. Ask for advice or help if you need it. It's difficult to take on your partner's role as well as your own.

- Children are often called the forgotten mourners. Share with them, and support each other. Seek additional support for them and yourself if you feel overwhelmed.

- There is no substitute for yourself. Don't avoid social contact, but try to accept people for who they are. Remember that new relationships can be comforting, but hard to judge objectively.

Few events in life are as painful as the death of a spouse. Losing your companion, the person with whom you shared your life, feels like losing a part of yourself.

Remember:

- Your feeling of emptiness is normal.

- Grief is a long process.

- You will be able to laugh again.

- Give yourself time.

Chapter 34

Cognitive Changes and Aging

Chapter Contents

Section 34.1

How Aging Changes the Brain

Excerpted from "Research on How Changes in the Aging Brain Are Related to Cognitive Decline," Infoaging (www.infoaging.org), a website of the American Federation for Aging Research, February 18, 2004.

The brains of older adults show a patchwork pattern of declines and preservation. Given the complexity of the changes, it is unlikely that only one factor is responsible for the changes in mental activity that accompany aging. It's more likely a combination of factors. However, some theories have been proposed for some of the changes seen.

The slowing of mental processing may be caused by the deterioration of neurons, whether they are lost, shrink, or lose connections. This depletion of fully functioning neurons makes it necessary to recruit additional networks of neurons to manage mental tasks that would otherwise be simple or automatic. Thus, the process is slowed down. Evidence also suggests that myelin, which forms a protective sheath around nerve fibers, breaks down during the aging process, possibly contributing to cognitive decline by slowing down the relaying of nerve signals.

A portion of the frontal lobe, called the prefrontal cortex, is involved in monitoring and controlling thoughts and actions. The atrophy that occurs in this brain region may account for the word-finding difficulties many older adults experience. It may also account for forgetting where you put your car keys or for general absentmindedness.

The shrinkage of both the frontal lobe and the hippocampus, an area of the brain crucial for memory, are thought to be responsible for memory difficulties. Numerous studies that have imaged the brains of persons with Alzheimer disease and other memory disorders have found atrophy in those regions.

Many of the neurons involved in motor function utilize the neurotransmitter dopamine, and dopamine is one of the neurotransmitters that declines with age. Therefore, it's been suggested that the effects of aging on dopamine account for some of the decline in motor function. Specifically how this would happen has not been discovered.

A lack of dopamine may also be responsible for normal age-related cognitive decline. Scientists working at Washington University believe that dopamine acts in the prefrontal cortex to allow us to process context for thoughts, memories, and behavior. Context processing allows us to adapt our behavior to varied circumstances and to interpret auditory and visual input. In a series of experiments comparing the context processing abilities of young (under thirty) and older (over sixty-five) adults, the researchers found that the older adults showed impaired context processing as compared to younger adults.

Several researchers have suggested that high blood pressure in the brain may be responsible for some of the detrimental effects of aging. A paper published in the March 23, 2003, issue of *Psychology and Aging* found that older adults with hypertension are more likely to develop white-matter lesions in the brain, which appear as bright patches on magnetic resonance imaging (MRI) brain scans. The study also found that the number of these white-matter lesions in the brain correlated directly with a person's level of cognitive impairment.

High blood sugar levels may also contribute to age-related memory decline. Researchers have noted for several years that diabetics tend to have memory and learning problems. Researchers at the New York University School of Medicine evaluated thirty older adults for glucose tolerance and memory and obtained MRI scans of their brains. They found that decreased ability to regulate glucose levels was associated with poorer cognitive performance, memory problems, and atrophy of the hippocampus.

Section 34.2

Understanding Memory Loss

Excerpted from Alzheimer's Disease Education and Referral (ADEAR)
Center, National Institute on Aging, National Institutes of Health,
NIH Publication No. 06-5442, March 2006.

We've all forgotten a name, where we put our keys, or if we locked
the front door. It's normal to forget things once in a while. However,
forgetting how to make change, use the telephone, or find your way
home may be signs of a more serious memory problem.

This section will help you understand:

- The difference between mild forgetfulness and more serious
  memory problems;

- The medical causes of memory problems and how they can be
  treated;

- How to cope with serious memory problems.

Differences between Mild Forgetfulness and More Serious Memory Problems

What Is Mild Forgetfulness?

It is true that some of us get more forgetful as we age. It may take
longer to learn new things, remember familiar names and words, or
find our glasses. These are usually signs of mild forgetfulness, not
serious memory problems. If you're worried about your forgetfulness,
see your doctor. You also can do many things to help keep your memory
sharp. Finding a hobby, spending time with friends, eating well, and
exercising may help you stay alert and clear-headed.

Here are some ways to help your memory:

- Learn a new skill.

- Volunteer in your community, school, or place of worship.

- Spend time with friends and family whenever possible.

- Use memory tools such as big calendars, to-do lists, and notes to yourself.
- Put your wallet or purse, keys, and glasses in the same place each day.
- Get lots of rest.
- Exercise and eat well.
- Don't drink a lot of alcohol.
- Get help if you feel depressed for weeks at a time.

What Is a Serious Memory Problem?

Serious memory problems affect your ability to carry out everyday life activities such as driving a car, shopping, or handling money. Signs of serious memory problems may include the following:

- Asking the same questions over and over again
- Becoming lost in places you know well
- Not being able to follow directions
- Getting very confused about time, people, and places
- Not taking care of yourself —eating poorly, not bathing, or being unsafe

What to Do about Serious Memory Problems

If you are having any of the problems listed previously, see your doctor. It's important to find out what might be causing a serious memory problem. Your treatment depends on the cause of the problem.

Medical Causes of Memory Problems

Medical Conditions

Certain medical conditions can cause serious memory problems. These problems should go away once you get treatment. Here's a list of things that cause memory problems:

- Bad reaction to certain medicines
- Depression
- Not having enough fluids in your body, also called dehydration

- Not eating enough healthy foods, or too few vitamins and minerals in your body

- Minor head injuries

- Thyroid problems

These medical conditions are serious and should be treated by a doctor.

Emotional Problems

Some emotional problems in older people can cause serious memory problems. Feeling sad, lonely, worried, or bored can cause you to be confused and forgetful. Being active, spending more time with family and friends, and learning new skills can help. You may need to see a doctor or counselor for treatment. Once you get help, your memory problems should get better.

Alzheimer Disease

Alzheimer disease also causes serious memory problems. The signs of Alzheimer disease begin slowly and get worse over time. This is because nerve cell changes in the brain cause large numbers of brain cells to die. It may look like simple forgetfulness at first, but over time, people with Alzheimer disease have trouble thinking clearly. They find it hard to do everyday things like shopping, driving, cooking, and having a conversation. As the illness gets worse, people with Alzheimer disease may need someone to take care of all their needs (feeding, bathing, etc.) at home or in a nursing home.

Medication can help. If you are in the early or middle stages of Alzheimer disease, taking medications can help. Some medicines keep symptoms, such as memory loss, from getting worse for a time. Medications also can help if you are worried, depressed, or are having problems sleeping.

Multi-Infarct Dementia

Many people have never heard of multi-infarct dementia. Like Alzheimer disease, it is a medical condition that causes serious memory problems. Unlike Alzheimer disease, signs of multi-infarct dementia may appear suddenly. This is because the memory loss and confusion are caused by small strokes or changes in the blood supply to the brain.

If the strokes stop, you can get better or stay the same for a long time. If you have more strokes, you can get worse. Taking care of your high blood pressure can lower your chances of getting this illness.

How to Cope with Serious Memory Problems

What Should I Do If I'm Worried about My Memory?

See your doctor. If your doctor thinks it's serious, you may need to have a complete checkup, including blood and urine tests. You also may need to take tests that check your memory, problem solving, counting, and language skills. In addition, you may need a computed axial tomography (CAT) scan of the brain. These pictures can show normal and problem areas in the brain. Once the doctor finds out what is causing your memory problems, ask about what is the best treatment for you.

What Can Family Members Do to Help?

Family members and friends can help you live as normal a life as possible. They can help you exercise, visit with friends, and keep up your daily routines. They can remind you of the time of day, where you live, and what is happening at home and in the world.

Some families use the following things to help with memory:

- Big calendars
- Lists of the plans for each day
- Notes about safety in the home
- Written directions for using common household items

See your doctor if you are worried about your memory. It's important to find out what is causing your memory problems.

Section 34.3

Keeping Your Mind Sharp

Whether you are calculating multivariate statistics or simply trying to stay alert during a long meeting, keeping your mind sharp matters. Luckily, the steps to exercising your brain are easier than you may think.

"Exercise is just as healthy for your mind as it is for your body," explains Christine Blue, D.O., an osteopathic psychiatrist specializing in general and geriatric psychiatry from Lewisburg, West Virginia. "Regular physical exercise will not only help your cardiovascular health, but it will increase blood flow to the brain and help with your creativity and memory."

In addition, the calming benefits of exercising will reduce stress, which can cause memory problems. Physical activity can also prevent depression, which slows thinking. Exercise will clear the mind and allow for creative thinking and a problem-solving state of mind. For example, studies have shown that after walking for fifteen minutes, individuals will increase their memory and ability to multitask by more than 15 percent. Relaxation techniques, such as yoga and meditation, are also beneficial for the brain.

Keep Your Mind Sharp with These Six Simple Tips

- Stay curious and involved
- Work crosswords or other puzzles
- Attend lectures and plays
- Continue your education
- Play games
- Try memory exercises

There are several different memory techniques and exercises. One technique is called over-learning. This means that the individual would repeat and study something more than the topic might normally require. This technique might be employed when meeting new people. Oftentimes repeating the new name several times will help with remembering the person's name later.

Another memory technique that helps with remembering short lists of items is called the link or story method. "Using this method, you would simply make up a story that links together the different items you want to remember," explains Dr. Blue.

Dr. Blue further explains that memory exercises can help fight age-related memory loss such as dementia. "There has been a growing amount of research indicating mental exercises can help prevent memory loss associated with dementia."

Dementia is a neurological disorder that affects the ability to think, speak, reason, remember, and move. The most common form of dementia, Alzheimer disease, involves a loss of nerve cells in the areas of the brain that control memory and other mental functions. The first sign of Alzheimer disease is usually forgetfulness. As the disease progresses, it affects language, reasoning, and understanding.

The precise cause of Alzheimer disease is unknown, but risk increases with age. Ten percent of the population over the age of sixty-five has Alzheimer, and nearly half of the population over eighty-five has the disease.

"It is important to make decisions today that will help you later in life," explains Dr. Blue. "Keeping both your mind and body active is a great start."

In addition to exercise for the brain and body, Dr. Blue also recommends including these healthy vitamins and minerals in your diet:

- **Vitamin E:** Vitamin E is found in all cells, including the cells of the brain. Damage to nerve tissue may result from a vitamin E deficiency in the cells. You can eat foods like almonds, green leafy vegetables, and whole-grain flour to benefit from the different forms of this vitamin.

- **Vitamin B:** Every type of Vitamin B helps in preserving brain function and sharpness. Early brain development, declining memory, and inability to focus have been linked with low levels of folic acid and Vitamins B_{12} and B_6.

- **Vitamin C:** Eating plenty of broccoli, legumes, oranges, potatoes, and strawberries will give you a large dose of this vitamin, which helps keep the brain healthy.

- **Magnesium:** Approximately 300 milligrams one to three times a day will help protect the brain from many substances that damage nerve cells.

"It's important that you consult your doctor if forgetfulness or mind lapses ever become disruptive in your daily routine and before taking any supplements," Dr. Blue cautions.

Chapter 35

Sensory Changes

Chapter Contents

Section 35.1

Aging and Your Eyes

Reprinted from the National Institute on Aging, National Institutes of Health, October 2005.

Are you holding the newspaper farther away from your eyes than you used to? Join the crowd—age can bring changes that affect your eyesight. Some changes are more serious than others, but no matter what the problem, there are things you can do to protect your vision. The keys are regular eye exams and finding problems early.

Five Steps to Protect Your Eyesight

- Have your eyes checked every one or two years by an eye care professional. This can be an ophthalmologist or optometrist. He or she should put drops in your eyes to enlarge (dilate) your pupils. This is the only way to find some eye diseases, such as diabetic retinopathy, that have no early signs or symptoms. If you wear glasses, they should be checked too.

- Find out if you are at high risk for eye disease. Are you over age sixty-five? Are you African American and over age forty? Do you or people in your family have diabetes or eye disease? If so, you need to have a dilated eye exam.

- Have regular physical exams to check for diseases like diabetes and high blood pressure. These diseases can cause eye problems if not treated.

- See an eye care professional right away if you suddenly cannot see or everything looks dim or if you see flashes of light. Also see an eye care professional if you have eye pain, fluid coming from the eye, double vision, redness, or swelling of your eye or eyelid.

- Wear sunglasses that block ultraviolet (UV) radiation and a hat with a wide brim when outside. This will protect your eyes from too much sunlight, which can raise your risk of getting cataracts.

Eye Problems

Some eye problems do not threaten your eyesight. Others are more serious diseases and can lead to blindness.

Common Eye Problems

The following common eye complaints, which can sometimes be signs of more serious problems, can be treated easily:

- **Presbyopia:** This is a slow loss of ability to see close objects or small print. It is a normal process that happens as you get older. Holding the newspaper at arm's length is a sign of presbyopia. You might also get headaches or tired eyes when you read or do other close work. Reading glasses usually fix the problem.

- **Floaters:** These are tiny specks or "cobwebs" that seem to float across your eyes. You might notice them in well-lit rooms or outdoors on a bright day. Floaters can be a normal part of aging. Sometimes they are a sign of a more serious eye problem such as retinal detachment. If you see many new floaters or flashes of light, see your eye care professional right away. This is considered a medical emergency.

- **Tearing (or having too many tears):** This can come from being sensitive to light, wind, or temperature changes. Protecting your eyes, by wearing sunglasses for example, may solve the problem. Sometimes, tearing may mean a more serious eye problem, such as an infection or a blocked tear duct. Your eye care professional can treat both of these conditions.

- **Eyelid problems:** These can come from different diseases or conditions. Common eyelid problems include red and swollen eyelids, itching, tearing, being sensitive to light, and crusting of eyelashes during sleep. This condition is called blepharitis and may be treated with warm compresses. Other less common eyelid problems, such as swelling or growths, can be treated with medicine or surgery.

Eye Diseases and Disorders

Some eye problems can lead to vision loss and blindness. Often they have few or no symptoms. Having regular eye exams is the best way to protect yourself. If your eye care professional finds a problem early there are things you can do to keep your eyesight. Following are some of the more serious eye problems:

- **Cataracts:** These are cloudy areas in the eye's lens causing loss of eyesight. Cataracts often form slowly without any symptoms. Some stay small and don't change eyesight very much. Others may become large or dense and harm vision. Cataract surgery can help. Your eye care professional can watch for changes in your cataract over time to see if you need surgery. Cataract surgery is very safe. It is one of the most common surgeries done in the United States.

- **Corneal diseases and conditions:** These can cause redness, watery eyes, pain, lower vision, or a halo effect. The cornea is the clear, dome-shaped "window" at the front of the eye. Disease, infection, injury, and other things can hurt the cornea. Some corneal conditions are more common in older people. Treatments for corneal problems can be simple. You may just need to change your eyeglass prescription and use eye drops. In severe cases, corneal transplantation is the treatment. It generally works well and is safe.

- **Dry eye:** This happens when tear glands don't work well. You may feel itching, burning, or have some vision loss. Dry eye is more common as people get older, especially among women. Your eye care professional may tell you to use a home humidifier, special eye drops (artificial tears), or ointments to treat dry eye. In serious cases special contact lenses or surgery may help.

- **Glaucoma:** This comes from too much fluid pressure inside the eye. Over time, the pressure can hurt the optic nerve. This leads to vision loss and blindness. Most people with glaucoma have no early symptoms or pain from the extra pressure. You can protect yourself by having regular eye exams through dilated pupils. Treatment may be prescription eye drops, medicines that you take by mouth, laser treatment, or surgery.

- **Retinal disorders:** These are a leading cause of blindness in the United States. The retina is a thin tissue that lines the back of the eye and sends light signals to the brain. Retinal disorders that affect aging eyes include:

  - *Age-related macular degeneration (AMD):* AMD affects the part of the retina (the macula) that gives you sharp central vision. Over time, AMD can ruin the sharp vision needed to see objects clearly and to do common tasks like driving and reading. In some cases, AMD can be treated with lasers. Photo-dynamic therapy uses a drug and strong light to slow the progress of AMD. Another treatment uses injections. Ask your eye care professional if you have signs of AMD. Also ask if you should be taking special dietary supplements that may lower your chances of it getting worse.

- *Diabetic retinopathy:* This is a problem that may appear if you have diabetes. It happens when small blood vessels stop feeding the retina as they should. It develops slowly and there are no early warning signs. Laser surgery and a treatment called vitrectomy can help. Studies show that keeping blood sugar under control can prevent diabetic retinopathy or slow its progress. If you have diabetes be sure to have an eye exam through dilated pupils at least once a year.

- *Retinal detachment:* This is when the retina separates from the back of the eye. When this happens, you may see more floaters or light flashes in your eye, either all at once or over time. Or it may seem as though there is a curtain in front of your eyes. If you have any of these symptoms, see your eye care professional at once. This is a medical emergency. With surgery or laser treatment, doctors often can bring back all or part of your eyesight.

Low Vision

Low vision affects some people as they age. Low vision means you cannot fix your eyesight with glasses, contact lenses, medicine, or surgery. It can get in the way of your normal daily routine. You may have low vision if the following are true:

- You have trouble seeing well enough to do everyday tasks like reading, cooking, or sewing.

- You can't recognize the faces of friends or family.

- You have trouble reading street signs.

- You find that lights don't seem as bright as usual.

If you have any of these problems, ask your eye care professional to test you for low vision. There are special tools and aids to help people with low vision read, write, and manage daily living tasks. Lighting can be changed to suit your needs. You also can try large-print reading materials, magnifying aids, closed-circuit televisions, audiotapes, electronic reading machines, and computers that use large print and speech.

Other simple changes also may help:

- Write with bold, black felt-tip markers.

- Use paper with bold lines to help you write in a straight line.

- Put colored tape on the edge of your steps to help you keep from falling.

- Install dark-colored light switches and electrical outlets that you can see easily against light-colored walls.

- Use motion lights that turn on by themselves when you enter a room. These may help you avoid accidents caused by poor lighting.

- Use telephones, clocks, and watches with large numbers; put large-print labels on the microwave and stove.

Section 35.2

Hearing Loss

Reprinted from the National Institute on Aging, National Institutes of Health, August 2005.

About one-third of Americans between the ages of sixty-five and seventy-four have hearing problems. About half the people who are eighty-five and older have hearing loss. Whether a hearing loss is small (missing certain sounds) or large (being profoundly deaf), it is a serious concern. If left untreated, problems can get worse.

Hearing loss can affect your life in many ways. You may miss out on talks with friends and family. On the telephone, you may find it hard to hear what the caller is saying. At the doctor's office, you may not catch the doctor's words.

Sometimes hearing problems can make you feel embarrassed, upset, and lonely. It's easy to withdraw when you can't follow a conversation at the dinner table or in a restaurant. It's also easy for friends and family to think you are confused, uncaring, or difficult, when the problem may be that you just can't hear well.

If you have trouble hearing, there is help. Start by seeing your doctor. Depending on the type and extent of your hearing loss, there are many treatment choices that may help. Hearing loss does not have to get in the way of your ability to enjoy life.

How do I know if I have a hearing loss?

See your doctor if any of the following are true:

- You have trouble hearing over the telephone.
- You find it hard to follow conversations when two or more people are talking.
- You need to turn up the TV volume so loud that others complain.
- You have a problem hearing because of background noise.
- You sense that others seem to mumble.
- You can't understand when women and children speak to you.

What should I do?

If you have trouble hearing, see your doctor. Sometimes the diagnosis and treatment can take place in the doctor's office. Or your doctor may refer you to an otolaryngologist, a doctor who specializes in the ear, nose, and throat. The otolaryngologist will take a medical history, ask if other family members have hearing problems, do a thorough exam, and suggest any needed tests. You may be referred to an audiologist. Audiologists are healthcare professionals trained to measure hearing. The audiologist will use an audiometer to test your ability to hear sounds of different pitch and loudness. These tests are painless. Audiologists can help if you need a hearing aid. They can help select the best hearing aid for you and help you learn to get the most from it.

What causes hearing loss?

Hearing loss can have many different causes, including the aging process, ear wax buildup, exposure to very loud noises over a long period of time, viral or bacterial infections, heart conditions or stroke, head injuries, tumors, certain medicines, and heredity.

What different types of hearing loss are there?

Presbycusis: This is age-related hearing loss. It becomes more common in people as they get older. People with this kind of hearing loss may have a hard time hearing what others are saying or may be unable to stand loud sounds. The decline is slow. Just as hair turns gray at different rates, presbycusis can develop at different rates. It can be caused by sensorineural hearing loss. This type of hearing loss results from damage to parts of the inner ear, the auditory nerve, or hearing pathways in the brain. Presbycusis may be caused by aging, loud noise, heredity, head injury, infection, illness, certain prescription drugs, and circulation problems such as high blood pressure. The degree of hearing loss varies from person to person. Also, a person can have a different amount of hearing loss in each ear.

Tinnitus: This accompanies many forms of hearing loss, including those that sometimes come with aging. People with tinnitus may hear a ringing, roaring, or some other noise inside their ears. Tinnitus may be caused by loud noise, hearing loss, certain medicines, and other health problems, such as allergies and problems in the heart and blood vessels. Often it is unclear why the ringing happens. Tinnitus can come and go, it can stop completely, or it can stay. Some medicines may help ease the problem. Wearing a hearing aid makes it easier for some people to hear the sounds they need to hear by making them louder. Maskers, small devices that use sound to make tinnitus less noticeable, help other people. Music also can be soothing and can sometimes mask the sounds caused by the condition. It also helps to avoid things that might make tinnitus worse, like smoking, alcohol, and loud noises.

Conductive hearing loss: This happens when something blocks the sounds that are carried from the eardrum (tympanic membrane) to the inner ear. Earwax buildup, fluid in the middle ear, abnormal bone growth, a punctured eardrum, or a middle ear infection can cause this type of hearing loss. If earwax blockage is a problem for you, the American Academy of Otolaryngology-Head and Neck Surgery suggests using mild treatments, such as mineral oil, baby oil, glycerin, or commercial eardrops to soften earwax. If you think you may have a hole in your eardrum, however, you should see your doctor.

How can I help a person with hearing loss?

Here are some tips you can use when talking with someone who has a hearing problem:

- Face the person and talk clearly.

- Speak at a reasonable speed; do not hide your mouth, eat, or chew gum.

- Stand in good lighting and reduce background noises.

- Use facial expressions or gestures to give useful clues.

- Repeat yourself if necessary, using different words.

- Include the hearing-impaired person when talking. Talk with the person, not about the person, when you are with others. This helps keep the hearing-impaired person from feeling alone and excluded.

- Be patient; stay positive and relaxed.

- Ask how you can help.

What can I do if I have trouble hearing?

- Let people know that you have trouble hearing.

- Ask people to face you, and to speak more slowly and clearly; also ask them to speak without shouting.

- Pay attention to what is being said and to facial expressions or gestures.

- Let the person talking know if you do not understand.

- Ask people to reword a sentence and try again.

What devices or treatments can help?

What will help you depends on your hearing problem. Some common solutions are listed here.

Hearing aids: These are small devices you wear in or behind your ear. Hearing aids can help some kinds of hearing loss by making sounds louder. However, they sometimes pick up background noises—for example, traffic noise in the street or people talking at other tables in a crowded restaurant. This can affect how well you hear in certain situations. Before buying a hearing aid, check to find out if your insurance will cover the cost.

There are many kinds of hearing aids. An audiologist can help fit you with the hearing aid that will work best for you. You can ask the audiologist about having a trial period to try out a few different aids.

Remember, when you buy a hearing aid, you are buying a product and a service. Find a hearing aid dealer (called a dispenser) who has the patience and skill to help you during the month or so it takes to get used to the new hearing aid.

You may need to have several fittings of your hearing aid, and you will need to get directions on how to use it. Hearing aids use batteries, which you will need to change on a regular basis. They also may need repairs from time to time. Buy a hearing aid that has only the features you need.

Assistive/adaptive devices: There are many products that can help you live well with less-than-perfect hearing. The list below includes some examples of the many choices:

- Telephone amplifying devices range from a special type of telephone receiver that makes sounds louder to special phones that work with hearing aids.

- TV and radio listening systems can be used with or without hearing aids. You do not have to turn the volume up high.

- Assistive listening devices are available in some public places such as auditoriums, movie theaters, churches, synagogues, and meeting places.

- Alerts such as doorbells, smoke detectors, and alarm clocks can give you a signal that you can see or a vibration that you can feel. For example, a flashing light could let you know someone is at the door or that the phone is ringing.

Cochlear implants: If your deafness is severe, a doctor may suggest cochlear implants. In this surgery, the doctor puts a small electronic device under the skin behind the ear. The device sends the message past the nonworking part of the inner ear and on to the brain. This process helps some people hear. These implants are not helpful for all types of deafness or hearing loss.

Section 35.3

Aging Changes in the Senses

Excerpted from "Aging Changes in the Senses," © 2007 A.D.A.M., Inc.
Reprinted with permission.

When you age, the way your senses (taste, smell, touch, vision, and hearing) are able to give you information about the world changes. Your senses become less acute, and you may have trouble distinguishing details.

Sensory changes can have a tremendous impact on your lifestyle. You may have problems with communication, enjoyment of activities, and social interactions. Sensory changes can contribute to a sense of isolation.

All of the senses receive information of some type from the environment (light, sound vibrations, and so on). This is converted to a nerve impulse and carried to the brain, where it is interpreted into a meaningful sensation.

Everyone requires a certain minimum amount of stimulation before a sensation is perceived. This minimum level is called the threshold. Aging increases this threshold, so the amount of sensory input needed to be aware of the sensation becomes greater. Changes in the body part related to the sensation account for most of the other sensation changes.

Hearing and vision changes are the most dramatic, but all senses can be affected by aging. Fortunately, many of the aging changes in the senses can be compensated for with equipment such as glasses and hearing aids or by minor changes in lifestyle.

Hearing

Your ears have two jobs. One is hearing and the other is maintaining balance. Hearing occurs after vibrations cross the eardrum to the inner ear. They are changed into nerve impulses and carried to the brain by the auditory nerve.

Balance (equilibrium) is controlled in a portion of the inner ear. Fluid and small hairs in the semicircular canal (labyrinth) stimulate the nerve that helps the brain maintain balance.

As you age, your ear structures deteriorate. The eardrum often thickens and the inner ear bones and other structures are affected. It often becomes increasingly difficult to maintain balance.

Hearing may decline slightly, especially that of high-frequency sounds, particularly in people who have been exposed to a lot of noise when younger. This age-related hearing loss is called presbycusis.

The sharpness (acuity) of hearing may decline slightly beginning about age fifty, possibly caused by changes in the auditory nerve. In addition, the brain may have a slightly decreased ability to process or translate sounds into meaningful information. Impacted earwax is another cause of trouble hearing and is more common with increasing age. Impacted earwax may be removed in your doctor's office.

Some hearing loss is almost inevitable. It is estimated that 30 percent of all people over sixty-five have significant hearing impairment.

Conductive hearing loss occurs when sound has problems getting through the external and middle ear. Surgery or a hearing aid may be helpful for this type of hearing loss, depending on the specific cause.

Sensorineural hearing loss involves damage to the inner ear, auditory nerve, or the brain. This type of hearing loss may or may not respond to treatment.

Persistent, abnormal ear noise (tinnitus) is another fairly common hearing problem, especially for older adults.

Vision

Vision occurs when light is processed by your eye and interpreted by your brain. Light passes through the transparent eye surface (cornea).

Your pupil is an opening to the eye interior. It becomes larger or smaller to regulate the amount of light that enters your eye. The colored portion (iris) is a muscle that controls the pupil size.

The inside of your eye is filled with a gel-like fluid. There is a flexible, transparent lens that focuses light on your retina (the back of the eye). Your retina converts light energy into a nerve impulse that is carried to the brain and interpreted.

Some age-related eye changes may begin as early as your thirties. Aging eyes produce less tears. Dry eyes can be quite uncomfortable. Many people find relief by using eye drops or artificial tears solutions.

All of the eye structures change with aging. The cornea becomes less sensitive, so injuries may not be noticed. By the time you turn sixty, your pupils decrease to about one-third of the size they were when you were twenty.

The pupil may also react more slowly in response to darkness or bright light. The lens becomes yellowed, less flexible, and slightly cloudy. The fat pads supporting the eye decrease and the eye sinks back into the socket. The eye muscles become less able to fully rotate the eye.

As you age, the sharpness of your vision (visual acuity) may gradually decline. Glasses or contact lenses may help correct age-related vision changes. You may eventually need bifocals.

Almost everyone older than fifty-five needs glasses at least part of the time. However, the amount of change is not universal. Only 15 to 20 percent of older people have bad enough vision to impair driving ability, and only 5 percent become unable to read. The most common problem is difficulty focusing the eyes (a condition called presbyopia).

You may be less able to tolerate glare, and you may find that you have more trouble adapting to darkness or bright light. Many older people find that although their vision is good enough to drive during the day, they must give up night driving because of problems with glare, brightness, and darkness. Significant difficulty with night driving may be the first sign of a cataract (a clouding of the eye lens).

Indoor glare, such as glare from a shiny floor in a sunlit room, can also make it difficult to get around inside.

For people of all ages, it is harder to distinguish blues and greens than it is to distinguish reds and yellows. This becomes even more pronounced with aging. As your age increases, using warm contrasting colors (yellow, orange, and red) in your home can improve your ability to tell where things are and make it easier to perform daily activities.

Many older people find that keeping a red light on in darkened rooms (such as the hallway or bathroom) makes it easier to see than using a "regular" night light. Red light produces less glare than a regular incandescent bulb.

With aging, the fluid inside your eye may change. Small particles can create "floaters" in your vision. Although annoying, floaters oftentimes do not indicate a dangerous condition and usually do not reduce vision. If you suddenly develop floaters or experience a rapid increase in the number of them, you should definitely have your eyes checked by a professional.

When your eyes are examined, you may not be able to move your eye in all directions. Your upward gaze may be limited. The area in which objects can be seen (visual field) gets smaller.

Reduced peripheral vision is common and can limit social interaction and activity. Older people may not communicate with people sitting next to them because they cannot see them well—or perhaps at all. Food and drinks may be spilled. Driving can become dangerous.

Common eye disorders in the elderly (changes that are *not* normal) include cataracts, glaucoma, senile macular degeneration, and diabetic and hypertensive retinopathy.

Taste and Smell

The senses of taste and smell interact closely, helping you appreciate food. Most taste really comes from odors. The sense of smell begins at nerve receptors high in the membranes of the nose.

You have approximately nine thousand taste buds. Your taste buds are primarily responsible for sensing sweet, salty, sour, and bitter tastes.

Smell (and to a lesser extent, taste) also play a role in both safety and enjoyment. We detect certain dangers, such as spoiled food, noxious gases, and smoke with taste and smell. A delicious meal or pleasant aroma can improve social interaction and enjoyment of life.

The number of taste buds decreases beginning at about age forty to fifty in women and at fifty to sixty in men. Each remaining taste bud also begins to atrophy (lose mass). The sensitivity to the four taste sensations does not seem to decrease until after age sixty, if at all. If taste sensation is lost, usually salty and sweet tastes are lost first, with bitter and sour tastes lasting slightly longer.

Additionally, your mouth produces less saliva as you age. This causes dry mouth, which can make swallowing more difficult. It also makes digestion slightly less efficient and can increase dental problems.

The sense of smell may diminish, especially after age seventy. This may be related to loss of nerve endings in the nose.

Studies about the cause of decreased sense of taste and smell with aging have conflicting results. Some studies have indicated that normal aging by itself produces very little change in taste and smell. Rather, changes may be related to diseases, smoking, and environmental exposures over a lifetime.

Regardless of the cause, decreased taste and smell can lessen your interest and enjoyment in eating. Some people become less aware of personal hygiene when the sense of smell is decreased. Enjoyment of your environment may be diminished.

Sometimes changes in the way food is prepared, such as a change in the spices used, may help.

For some people, there is an increased risk of asphyxia because they cannot detect the odor of natural gas from the stove, furnace, or other appliance. A visual gas detector that changes appearance when natural gas is present may be helpful.

Touch, Vibration, and Pain

The sense of touch also includes awareness of vibrations and pain. The skin, muscles, tendons, joints, and internal organs have receptors that detect touch, temperature, or pain.

Your brain interprets the type and amount of touch sensation. It also interprets the sensation as pleasant (such as being comfortably warm), unpleasant (such as being very hot), or neutral (such as being aware that you are touching something).

Medications, brain surgery, problems in the brain, confusion, and nerve damage from trauma or chronic diseases such as diabetes can change this interpretation without changing awareness of the sensation. For example, you may feel and recognize a painful sensation, but it does not bother you.

Some of the receptors give the brain information about the position and condition of internal organs. Even though you may not be consciously aware of this information, it helps to identify changes (for example, the pain of appendicitis).

Many studies have shown that with aging, you may have reduced or changed sensations of pain, vibration, cold, heat, pressure, and touch. It is hard to tell whether these changes are related to aging itself or to the disorders that occur more often in the elderly.

It may be that some of the normal changes of aging are caused by decreased blood flow to the touch receptors or to the brain and spinal cord. Minor dietary deficiencies, such as decreased thiamine levels, may also be a cause of changes.

Regardless of the cause, many people experience changes in the touch-related sensations as they age. You may find it harder, for example, to tell the difference between cool and cold. Decreased temperature sensitivity increases the risk of injuries such as frostbite, hypothermia, and burns.

Reduced ability to detect vibration, touch, and pressure increases the risk of injuries, including pressure ulcers. After age fifty, many people have reduced sensitivity to pain. You may develop problems with walking because of reduced ability to perceive where your body is in relation to the floor.

Fine touch may decrease. However, some people develop an increased sensitivity to light touch because of thinner skin (especially people older than seventy).

To increase safety, make allowances for changes in touch-related sensations:

- Limit the maximum water temperature in your house (there is an adjustment on the water heater) to reduce the risk of burns.

- Look at the thermometer to decide how to dress rather than waiting until you feel overheated or chilled.

- Inspect your skin (especially your feet) for injuries, and if you find an injury, treat it. Don't assume that just because an area is not painful, the injury is not significant.

Chapter 36

Changes in the
Hair, Nails, and Skin

Chapter Contents

Section 36.1

Aging Changes in the Hair and Nails

Copyright 2007, A.D.A.M., Inc. Reprinted with permission.

Hair color change is probably one of the most obvious signs of aging. Hair color is caused by a pigment (melanin) produced by hair follicles. With aging, the follicle produces less melanin.

Graying often begins in the thirties, although this varies widely. Graying usually begins at the temples and extends to the top of the scalp. Hair becomes progressively lighter, eventually turning white.

Many people have some gray scalp hair by the time they are in their forties. Body and facial hair also turn gray, but usually later than scalp hair. The hair in the armpit, chest, and pubic area may gray less or not at all.

Graying is genetically determined. Gray hair tends to occur earlier in Caucasians and later in Asian races. Nutritional supplements, vitamins, and other products will not stop or decrease the rate of graying.

Hair Thickness Changes

Hair is a protein strand that grows through an opening (follicle) in the skin. A single hair has a normal life of about four or five years. That hair then falls out and is replaced with a new hair.

How much hair you have on your body and head is determined by your genes. However, almost everyone experiences some hair loss with aging. The rate of hair growth slows.

The hair strands become smaller and have less pigment, so the thick, coarse hair of a young adult eventually becomes thin, fine, light-colored hair. Many hair follicles stop producing new hairs altogether.

About a quarter of men begin to show signs of baldness by the time they are thirty years old, and about two-thirds of men have significant baldness by age sixty. Men develop a typical pattern of baldness associated with the male hormone testosterone (male-pattern baldness). Hair may be lost at the temples or at the top of the head.

Women may also develop a typical pattern of hair loss as they age (female-pattern baldness). The hair becomes less dense all over and the scalp may become visible.

Body and facial hair are also lost, but the hairs that remain may become coarser. Some women may notice a loss of body hair, but may find that they have coarse facial hair, especially on the chin and around the lips.

Men may find the hair of their eyebrows, ears, and nose becoming longer and coarser.

Nail Changes

The nails also change with aging. They grow slower and may become dull and brittle. They may become yellowed and opaque.

Nails, especially toenails, may become hard and thick. Ingrown toenails may be more common. The tips of the fingernails may fragment.

Sometimes, lengthwise ridges will develop in the fingernails and toenails. This can be a normal aging change. However, some nail changes can be caused by infections, nutritional deficiencies, trauma, and other problems.

Check with your healthcare provider if your nails develop pits, ridges, lines, changed shape, or other changes. These can be related to iron deficiency, kidney disease, and nutritional deficiencies.

Section 36.2

Male Pattern Baldness

It is estimated that thirty-five million men in the United States are affected by male pattern baldness or androgenic alopecia. "Andro" refers to the androgens (testosterone, dihydrotestosterone) necessary to produce male-pattern hair loss (MPHL). "Genic" refers to the inherited gene necessary for MPHL to occur. In men who develop male pattern baldness the hair loss may begin any time after puberty when blood levels of androgens rise. The first change is usually recession in the temporal areas, which is seen in 96 percent of mature Caucasian males, including those men not destined to progress to further hair loss.

Hamilton and later Norwood have classified the patterns of male pattern baldness. Although the density of hair in a given pattern of loss tends to diminish with age, there is no way to predict what pattern of hair loss a young man with early male pattern baldness will eventually assume. In general, those who begin losing hair in the second decade are those in whom the hair loss will be the most severe. In some men, initial male-pattern hair loss may be delayed until the late third to fourth decade. It is generally recognized that men in their twenties have a 20 percent incidence of male pattern baldness, in their thirties a 30 percent incidence of male pattern baldness, in their forties a 40 percent incidence of male pattern baldness, etc. Using these numbers one can see that a male in his nineties has a 90 percent chance of having some degree of male pattern baldness.

Hamilton first noted that androgens (testosterone, dihydrotestosterone) are necessary for the development of male pattern baldness. The amount of androgens present does not need to be greater than normal for male pattern baldness to occur. If androgens are present in normal amounts and the gene for hair loss is present, male pattern hair loss will occur. Axillary (under arm) and pubic hair are dependent on testosterone for growth. Beard growth and male pattern hair loss are dependent on dihydrotestosterone (DHT). Testosterone is converted to

DHT by the enzyme 5-alpha-reductase. Finasteride (Propecia®) acts by blocking this enzyme and decreasing the amount of DHT. Receptors exist on cells that bind androgens. These receptors have the greatest affinity for DHT followed by testosterone, estrogen, and progesterone. After binding to the receptor, DHT goes into the cell and interacts with the nucleus of the cell, altering the production of protein by the DNA in the nucleus of the cell. Ultimately growth of the hair follicle ceases.

The hair growth cycle is affected in that the percentage of hairs in the growth phase (anagen) and the duration of the growth phase diminish, resulting in shorter hairs. More hairs are in the resting state (telogen) and these hairs are much more subject to loss with the daily trauma of combing and washing. The hair shafts in male pattern baldness become progressively miniaturized, smaller in diameter and length, with time. In men with male pattern baldness all the hairs in an affected area may eventually (but not necessarily) become involved in the process and may with time cover the region with fine (vellus) hair. Pigment (color) production is also terminated with miniaturization so the fine hair becomes lighter in color. The lighter color, miniaturized hairs cause the area to first appear thin. Involved areas in men can completely lose all follicles over time. Male pattern baldness is an inherited condition and the gene can be inherited from either the mother or father's side. There is a common myth that inheritance is only from the mother's side. This is not true.

In summary, male pattern hair loss (androgenic alopecia) is an inherited condition manifested when androgens are present in normal amounts. The gene can be inherited from the mother or father's side. The onset, rate, and severity of hair loss are unpredictable. The severity increases with age and if the condition is present it will be progressive and relentless.

Hair loss in men is likely to occur primarily between the late teenage years and age forty to fifty, in a generally recognizable "male-pattern" baldness known as androgenic alopecia. Men with male-pattern hair loss may have an expectation of hair loss if they have male relatives who lost hair in a recognizably male pattern.

Section 36.3

Female Pattern Baldness

"Female Hair Loss and Pattern Baldness in Women," © 2005 International Society of Hair Restoration Surgery. Reprinted with permission. For additional information, visit www.ishrs.org, or call toll-free 800-444-2737.

Female hair loss occurs in more than one pattern. If you are a woman with loss of scalp hair, you should seek professional advice from a physician hair restoration specialist.

In most cases, female hair loss can be effectively treated. If you are a woman who has started to lose scalp hair, you are not alone if:

- You are unpleasantly surprised by the hair loss.

- You don't understand why you are losing hair.

The patterns of hair loss in women are not as easily recognizable as those in men.

Unlike hair loss in men, female scalp hair loss may commonly begin at any age through fifty or later, may not have any obvious hereditary association, and may not occur in a recognizable "female-pattern alopecia" of diffuse thinning over the top of the scalp. A woman who notices the beginning of hair loss may not be sure if the loss is going to be temporary or permanent—for example, if there has been a recent event such as pregnancy or illness that may be associated with temporary hair thinning.

If you are a woman who is worried about loss of scalp hair, you should consult a physician hair restoration specialist for an evaluation and diagnosis.

Self-diagnosis is often ineffective. Women tend to have less obvious patterns of hair loss than men, and non-pattern types of hair loss are more frequent in women than in men. Diagnosis of hair loss in a woman should be made by a trained and experienced physician.

In women, as in men, the most likely cause of scalp hair loss is androgenic alopecia—an inherited sensitivity to the effects of androgens (male hormones) on scalp hair follicles. However, women with hair loss due to this cause usually do not develop true baldness in the patterns that occur in men—for example, women rarely develop the "cue-ball" appearance often seen in male-pattern androgenic alopecia.

Patterns of female androgenic alopecia can vary considerably in appearance. Patterns that may occur include:

- Diffuse thinning of hair over the entire scalp, often with more noticeable thinning toward the back of the scalp;

- Diffuse thinning over the entire scalp, with more noticeable thinning toward the front of the scalp but not involving the frontal hairline;

- Diffuse thinning over the entire scalp, with more noticeable thinning toward the front of the scalp, involving and sometimes breaching the frontal hairline.

Unlike the case for men, thinning scalp hair in women due to androgenic alopecia does not uniformly grow smaller in diameter (miniaturize). Women with hair loss due to androgenic alopecia tend to have miniaturizing hairs of variable diameter over all affected areas of the scalp. While miniaturizing hairs are a feature of androgenic alopecia, miniaturization may also be associated with other causes and is not in itself a diagnostic feature of androgenic alopecia. In postmenopausal women, for example, hair may begin to miniaturize and become difficult to style. The precise diagnosis should be made by a physician hair restoration specialist.

It is important to note that female pattern hair loss can begin as early as the late teens to the early twenties in women who have experienced early puberty. If left untreated, this hair loss associated with early puberty can progress to more advanced hair loss.

Non-Pattern Causes of Hair loss in Women

In women more often than in men, hair loss may be due to conditions other than androgenic alopecia. Some of the most common of these causes are as follows:

- **Trichotillomania:** Compulsive hair pulling. Hair loss due to trichotillomania is typically patchy, as compulsive hair pullers tend to concentrate the pulling in selected areas. Hair loss due to this cause cannot be treated effectively until the psychological or emotional reasons for trichotillomania are effectively addressed.

- **Alopecia areata:** A possibly autoimmune disorder that causes patchy hair loss that can range from diffuse thinning to extensive areas of baldness with "islands" of retained hair. Medical examination is necessary to establish a diagnosis.

- **Triangular alopecia:** Loss of hair in the temporal areas that sometimes begins in childhood. Hair loss may be complete, or a few fine, thin-diameter hairs may remain. The cause of triangular alopecia is not known, but the condition can be treated medically or surgically.

- **Scarring alopecia:** Hair loss due to scarring of the scalp area. Scarring alopecia typically involves the top of the scalp and occurs predominantly in women. The condition frequently occurs in African American women and is believed to be associated with persistent tight braiding or "corn-rowing" of scalp hair. A form of scarring alopecia also may occur in postmenopausal women, associated with inflammation of hair follicles and subsequent scarring.

- **Telogen effluvium:** A common type of hair loss caused when a large percentage of scalp hairs are shifted into "shedding" phase. The causes of telogen effluvium may be hormonal, nutritional, drug-associated, or stress-associated.

- **Loose-anagen syndrome:** A condition occurring primarily in fair-haired persons in which scalp hair sits loosely in hair follicles and is easily extracted by combing or pulling. The condition may appear in childhood, and may improve as the person ages.

Diagnosis and Treatment

If you are a woman with thinning or lost scalp hair, your first necessary step is to have the condition correctly diagnosed by a physician hair restoration specialist. After a diagnosis is made, the physician will recommend an approach to effective medical or surgical treatment.

References

Olsen EA (ed). Female Pattern Hair loss: Clinical Features and Potential Hormonal Factors. *J Amer Acad Dermatol* 2001; 45:S70–S80.

Olsen EA. Hair disorders. In: Freedberg IM et al (eds.) *Fitzpatrick's Dermatology in General Medicine*, 5th ed. New York: McGraw-Hill, 1999:729–51.

Section 36.4

Aging Changes in the Skin

Skin changes are among the most visible signs of aging. Evidence of increasing age includes wrinkles and sagging skin. Whitening or graying of the hair is another obvious sign of aging.

Your skin does many things. It protects you from the environment, helps regulate your body temperature, helps with fluid and electrolyte balance, and provides receptors for sensations such as touch, pain, and pressure.

Although skin has many layers, it can be generally divided into three main portions. The outer portion (epidermis) contains skin cells, pigment, and proteins. The middle portion (dermis) contains blood vessels, nerves, hair follicles, and oil glands. The dermis provides nutrients to the epidermis.

The layer under the dermis (the subcutaneous layer) contains sweat glands, some hair follicles, blood vessels, and fat. Each layer also contains connective tissue with collagen fibers to give support and elastin fibers to provide flexibility and strength.

Skin changes are related to environmental factors, genetic makeup, nutrition, and other factors. The greatest single factor, though, is sun exposure. This can be seen by comparing areas of your body that have regular sun exposure with areas that are protected from sunlight.

Natural pigments seem to provide some protection against sun-induced skin damage. Blue-eyed, fair-skinned people show more aging skin changes than people with darker, more heavily pigmented skin.

Aging Changes

With aging, the outer skin layer (epidermis) thins even though the number of cell layers remains unchanged.

The number of pigment-containing cells (melanocytes) decreases, but the remaining melanocytes increase in size. Aging skin thus appears thinner, more pale, and translucent. Large pigmented spots (called age spots, liver spots, or lentigos) may appear in sun-exposed areas.

Changes in the connective tissue reduce the skin's strength and elasticity. This is known as elastosis and is especially pronounced in sun-exposed areas (solar elastosis). Elastosis produces the leathery, weather-beaten appearance common to farmers, sailors, and others who spend a large amount of time outdoors.

The blood vessels of the dermis become more fragile, which in turn leads to bruising, bleeding under the skin, cherry angiomas, and similar conditions.

Sebaceous glands produce less oil as you age. Men experience a minimal decrease, usually after the age of eighty. Women gradually produce less oil beginning after menopause. This can make it harder to keep the skin moist, resulting in dryness and itchiness.

The subcutaneous fat layer, which provides insulation and padding, thins. This increases your risk of skin injury and reduces your ability to maintain body temperature. Because you have less natural insulation, in cold weather hypothermia can result.

Some medications are absorbed by the fat layer, and loss of this layer changes the way that these medications work.

The sweat glands produce less sweat. This makes it harder to keep cool, and you become at increased risk for becoming overheated or developing heat stroke.

Growths such as skin tags, warts, and other blemishes are more common in older people.

Effect of Changes

As you age, you are at increased risk for skin injury. Your skin is thinner, more fragile, and the protective subcutaneous fat layer is lost. In addition, your ability to sense touch, pressure, vibration, heat, and cold may be reduced. Thus, your aging skin is at higher risk for injury.

Rubbing or pulling on the skin can cause skin tears. Fragile blood vessels are easily broken. Bruises, flat collections of blood (purpura), and raised collections of blood (hematomas) may form after even a minor injury.

This is most easily seen on the outside surface of the forearms, but can occur anywhere on the body. Skin changes and loss of subcutaneous fat, combined with a tendency to be less active, as well as some nutritional deficiencies and other illnesses contribute to pressure ulcers.

Aging skin repairs itself more slowly than younger skin. Wound healing may be up to four times slower. This contributes to pressure ulcers and infections. Diabetes, blood vessel changes, lowered immunity, and similar factors also affect healing.

Common Problems

Skin disorders are so common among older people that it is often difficult to tell normal changes from those related to a disorder. More than 90 percent of all older people have some type of skin disorder.

Skin disorders can be caused by many diseases, including diabetes, liver disease, heart disease, and blood vessel diseases such as arteriosclerosis. Stress, reactions to medications, obesity, and nutritional deficiencies can be other causes.

Climate, exposures to industrial and household chemicals, indoor heating, clothing, allergies to plants and other allergies, and many other common exposures can also cause skin changes.

Sunlight can cause elastosis (loss of elasticity), keratoacanthomas (noncancerous skin growths), thickening of the skin, pigment changes such as liver spots, and other conditions.

Sun exposure has also been directly linked to skin cancers, including basal cell epithelioma, squamous cell carcinoma, and melanoma.

Prevention

Because most skin changes are related to sun exposure, prevention is a lifelong process:

- Prevent sunburn if at all possible.

- Use a good quality sunscreen when outdoors, even in the winter.

- Wear protective clothing and hats as necessary.

Good nutrition and adequate fluids are also helpful. Dehydration increases the risk of skin injury. Sometimes minor nutritional deficiencies can cause rashes, skin lesions, and other skin changes even if no other symptoms are present.

Keep skin moist with lotions and do not use soaps that are heavily perfumed. Bath oils are not recommended because they can cause you to slip and fall.

Moist skin is more comfortable and may heal better.

Section 36.5

What Are Wrinkles?

This information was provided by KidsHealth, one of the largest resources online for medically reviewed health information written for parents, kids, and teens. For more articles like this one, visit www.KidsHealth.org, or www.TeensHealth.org. © 2004 The Nemours Foundation.

You can often get an idea of how old someone is by looking at his or her face—specifically the skin. As people age, it's normal to get wrinkles. And if the person has spent a lot of time in the sun, at tanning salons, or smoking cigarettes, he or she might have a lot of them. The skin is made up of three layers:

- The outermost layer everyone can see, called the epidermis
- The middle layer, called the dermis
- The innermost layer, called the subcutaneous layer

When a person is young, he or she doesn't have wrinkles because the skin does a great job of stretching and holding in moisture. The dermis has an elastic quality thanks to fibers called elastin that keep the skin looking and feeling young. A protein in the dermis called collagen also plays a part in preventing wrinkles.

However, over time, the dermis loses both collagen and elastin, so skin gets thinner and has trouble getting enough moisture to the epidermis. The fat in the subcutaneous layer that gives skin a plump appearance also begins to disappear, the epidermis starts to sag, and wrinkles form.

There's not a magic age (like forty) when everyone suddenly gets wrinkles. Some people in their twenties have little wrinkles around their eyes (called "crow's feet") from squinting or spending too much time in the sun.

Other people may be in their fifties or sixties before you can even see a wrinkle. This is usually because they have taken good care of their skin over the years and may have more sebum, the skin's natural oil. They may also have "good genes"—which means their family members don't have many wrinkles. Eventually, however, everyone will have at least a few wrinkles. It's a natural part of the aging process.

Here are some things people can do to prevent getting many wrinkles at an early age:

- Avoid spending too much time in the direct sun, especially during the hours when the sun's rays are harshest (between 10:00 A.M. and 4:00 P.M.). Ultraviolet (UV) rays cause many wrinkles. Sun block helps, but it doesn't block out all the damaging UV rays that cause wrinkles to the skin. Still, if you are outside a lot, be sure to wear a sun block with sun protection factor (SPF) 15 or higher and reapply often (every two to three hours). Always reapply after swimming or playing sports that make you sweaty!

- Don't go to the tanning salon. The UV light from tanning booths is just as damaging as the sun's—and sometimes worse.

- Don't smoke! Smoking robs your skin of precious moisture and causes premature (early) wrinkles. (Did you ever notice that most heavy smokers have wrinkles around their mouths?)

- Drink water.

- Moisturize dry skin, especially during months when the air is drier.

Chapter 37

Sleep and Aging

About Sleep

We all look forward to a good night's sleep. Sleep allows our body to rest and to restore its energy levels. Without enough restful sleep, not only can we become grumpy and irritable, but also inattentive and more prone to accidents. Like food and water, adequate sleep is essential to good health and quality of life.

There are two types of sleep: non-rapid eye movement—or NREM sleep—and rapid eye movement—or REM sleep. NREM sleep includes four stages, ranging from light to deep sleep. We cycle through these four stages of sleep approximately every ninety minutes. Then we go into REM sleep, the most active stage of sleep when dreaming often occurs. During REM sleep, the eyes move back and forth beneath the eyelids and muscles become immobile.

Researchers believe that two body systems—the sleep-wake process and our circadian biologic clock—regulate our sleep. They program our bodies to feel sleepy at night and awake during the day.

The sleep-wake process works by balancing the amount of sleep a person needs based on the time spent awake. Our circadian biologic clock is a twenty-four-hour body rhythm affected by sunlight. It regulates hormones such as melatonin, which is secreted during the night and promotes sleep, and other processes like body temperature. Sleeping at a time that is in sync with this rhythm is important for healthy sleep.

Excerpted from "Sleep and Aging," NIH Senior Health, National Institutes of Health, April 12, 2005

Sleep needs change over a person's lifetime. Children and adolescents need more sleep than adults. Interestingly, older adults need about the same amount of sleep as younger adults—seven to nine hours of sleep per night.

Unfortunately, many older adults often get less sleep than they need. One reason is that they often have more trouble falling asleep. A study of adults over sixty-five found that 13 percent of men and 36 percent of women take more than thirty minutes to fall asleep.

Also, older people often sleep less deeply and wake up more often throughout the night, which may be why they may nap more often during the daytime. Nighttime sleep schedules may change with age too. Many older adults tend to get sleepier earlier in the evening and awaken earlier in the morning.

There are many possible explanations for these changes. Older adults may produce and secrete less melatonin, the hormone that promotes sleep. They may also be more sensitive to—and may awaken because of—changes in their environment, such as noise.

Older adults may also have other medical and psychiatric problems that can affect their nighttime sleep. Researchers have noted that people without major medical or psychiatric illnesses report better sleep.

Not sleeping well can lead to a number of problems. Older adults who have poor nighttime sleep are more likely to have a depressed mood, attention and memory problems, excessive daytime sleepiness, more nighttime falls, and use more over-the-counter or prescription sleep aids. Poor sleep is also associated with a poorer quality of life.

Many people believe that poor sleep is a normal part of aging, but it is not. In fact, many healthy older adults report few or no sleep problems. Sleep patterns change as we age, but disturbed sleep and waking up tired every day are not part of normal aging. If you are having trouble sleeping, see your doctor or a sleep specialist. There are treatments that can help.

Sleep Disorders

If you have a sleep disorder it can be hard to get a good night's sleep. Sleep disorders can make it hard to fall asleep or stay asleep during the night and can make you drowsy during the day. The most common sleep disorders among older adults are insomnia, sleep-disordered breathing, such as snoring and sleep apnea, and movement disorders like restless legs syndrome.

Insomnia

Insomnia is the most common sleep complaint at any age. It affects almost half of adults sixty and older.

If you have insomnia, you may experience any one or any combination of the following symptoms:

- Taking a long time—more than thirty to forty-five minutes—to fall asleep

- Waking up many times each night

- Waking up early and being unable to get back to sleep

- Waking up feeling tired

Short-term insomnia, lasting less than one month, may result from a medical or psychiatric condition. Or it may occur after a change in personal circumstances like losing a loved one, relocating, or being hospitalized. If insomnia lasts longer than a month, it is considered chronic, even if the original cause has been resolved.

Many factors can cause insomnia. However, the most common reason older adults wake up at night is to go to the bathroom. Prostate enlargement in men and continence problems in women are often the cause. Unfortunately, waking up to go to the bathroom at night also places older adults at greater risk for falling.

Disorders that cause pain or discomfort during the night such as heartburn, arthritis, menopause, and cancer also can cause you to lose sleep. Medical conditions such as heart failure and lung disease may make it more difficult to sleep through the night, too.

Neurological conditions such as Parkinson disease and dementia are often a source of sleep problems, as are psychiatric conditions, such as depression. Although depression and insomnia are often related, it is currently unclear whether one causes the other.

Many older people also have habits that make it more difficult to get a good night's sleep. They may nap more frequently during the day or may not exercise as much. Spending less time outdoors can reduce their exposure to sunlight and upset their sleep cycle. Drinking more alcohol or caffeine can keep them from falling asleep or staying asleep.

Also, as people age, their sleeping and waking patterns tend to change. Older adults usually become sleepier earlier in the evening and wake up earlier in the morning. If they don't adjust their bedtimes to these changes, they may have difficulty falling and staying asleep.

Lastly, many older adults take a variety of different medications that may negatively affect their sleep. Many medications have side effects that can cause sleepiness or affect daytime functioning.

Sleep-Disordered Breathing

Sleep apnea and snoring are two examples of sleep-disordered breathing—conditions that make it more difficult to breathe during sleep. When severe, these disorders may cause people to wake up often at night and be drowsy during the day.

Snoring is a very common condition affecting nearly 40 percent of adults. It is more common among older people and those who are overweight. When severe, snoring not only causes frequent awakenings at night and daytime sleepiness, it can also disrupt a bed partner's sleep.

Snoring is caused by a partial blockage of the airway passage from the nose and mouth to the lungs. The blockage causes the tissues in these passages to vibrate, leading to the noise produced when someone snores.

There are two kinds of sleep apnea: obstructive sleep apnea and central sleep apnea. Obstructive sleep apnea occurs when air entering from the nose or mouth is either partially or completely blocked, usually because of obesity or extra tissue in the back of the throat and mouth. If these episodes occur frequently or are severe, they may cause a person to awaken frequently throughout the night. This may disrupt their sleep and make them sleepy during the day.

Central sleep apnea is less common. It occurs when the brain doesn't send the right signals to start the breathing process. Often, both types of sleep apnea occur in the same person.

Obstructive sleep apnea is more common among older adults and among people who are significantly overweight. Obstructive sleep apnea can increase a person's risk for high blood pressure, strokes, heart disease, and cognitive problems. However, more research is needed to understand the long-term consequences of obstructive sleep apnea in older adults.

Movement Disorders

Two movement disorders that can make it harder to sleep include restless legs syndrome, or RLS, and periodic limb movement disorder, or PLMD. Both of these conditions cause people to move their limbs when they sleep, leading to poor sleep and daytime drowsiness. Often, both conditions occur in the same person.

Restless legs syndrome is a common condition in older adults and affects more than 20 percent of people eighty years and older. People with RLS experience uncomfortable feelings in their legs such as tingling, crawling, or pins and needles. This often makes it hard for them to fall asleep or stay asleep, and causes them to be sleepy during the day.

Although scientists do not fully understand what causes restless legs syndrome, it has been linked to a variety of conditions. Some of these conditions include iron deficiency, kidney failure and dialysis, pregnancy, and nerve abnormalities.

Periodic limb movement disorder, or PLMD, is a condition that causes people to jerk and kick their legs every twenty to forty seconds during sleep. As with RLS, PLMD often disrupts sleep—not only for the patient but the bed partner as well. One study found that roughly 40 percent of older adults have at least a mild form of PLMD.

Another condition that may make it harder to get a good night's sleep is rapid eye movement sleep behavior disorder, also known as REM sleep behavior disorder. It is somewhat more common in men over the age of fifty.

REM sleep, or rapid eye movement sleep, is the most active stage of sleep, where dreaming often occurs. During normal REM sleep, the eyes move back and forth beneath the eyelids, and muscles cannot move. In more severe forms of REM sleep behavior disorder, the muscles become quite mobile and sufferers often act out their dreams.

Diagnosis and Treatment

If you are often tired during the day and don't feel that you sleep well, you should discuss this with your doctor or healthcare provider. Many primary care providers can diagnose sleep disorders and offer suggestions and treatments that can improve your sleep.

Diagnosis

Before you visit the doctor, it may be very helpful for you to ask for and keep a sleep diary for a week or more. A sleep diary will give you and your doctor a picture of your sleep habits and schedules and help determine whether they may be affecting your sleep.

During your appointment your doctor will ask you about your symptoms and may have you fill out questionnaires that measure the severity of your sleep problem. It is also helpful to have your bed partner come with you to your appointment since he or she may be able to report symptoms unknown to you like loud snoring, breathing pauses, or movements during sleep.

Since older people are more likely to take medications and to have medical problems that may affect sleep, it is important for your doctor to be aware of any health condition or medication you are taking. Don't forget to mention over-the-counter medications, coffee or caffeine use, and alcohol since these also may have an impact on your sleep.

The doctor will then perform a physical examination. During the exam the doctor will look for signs of other diseases that may affect sleep, such as Parkinson disease, stroke, heart disease, or obesity. If your doctor feels more information is needed, he or she may refer you to a sleep center for more testing.

Sleep centers employ physicians and others who are experts in problems that affect sleep. If the sleep specialist needs more information, he or she may ask you to undergo an overnight sleep study, also called a polysomnogram, and/or a sleepiness or a nap test. A polysomnogram is a test that measures brain waves, heart rate, breathing patterns, and body movements.

A common sleepiness test is the multiple sleep latency test. During this test, the person has an opportunity to nap every two hours during the daytime. If the person falls asleep too quickly it may mean that he or she has too much daytime sleepiness.

Treatment

Based on your sleep evaluation, your doctor or sleep specialist may recommend individual treatment options. It is important to remember that there are effective treatments for most sleep disorders.

If you are diagnosed with a sleep disorder, your doctor may suggest specific treatments. You should ask for information to find out more about your condition and ways to improve your sleep.

There are a number of therapies available to help you fall asleep and stay asleep. You may want to try limiting excessive noise and/or light in your sleep environment. Or, you could limit the time spent in bed while not sleeping, and use bright lights to help with circadian rhythm problems. Circadian rhythm is our twenty-four-hour internal body clock that is affected by sunlight.

Some specialists believe medications also can be useful early in your treatment, and if necessary, you can use them from time to time if you have trouble falling asleep.

People who are diagnosed with sleep apnea should try to lose weight if possible, but often they may need other treatments as well. Adjusting your body position during the night may benefit you if you experience sleep apnea more often when you lie on your back.

The most effective and popular treatment for sleep apnea is nasal continuous positive airway pressure, or CPAP. This device keeps your air passages open by supplying a steady stream of air pressure through your nose while you sleep.

To use the CPAP, the patient puts on a small mask that fits around the nose. Air pressure is delivered to the mask from a small, quiet air pump that sits at the bedside. The patient not only wears the mask at night but also during naps, since obstructions can occur during these times as well.

If you have a mild case of sleep apnea, sometimes a dental device or appliance can be helpful. If your condition is more severe and you don't tolerate other treatments, your doctor may suggest surgery to increase the airway size in the mouth and throat. One common surgical method removes excess tissue from the back of the throat.

Very often, people who suffer from movement disorders during sleep such as restless legs syndrome or periodic limb movement disorder are successfully treated with the same medications used for Parkinson disease. People with restless legs syndrome often have low levels of iron in their blood. In such cases doctors often prescribe supplements.

Medications can also treat people with REM behavior disorder. If there are reports of dangerous activities such as hitting or running during these episodes, it may be necessary to make changes to the person's sleeping area to protect sufferers and their bed partners from injury.

Sleeping Well

A good night's sleep can make a big difference in how you feel. Here are some suggestions to help you:

- Follow a regular schedule. Go to sleep and wake up at the same time, even on weekends. Sticking to a regular bedtime and wake time schedule helps keep you in sync with your body's circadian clock, a twenty-four-hour internal rhythm affected by sunlight.

- Try not to nap too much during the day. You might be less sleepy at night.

- Try to exercise at regular times each day. Exercising regularly improves the quality of your nighttime sleep and helps you sleep more soundly. Try to finish your workout at least three hours before bedtime.

- Try to get some natural light in the afternoon each day.

- Be careful about what you eat. Don't drink beverages with caffeine late in the day. Caffeine is a stimulant and can keep you awake. Also, if you like a snack before bed, a warm beverage and a few crackers may help.

- Don't drink alcohol or smoke cigarettes to help you sleep. Even small amounts of alcohol can make it harder to stay asleep. Smoking is dangerous for many reasons, including the hazard of falling asleep with a lit cigarette. Also, the nicotine in cigarettes is a stimulant.

- Create a safe and comfortable place to sleep. Make sure there are locks on all doors and smoke alarms on each floor. A lamp that's easy to turn on and a phone by your bed may be helpful. The room should be dark, well ventilated, and as quiet as possible.

- Develop a bedtime routine. Do the same things each night to tell your body that it's time to wind down. Some people watch the evening news, read a book, or soak in a warm bath.

- Use your bedroom only for sleeping. After turning off the light, give yourself about fifteen minutes to fall asleep. If you are still awake and not drowsy, get out of bed. When you get sleepy, go back to bed.

- Try not to worry about your sleep. Some people find that playing mental games is helpful. For example, think black—a black cat on a black velvet pillow on a black corduroy sofa, etc. Or, tell yourself it's five minutes before you have to get up and you're just trying to get a few extra winks.

- If you are so tired during the day that you cannot function normally and if this lasts for more than two to three weeks, you should see your family doctor or a sleep disorders specialist.

Chapter 38

Sexuality and Aging

People seem to want and need to be close to others. As we grow older, many of us also want to continue an active, satisfying sex life. But the aging process may cause some changes.

What are normal changes?

Normal aging brings physical changes in both men and women. These changes sometimes affect one's ability to have and enjoy sex with another person. Some women enjoy sex more as they grow older. After menopause or a hysterectomy, they may no longer fear an unwanted pregnancy. They may feel freer to enjoy sex.

Some women do not think things like gray hair and wrinkles make them less attractive to their sexual partner. But if a woman believes that looking young or being able to give birth makes her more feminine, she may begin to worry about how desirable she is no matter what her age is. That might make sex less enjoyable for her.

A woman may notice changes in her vagina. As she ages, her vagina shortens and narrows. The walls become thinner and also a little stiffer. These changes do not mean she can't enjoy having sex. However, most women will also have less vaginal lubrication. This could affect sexual pleasure.

As men get older, impotence becomes more common. Impotence is the loss of ability to have and keep an erection hard enough for sexual

Reprinted from "Sexuality in Later Life," National Institute on Aging, National Institutes of Health, July 2005.

intercourse. By age sixty-five, about 15 to 25 percent of men have this problem at least one out of every four times they are having sex. This may happen in men with heart disease, high blood pressure, or diabetes—either because of the disease or because of the medicines used to treat it.

A man may find it takes longer to get an erection. His erection may not be as firm or as large as it used to be. The amount of ejaculate may be smaller. The loss of erection after orgasm may happen more quickly, or it may take longer before an erection is again possible. Some men may find they need more foreplay.

What causes sexual problems?

Illness, disability, or the drugs you take to treat a health problem can affect your ability to have and enjoy sex. But even the most serious health problems usually don't have to stop you from having a satisfying sex life.

Arthritis: Joint pain due to arthritis can make sexual contact uncomfortable. Joint replacement surgery and drugs may relieve this pain. Exercise, rest, warm baths, and changing the position or timing of sexual activity can be helpful.

Chronic pain: In addition to arthritis, pain that continues for more than a month or comes back on and off over time can be caused by other bone and muscle conditions, shingles, poor blood circulation, or blood vessel problems. This discomfort can, in turn, lead to sleep problems, depression, isolation, and difficulty moving around. These can interfere with intimacy between older people. Chronic pain does not have to be part of growing older and can often be treated.

Diabetes: Many men with diabetes do not have sexual problems, but this is one of the few illnesses that can cause impotence. In most cases medical treatment can help.

Heart disease: Narrowing and hardening of the arteries known as atherosclerosis can change blood vessels so that blood does not flow freely. This can lead to trouble with erections in men, as can high blood pressure (hypertension). Some people who have had a heart attack are afraid that having sex will cause another attack. The chance of this is very low. Most people can start having sex again three to six weeks after their condition becomes stable following an attack, if their doctor agrees. Always follow your doctor's advice.

Incontinence: Loss of bladder control or leaking of urine is more common as we grow older, especially in women. Stress incontinence happens during exercise, coughing, sneezing, or lifting, for example. Because of the extra pressure on your abdomen during sex, incontinence might cause some people to avoid sex. The good news is that this can usually be treated.

Stroke: The ability to have sex is rarely damaged by a stroke, but problems with erections are possible. It is unlikely that having sex will cause another stroke. Someone with weakness or paralysis caused by a stroke might try using different positions or medical devices to help them continue having sex.

What about surgery and drugs?

Surgery: Many of us worry about having any kind of surgery—it is especially troubling when the genital area is involved. Happily, most people do return to the kind of sex life they enjoyed before having surgery.

Hysterectomy is surgery to remove the uterus. It does not interfere with sexual functioning. If a hysterectomy seems to take away from a woman's ability to enjoy sex, a counselor may be helpful. Men who feel their partners are "less feminine" after a hysterectomy may also be helped by counseling.

Mastectomy is surgery to remove all or part of a woman's breast. Your body is as capable of sexual response as ever, but you may lose your sexual desire or sense of being desired. Sometimes it is useful to talk with other women who have had this surgery. Programs like the American Cancer Society's (ACS) "Reach to Recovery" can be helpful for both women and men. Rebuilding of the breast (reconstruction) is also a possibility to discuss with your surgeon.

About 1,500 American men develop breast cancer each year. In them the disease can make their bodies make extra "female" hormones. These can greatly lower their sex drive.

Prostatectomy is surgery that removes all or part of a man's prostate. Sometimes this procedure is done because of an enlarged prostate. It may cause urinary incontinence or impotence. If removal of the prostate gland (radical prostatectomy) is needed, doctors can often save the nerves going to the penis. An erection may still be possible.

Talk to your doctor before surgery to make sure you will be able to lead a fully satisfying sex life.

Medications: Some drugs can cause sexual problems. These include some blood pressure medicines, antihistamines, antidepressants, tranquilizers, appetite suppressants, diabetes drugs, and some ulcer drugs like ranitidine. Some can lead to impotence or make it hard for men to ejaculate. Some drugs can reduce a woman's sexual desire. Check with your doctor. She or he can often prescribe a different drug without this side effect.

Alcohol: Too much alcohol can cause erection problems in men and delay orgasm in women.

Am I too old to worry about safe sex?

Having safe sex is important for people at any age. As a woman gets closer to menopause, her periods may be irregular. But, she can still get pregnant. In fact, pregnancy is still possible until your doctor says you are past menopause—you have not had a menstrual period for twelve months.

Age does not protect you from sexually transmitted diseases. Young people are most at risk for diseases such as syphilis, gonorrhea, chlamydial infection, genital herpes, hepatitis B, genital warts, and trichomoniasis. But these diseases can and do happen in sexually active older people.

Almost anyone who is sexually active is also at risk for being infected with human immunodeficiency virus (HIV), the virus that causes AIDS. The number of older people with HIV/AIDS is growing. One out of every ten people diagnosed with AIDS in the United States is over age fifty. You are at risk if you have more than one sexual partner or are recently divorced or widowed and have started dating and having unprotected sex again. Always use a latex condom during sex, and talk to your doctor about ways to protect yourself from all sexually transmitted diseases. You are never too old to be at risk.

Can emotions play a part?

Sexuality is often a delicate balance of emotional and physical issues. How you feel may affect what you are able to do. For example, men may fear that impotence will become a more common problem as they age. But if you are too concerned with that possibility, you can cause enough stress to trigger impotence. A woman who is worried about how her looks are changing as she ages may think her partner will no longer find her attractive. This focus on youthful physical beauty may get in the way of her enjoyment of sex.

Older couples face the same daily stresses that affect people of any age. But they may also have the added concerns of age, illness, and retirement and other lifestyle changes. These worries can cause sexual difficulties. Talk openly with your doctor, or see a counselor. These health professionals can often help.

Don't blame yourself for any sexual difficulties you and your partner are having. You might want to talk with a therapist about them. If your male partner is troubled by impotence or your female partner seems less interested in sex, don't assume he or she doesn't find you attractive anymore. There can be many physical causes for these problems.

What can I do?

There are several things you can do on your own to keep an active sexual life. Remember that sex does not have to include intercourse. Make your partner a high priority. Pay attention to his or her needs and wants. Take time to understand the changes you both are facing. Try different positions and new times, like having sex in the morning when you both may have more energy. Don't hurry—you or your partner may need to spend more time touching to become fully aroused. Masturbation is a sexual activity that some older people, especially unmarried, widowed, or divorced people and those whose partners are ill or away, may find satisfying.

Some older people, especially women, may have trouble finding a partner with whom they can share any type of intimacy. Women live longer than men, so there are more of them. In 2000 women over age sixty-five outnumbered older men by 100 to 70. Doing activities that other seniors enjoy or going places where older people gather are ways to meet new people. Some ideas include mall walking, senior centers, adult education classes at a community college, or day trips sponsored by your city or county recreation department.

If you do seem to have a problem that affects your sex life, talk to your doctor. He or she can suggest a treatment depending on the type of problem and its cause. For example, the most common sexual difficulty of older women is dyspareunia, painful intercourse caused by poor vaginal lubrication. Your doctor or a pharmacist can suggest over-the-counter, water-based vaginal lubricants to use. Or, your doctor might suggest estrogen supplements or an estrogen vaginal insert.

If impotence is the problem, it can often be managed and perhaps even reversed. There is a pill that can help. It is called sildenafil and should not be taken by men taking medicines containing nitrates, such as nitroglycerin. This pill does have possible side effects. Other available treatments include vacuum devices, self-injection of a drug (either papaverine or prostaglandin E1), or penile implants.

There is a lot you can do to continue an active sex life. Follow a healthy lifestyle—exercise, eat good food, drink plenty of fluids like water or juices, don't smoke, and avoid alcohol. Try to reduce the stress in your life. See your doctor regularly. And keep a positive outlook on life.

Chapter 39

Changes in the Coronary and Vascular Systems

Chapter Contents

Section 39.1

How Aging Changes the Heart and Blood Vessels

From "Aging Changes in the Heart and Blood Vessels," © 2007 A.D.A.M., Inc. Reprinted with permission.

Some changes in the heart and blood vessels normally occur with age, but many others are modifiable factors that, if not treated, can lead to heart disease.

Aging Changes

Heart

Normal changes in the heart include deposits of the "aging pigment," lipofuscin. The heart muscle cells degenerate slightly. The valves inside the heart, which control the direction of blood flow, thicken and become stiffer. A heart murmur caused by valve stiffness is fairly common in the elderly.

The heart has a natural pacemaker system that controls heartbeat. Some of the pathways of this system may develop fibrous tissue and fat deposits. The natural pacemaker (the sinoatrial, or SA, node) loses some of its cells. These changes may result in a slightly slower heart rate.

Heart changes cause the electrocardiogram (ECG) of a normal, healthy aged person to be slightly different than the ECG of a healthy younger adult. Abnormal rhythms (arrhythmias) such as atrial fibrillation are common in older people, which may be caused by heart disease.

A slight increase in the size of the heart, especially the left ventricle, is not uncommon. The heart wall thickens, so the amount of blood that the chamber can hold may actually decrease despite the increased overall heart size. The heart may fill more slowly.

Blood Vessels

The main artery from the heart (aorta) becomes thicker, stiffer, and less flexible. This is probably related to changes in the connective tissue of the blood vessel wall. This makes the blood pressure higher and makes the heart work harder, which may lead to hypertrophy (thickening of the heart muscle). The other arteries also thicken and stiffen. In general, most elderly people experience a moderate increase in blood pressure.

Receptors, called baroreceptors, monitor the blood pressure and make changes to help maintain a fairly constant blood pressure when a person changes positions or activities. The baroreceptors become less sensitive with aging. This may explain the relatively common finding of orthostatic hypotension, a condition in which the blood pressure falls when a person goes from lying or sitting to standing, resulting in dizziness.

The wall of the capillaries thickens slightly. This may cause a slightly slower rate of exchange of nutrients and wastes.

Blood

The blood itself changes slightly with age. Aging causes a normal reduction in total body water. As part of this, there is less fluid in the bloodstream, so blood volume decreases.

The number of red blood cells (and correspondingly, the hemoglobin and hematocrit levels) are reduced. This contributes to fatigue. Most of the white blood cells stay at the same levels, although certain white blood cells important to immunity (lymphocytes) decrease in number and ability to fight off bacteria. This reduces the ability to resist infection.

Effect of Changes

Under normal circumstances, the heart continues to adequately supply all parts of the body. However, an aging heart may be slightly less able to tolerate increased workloads, because changes reduce this extra pumping ability (reserve heart function).

Some of the things that can increase heart workload include illness, infections, emotional stress, injuries, extreme physical exertion, and certain medications.

Common Problems

- Heart and blood vessel diseases are fairly common in older people. Common disorders include high blood pressure and orthostatic hypotension.

- Arteriosclerosis (hardening of the arteries) is very common. Fatty plaque deposits inside the blood vessels cause it to narrow and can totally block blood vessels.

- Coronary artery disease is fairly common.

- Angina (chest pain caused by temporarily reduced blood flow to the heart muscle), shortness of breath with exertion and heart attack can result from coronary artery disease.

- Abnormal heart rhythms (arrhythmias) of various types can occur.

- Heart failure is also very common in the elderly. In people older than seventy-five, heart failure occurs ten times more often than in younger adults.

- Valve diseases are fairly common. Aortic stenosis, or narrowing of the aortic valve, is the most common valve disease in the elderly.

- Anemia may occur, possibly related to malnutrition, chronic infections, blood loss from the gastrointestinal tract, or as a complication of other diseases or medications.

- Transient ischemic attacks (TIA) or strokes can occur if blood flow to the brain is disrupted.

Other problems with the heart and blood vessels include the following:

- Peripheral vascular disease, resulting in claudication (intermittent pain in the legs with walking)

- Varicose veins

- Blood clots:
  - Thrombophlebitis
  - Deep vein thrombosis

Prevention

You can help your circulatory system (heart and blood vessels). Heart disease risk factors that you have some control over include high blood pressure, cholesterol levels, diabetes, obesity, and smoking.

Eat a heart-healthy diet with reduced amounts of saturated fat and cholesterol, and control your weight. Follow your healthcare provider's recommendations for treatment of high blood pressure, high choles-terol, or diabetes. Minimize or stop smoking.

Moderate exercise is one of the best things you can do to keep your heart, and the rest of your body, healthy. Consult with your healthcare provider before beginning a new exercise program. Exercise moder-ately and within your capabilities, but do it regularly.

People who exercise usually have less body fat and smoke less than people who do not exercise. They also tend to have fewer blood pres-sure problems and less heart disease.

Exercise may help prevent obesity and helps people with diabetes control their blood sugar.

Exercise may help you maintain your maximum abilities as much as possible and reduces stress.

Section 39.2

High Blood Pressure

Reprinted from the National Institute on Aging,
National Institutes of Health, July 2004.

You can have high blood pressure, or hypertension, and still feel just fine. That's because high blood pressure does not cause symptoms that you can see or feel. But high blood pressure, sometimes called "the silent killer," is a major health problem. If not treated, it can lead to stroke, heart disease, eye problems, or kidney failure. The good news is that there are ways you can prevent high blood pressure. And, if you already have high blood pressure, there are ways to control it and prevent its complications.

What Is Blood Pressure?

When your doctor checks your blood pressure and tells you the result, she or he will say two numbers. The numbers are written one above, or before, the other. The first, or top, number is your systolic pressure. This tells you how much the blood flowing through your blood vessels pushes against the vessel walls as your heart beats. The second, or bottom, number measures the pressure while the heart relaxes between beats. This is the diastolic pressure. If your blood pressure is normal, your systolic pressure is less than 120 and your diastolic pressure is less than 80—for example, 119/79.

Do You Have High Blood Pressure?

One reason to have regular checkups by your doctor is to check your blood pressure. If you have only a slightly higher reading—such as a top number between 120 and 139 or the bottom number between 80 and 89, you have prehypertension. You may be at risk for developing high blood pressure. Your healthcare provider will probably want you to make changes in your daily habits to try and lower those numbers.

Your doctor will say your blood pressure is high when it measures 140/90 or higher at two or more checkups. He or she may also ask you to check your blood pressure at home at different times of the day. If the numbers are still high after several checks, your healthcare provider will probably suggest medicine, changes in your diet, and exercise.

What If Just the First Number Is High?

For older people, the first number (systolic) often is high (greater than 140), but the second number (diastolic) is normal (less than 90). This problem is called isolated systolic hypertension. Isolated systolic hypertension is the most common form of high blood pressure in older people.

Isolated systolic hypertension can lead to serious health problems. It should be treated in the same way as regular high blood pressure. If your systolic pressure is over 140, ask your doctor how you can lower it.

Can You Prevent or Control High Blood Pressure?

More than half of Americans over age sixty have high blood pressure. But, that does not mean it is part of normal aging. Try these healthy habits to help you control or prevent high blood pressure:

- **Keep a healthy weight:** Being overweight adds to your risk of high blood pressure. Ask your doctor if you need to lose weight.

- **Exercise every day:** Moderate exercise can lower your risk of heart disease. Try to exercise at least thirty minutes a day, five days a week or more. Check with your doctor before starting a new exercise plan if you have a long-term health problem or if you are a man over forty or a woman over fifty.

- **Eat more fruits, vegetables, whole grains, and low-fat dairy foods:** A healthy diet is important. To control high blood pressure, eat a diet rich in these foods. Make sure you are getting enough potassium. Fresh fruits and vegetables are high in potassium. If using packaged foods, read the nutrition labels to choose those that have more potassium.

- **Cut down on salt and sodium:** Most Americans eat more salt and sodium than they need. A low-salt diet might help lower your blood pressure. Talk with your doctor about your salt intake.

- **Drink less alcohol:** Drinking alcohol can affect your blood pressure. The effect is different depending on body size. As a general rule, men shouldn't have more than two drinks a day; women not more than one drink a day.

- **Follow your doctor's orders:** If lifestyle changes alone do not control your high blood pressure, your doctor may tell you to take blood pressure pills. You may need to take your medicine for the rest of your life. If you have questions about it, talk to your doctor.

High Blood Pressure Facts

If you have high blood pressure, remember the following facts:

- High blood pressure may not make you feel sick, but it is serious. See a doctor to treat it.

- You can lower your blood pressure by changing your daily habits and, if needed, by taking medicine. If you need to take high blood pressure medicine, lifestyle changes may help lower the dose you need and reduce side effects.

- Are you already taking blood pressure medicine and your blood pressure is less than 120/80? That's good. It means the lifestyle changes and medicine are working. But if another doctor asks if you have high blood pressure, the answer is still "yes, but it is being treated."

- Tell your doctor about all the drugs you take. Don't forget to mention over-the-counter drugs, vitamins, and dietary supplements.

They may affect your blood pressure. They also can change how well your blood pressure medicine works.

- Blood pressure pills should be taken at the same time each day. For example, take your medicine in the morning with breakfast or in the evening after brushing your teeth. If you miss a dose, do not double the dose the next day. Call your doctor to find out what to do.

- If you have high blood pressure, test it at home between check-ups. Ask your doctor, the nurse, or your pharmacist to show you how. Make sure you are seated with your feet on the floor and your back has something to lean against. Relax quietly for five minutes before checking your blood pressure. Your arm should be resting on a support at the level of your heart. Keep a list of the results to share with the doctor, physician's assistant, or nurse.

Section 39.3

Spider and Varicose Veins

What are spider (telangiectatic) and varicose veins?

Spider veins are formed by the dilation of a small group of blood vessels located close to the surface of the skin. Although they can appear anywhere on the body, spider veins are most commonly found on the face and legs. They usually pose no health hazard, but may produce a dull aching in the legs after prolonged standing and indicate more severe venous disease.

Varicose veins are abnormally swollen or enlarged blood vessels caused by a weakening in the vein's wall. They can be harmful to a patient's health because they may be associated with the development of one or more of the following conditions: phlebitis or inflamed, tender vein; thrombosis or a clot in the vein; and venous stasis ulcers or open sores from inadequate tissue oxygen and fluid retention.

Who develops spider and varicose veins?

The exact cause of spider and varicose veins is unknown, although heredity, pregnancy, and hormonal influences are believed to be primary factors contributing to both conditions. More than 40 percent of women have some form of varicose conditions, with an increasing incidence of venous disease as one gets older, so that up to 80 percent of women have some form of venous disease by age eighty. Slightly more women than men have varicose and telangiectatic leg veins.

What is sclerotherapy?

Sclerotherapy is considered the gold standard treatment for removing spider and some varicose leg veins. It is a very cost-effective procedure that seldom leaves a scar or produces adverse effects. It is typically performed on an outpatient basis by a dermasurgeon. A concentrated saline or specially developed chemical solution is injected with a very small needle into the spider or varicose vein. The solution causes the vein to close up or collapse and become scar tissue that is eventually absorbed by the body. The work of carrying the blood is shifted to other healthy blood vessels nearby.

Sclerotherapy generally requires multiple treatment sessions. One to three injections are usually required to effectively treat any vein. The same area should not be retreated for four to six weeks to allow for complete healing, although other areas may undergo treatment during this time. Many dermasurgeons have found that treating all abnormal veins in one session gives the best results.

Post-treatment therapy includes wearing bandages and support hose for two days to three weeks (most commonly one week) following treatment. Walking and moderate exercise also helps speed recovery. Although sclerotherapy works for existing spider and varicose veins, it does not prevent new ones from developing, but may decrease this risk.

Are there side effects or complications?

Most patients report few, if any, minor side effects, which usually disappear in time. Temporary reactions can include a slight swelling of the leg or foot, minor bruising, pigmentation, the temporary appearance of new blood vessels, redness, and mild soreness.

What are other treatments for vein conditions?

Laser surgery: Laser and intense pulsed light (IPL) therapy may be effective for certain leg veins and facial blood vessels. The heat from the high-intensity laser or IPL beam selectively destroys the abnormal veins.

Electrodesiccation: The veins are sealed off with the application of electrical current. The treatment may leave scars.

Surgical ligation, and stripping and intravascular laser or radiofrequency ablation: Certain varicose veins may require an in-hospital procedure, usually performed by a vascular surgeon, which involves making an incision in the skin and either tying off or removing the damaged blood vessel. This procedure has been mostly replaced by intravascular laser or radiofrequency ablation of varicose veins. Intravascular laser or radiofrequency ablation, pioneered by dermasurgeons, is performed entirely under local anesthesia. A laser fiber or radiofrequency catheter is inserted into the abnormal vein, which is then sealed closed by thermal energy. Patients are awake during the procedure and can resume almost all normal activities immediately after the procedure.

Ambulatory phlebectomy: Removal of undesired veins through a series of tiny incisions along the path of an enlarged vein. This procedure, pioneered by dermasurgeons, is performed entirely under local anesthesia with patients being able to resume nearly all normal activities immediately after the procedure.

Combined approaches: Your dermasurgeon may utilize a combination of techniques and technologies to provide an optimal treatment program for your individual condition and lifestyle.

Chapter 40

Changes Affecting
the Bones and Joints

Chapter Contents

Section 40.1

Aging Changes in the
Bones, Muscles, and Joints

Excerpted from "Aging Changes in the Bones-Muscles-Joints," © 2007
A.D.A.M., Inc. Reprinted with permission.

Changes in posture and gait are as universally associated with aging as changes in the skin and hair.

The skeleton provides support and structure to the body. Joints are the areas where bones come together. They allow the skeleton to be flexible for movement. In a joint, bones do not directly contact each other. Instead, they are cushioned by cartilage, membranes, and fluid.

Muscles provide the force and strength to move the body. Coordination, although directed by the brain, is affected by changes in the muscles and joints. Changes in the posture and gait, weakness, and slowed movement are caused by changes in the muscles, joints, and bones.

Aging Changes

Bone mass or density is lost as people age, especially in women after menopause. The bones lose calcium and other minerals.

The spine is made up of bones called vertebrae. Between each bone is a gel-like cushion (intervertebral disk). The trunk becomes shorter as the disks gradually lose fluid and become thinner.

In addition, vertebrae lose some of their mineral content, making each bone thinner. The spinal column becomes curved and compressed (packed together). Bone spurs, caused by aging and overall use of the spine, may also form on the vertebrae.

The shoulder blades (scapulae) and other bones may become porous—on an x-ray they may look "moth-eaten." The foot arches become less pronounced, contributing to slight loss of height.

The long bones of the arms and legs, although more brittle because of mineral losses, do not change length. This makes the arms and legs look longer when compared to the shortened trunk.

The joints become stiffer and less flexible. Fluid in the joints may decrease, and the cartilage may begin to rub together and erode. Minerals may deposit in some joints (calcification). This is common in the shoulder.

Hip and knee joints may begin to lose structure (degenerative changes). The finger joints lose cartilage and the bones thicken slightly. Finger joint changes are more common in women and may be hereditary.

Some joints, such as the ankle, typically experience little change with aging.

Lean body mass decreases, caused in part by loss of muscle tissue (atrophy). The rate and extent of muscle changes seems to be genetically determined. Muscle changes often begin in the twenties in men and the forties in women.

Lipofuscin (an age-related pigment) and fat are deposited in muscle tissue. The muscle fibers shrink. Muscle tissue is replaced more slowly, and lost muscle tissue may be replaced with a tough fibrous tissue. This is most noticeable in the hands, which may appear thin and bony.

Muscle tissue changes, combined with normal aging changes in the nervous system, cause muscles to have reduced tone and contractility. Muscles may become rigid with age and may lose tone even if exercised regularly.

Effect of Changes

Bones become more brittle and may break more easily. Height decreases, primarily caused by shortening of the trunk and spine.

Inflammation, pain, stiffness, and deformity may result from breakdown of the joint structures. Almost all elderly people are affected by joint changes, ranging from minor stiffness to severe arthritis.

The posture may become progressively stooped (bent) and the knees and hips more flexed. The neck may become tilted, and the shoulders may narrow while the pelvis, on the other hand, may become wider.

Movement slows and may become limited. The walking pattern (gait) becomes slower and shorter. Walking may become unsteady, and there is less arm swinging. Fatigue occurs more readily, and overall energy may be reduced.

Strength and endurance change. Loss of muscle mass reduces strength. However, endurance may be enhanced by changes in the muscle fibers. Aging athletes with healthy hearts and lungs may find that performance improves in events that require endurance, and decreases slightly in events that require short bursts of high-speed performance.

Common Problems

Osteoporosis is a common problem, especially for older women. Broken bones occur more readily, and compression fractures of the vertebrae can cause pain and reduce mobility.

Muscle weakness contributes to fatigue, weakness, and reduced activity tolerance. Joint problems are extremely common. This may be anything from mild stiffness to debilitating arthritis.

Injury risk is greater because of falls related to gait changes, instability, and loss of balance.

Some elderly people have reduced reflexes. This is most often caused by changes in the muscles and tendons rather than changes in the nerves. Decreased knee jerk or ankle jerk is not unexpected.

Some changes, such as a positive Babinski reflex, are always considered abnormal.

Involuntary movements (muscle tremors and fine movements called fasciculations) are more common in the elderly. Inactive or immobile elderly people may experience weakness or abnormal sensations (paresthesias).

Muscle contractures may occur in those unable to move voluntarily or to have their muscles stretched through exercise. Restless leg syndrome may occur.

Prevention

Exercise is one of the best ways to slow or prevent problems with the muscles, joints, and bones. A moderate exercise program can help you maintain strength and flexibility. Exercise helps the bones to remain strong.

Consult with your healthcare provider before beginning a new exercise program.

A well-balanced diet with adequate amounts of calcium is important. Women need to be especially careful to get enough calcium as they age. Postmenopausal women need 1,200–1,500 mg of calcium per day. If you have osteoporosis, talk to your doctor about prescription treatments.

Section 40.2

Arthritis: Frequently Asked Questions

Excerpted from "Arthritis," NIH Senior Health, National
Institutes of Health, August 15, 2006.

What is arthritis?

Arthritis literally means joint inflammation, but it is often used
to identify a group of more than one hundred rheumatic diseases that
may cause pain, stiffness, and swelling in the joints and in areas close
to the joints. Joints are places in the body where two bones meet.

How many people have arthritis?

More than forty million people in the United States have some form
of arthritis, and many have chronic pain that limits daily activity.
Osteoarthritis is by far the most common form of arthritis, affecting
more than twenty million people.

Rheumatoid arthritis is the most disabling form of arthritis. More
than two million people have this disease. Gout occurs in approximately
840 out of every 100,000 people. It is rare in children and young adults.

What is osteoarthritis?

Osteoarthritis is the most common form of arthritis among older
people. It affects hands, low back, neck, and weight-bearing joints such
as knees, hips, and feet.

Osteoarthritis occurs when cartilage, the tissue that cushions the
ends of the bones within the joints, breaks down and wears away. This
causes bones to rub together, causing pain, swelling, and loss of motion of the joint.

How common is osteoarthritis in older adults?

The chance of developing osteoarthritis increases with age. By age
sixty-five, half of the population has x-ray evidence of osteoarthritis
in at least one joint, most often in the hips, knees, or fingers.

What causes osteoarthritis?

Osteoarthritis often results from years of wear and tear on joints. This wear and tear mostly affects the cartilage, the tissue that cushions the ends of bones within the joint. Osteoarthritis occurs when the cartilage begins to fray, wear away, and decay.

Putting too much stress on a joint that has been repeatedly injured may lead to the development of osteoarthritis, too. A person who is overweight is more likely to develop osteoarthritis because of too much stress on the joints. Also, improper joint alignment may lead to the development of osteoarthritis.

How can I reduce my chances of developing osteoarthritis?

Maintaining a healthy weight, avoiding injury, and engaging in moderate daily physical activity are all ways to decrease your chances of developing osteoarthritis.

What are some common symptoms of osteoarthritis?

Common symptoms of osteoarthritis include joint pain, swelling, or tenderness; stiffness after getting out of bed; and a crunching feeling or sound of bone rubbing on bone. Not everyone with osteoarthritis develops symptoms. In fact, only a third of people with x-ray evidence of osteoarthritis report pain or other symptoms.

How is osteoarthritis diagnosed?

No single test can diagnose osteoarthritis. When a person feels pain in his or her joints, it may or may not be osteoarthritis.

The doctor will use a combination of tests to try to determine if osteoarthritis is causing the symptoms. These may include a medical history, a physical examination, x-rays, and laboratory tests. A patient's attitudes, daily activities, and levels of anxiety or depression have a lot to do with how much the symptoms of osteoarthritis affect day-to-day living.

Is there a cure for osteoarthritis?

There is no cure for osteoarthritis and no way to reverse the joint damage once it occurs. However, current treatments can relieve symptoms.

Exercise is one of the best treatments. Exercise can improve mood and outlook, decrease pain, and assist in maintaining a healthy weight.

Warm towels, hot packs, or a warm bath or shower can provide temporary pain relief. Medications such as nonsteroidal anti-inflammatory drugs, or NSAIDs, help reduce pain and inflammation that result from osteoarthritis.

Can glucosamine and chondroitin sulfate relieve symptoms of osteoarthritis?

For some people, glucosamine and chondroitin sulfate may help relieve the symptoms of osteoarthritis. Scientific studies have shown that these supplements may have some benefit for people with osteoarthritis. However, the effectiveness of these supplements is still under investigation.

The NIH is currently funding the Glucosamine and Chondroitin Arthritis Intervention Trial, or GAIT, to test whether or not glucosamine or chondroitin have a beneficial effect for people with knee osteoarthritis. The results of the recently completed first phase of the study indicate that these supplements have a limited effectiveness for most patients with osteoarthritis.

What is rheumatoid arthritis?

Rheumatoid arthritis is an inflammatory disease that causes pain, swelling, stiffness, and loss of function in the joints. It can cause mild to severe symptoms.

People with rheumatoid arthritis may feel sick, tired, and sometimes feverish. Sometimes rheumatoid arthritis attacks tissue in the skin, lungs, eyes, and blood vessels.

The disease generally occurs in a symmetrical pattern. If one knee or hand is involved, usually the other one is, too. It can occur at any age, but often begins between ages forty and sixty. About two to three times as many women as men have rheumatoid arthritis.

What causes rheumatoid arthritis?

Scientists believe that rheumatoid arthritis results from the interaction of many factors such as genetics, hormones, and the environment. Although rheumatoid arthritis sometimes runs in families, the actual cause of rheumatoid arthritis is still unknown.

Research suggests that a person's genetic makeup is an important part of the picture, but not the whole story. Some evidence shows that infectious agents, such as viruses and bacteria, may trigger rheumatoid arthritis in people with an inherited tendency to develop the disease. The exact agent or agents, however, are not yet known.

It is important to note that rheumatoid arthritis is not contagious. A person cannot catch it from someone else.

What are some common symptoms of rheumatoid arthritis?

Rheumatoid arthritis is characterized by inflammation of the joint lining. This inflammation causes warmth, redness, swelling, and pain around the joints.

The pain of rheumatoid arthritis varies greatly from person to person. Factors that contribute to the pain include swelling within the joint, the amount of heat or redness present, or damage that has occurred within the joint.

How is rheumatoid arthritis diagnosed?

Rheumatoid arthritis can be difficult to diagnose in its early stages because the full range of symptoms develops over time, and only a few symptoms may be present in the early stages.

As part of the diagnosis, your doctor will look for symptoms such as swelling, warmth, pain, and limitations in joint motion throughout your body. Your doctor may ask you questions about the intensity of your pain symptoms, how often they occur, and what makes the pain better or worse.

There is no single, definitive test for rheumatoid arthritis. One common test is for rheumatoid factor, an antibody that is eventually present in the blood of most rheumatoid arthritis patients. An antibody is a special protein made by the immune system that normally helps fight foreign substances in the body. Not all people with rheumatoid arthritis test positive for rheumatoid factor, however, especially early in the disease.

Another test is the citrulline antibody test. Other common tests include one called the erythrocyte sedimentation rate that indicates the presence of inflammation in the body, a white blood cell count, and a blood test for anemia.

X-rays are often used to determine the degree of joint destruction. They are not useful in the early stages of rheumatoid arthritis before bone damage is evident, but they can be used later to monitor the progression of the disease.

How is rheumatoid arthritis treated?

Medication, exercise, and, in some cases, surgery are common treatments for this disease. Most people who have rheumatoid arthritis take medications. Some drugs only provide relief for pain; others reduce inflammation.

People with rheumatoid arthritis can also benefit from exercise, but they need to maintain a good balance between rest and exercise. They should get rest when the disease is active and get more exercise when it is not.

In some cases, a doctor will recommend surgery to restore function or relieve pain in a damaged joint. Several types of surgery are available to patients with severe joint damage. Joint replacement and tendon reconstruction are examples.

What are some nondrug therapies that can help people with rheumatoid arthritis?

Both rest and exercise can help people with rheumatoid arthritis. Rest helps reduce active joint inflammation and pain and fights tiredness. Exercise can help people sleep well, reduce pain, and maintain a positive attitude. An overall nutritious diet with the right amount of calories, protein, and calcium is important.

Some people find that using a splint for a short time around a painful joint reduces pain and swelling by supporting the joint and letting it rest. Assistive devices may help reduce stress and lessen pain in the joints. Examples include zipper pullers and aids to help with moving in and out of chairs and beds.

What kind of surgery is available for people with rheumatoid arthritis or osteoarthritis?

Several types of surgery, including joint replacement and tendon reconstruction, are available to people with rheumatoid arthritis and osteoarthritis. A doctor may perform surgery to smooth out, fuse, or reposition bones, or to replace joints.

The purpose of these procedures is to reduce pain, improve joint function, and improve a person's ability to perform activities of daily living. For people with arthritis, surgery is one way to help relieve pain and disability.

If you are considering surgery for osteoarthritis or rheumatoid arthritis, there are important factors to discuss with your doctor beforehand. These include your age and occupation, the extent of your disability and pain, and how much the disease interferes with your everyday life.

Today, most surgery for osteoarthritis involves replacing the hip or knee joint. Surgeons may replace affected joints with artificial ones called prostheses.

What is gout?

Gout is one of the most painful rheumatic diseases. It occurs when needle-like crystals of uric acid build up in connective tissue, in the joint space between two bones, or in both.

Sometime during the course of the disease, gout will affect the big toe in about 75 percent of patients. Gout frequently affects joints in the lower part of the body such as knees, ankles, or toes.

What causes gout?

Researchers have discovered several key risk factors for developing gout. In addition to inherited traits, diet, weight, and alcohol play a role in the development of gout. Up to 8 percent of people with gout have a family history of the disease.

Most people with gout have too much uric acid in their blood, a condition called hyperuricemia. Uric acid is a substance that results from the breakdown of purines, which are part of all human tissue and are found in many foods. Hyperuricemia occurs when high levels of uric acid build up in the bloodstream.

What are some common symptoms of gout?

Gout frequently first attacks the joints in the big toe. The affected joint may become swollen, red, or warm. Attacks usually occur at night.

How is gout diagnosed?

To confirm a diagnosis of gout, the doctor inserts a needle into the inflamed joint and draws a sample of synovial fluid, the substance that lubricates a joint. A laboratory technician places some of the fluid on a slide and looks for uric acid crystals under a microscope. If uric acid crystals are found in the fluid surrounding the joint, the person usually has gout.

What are the most common treatments for an acute attack of gout?

Physicians often prescribe high doses of nonsteroidal anti-inflammatory drugs, or NSAIDs, or steroids for a sudden attack of gout. NSAIDs are taken by mouth and corticosteroids are either taken by mouth or injected into the affected joint. Patients often begin to improve within a few hours of treatment, and the attack usually goes away completely within a week or so.

Section 40.3

Osteoporosis: Frequently Asked Questions

Excerpted from "Osteoporosis," NIH Senior Health,
National Institutes of Health, January 3, 2006.

What is osteoporosis?

Osteoporosis is a disease that thins and weakens the bones to the point that they break easily. Women and men with osteoporosis most often break bones in the hip, spine, and wrist, but osteoporosis can be the cause of bone fractures anywhere.

Why is osteoporosis called "the silent disease"?

Osteoporosis is often called "the silent disease" because the bone loss occurs without symptoms. People may not know that they have osteoporosis until a sudden strain, bump, or fall causes a bone to break.

How many people have osteoporosis?

In the United States, ten million people already have osteoporosis. Millions more have low bone mass, or osteopenia, placing them at increased risk for the disease. Osteoporosis can strike at any age, but it is most common among older people, especially older women. Eighty percent of the ten million Americans with osteoporosis are women.

Why are women at greater risk for osteoporosis than men?

Women have smaller bones, and they lose bone more rapidly than men because of hormone changes that occur after menopause. Therefore, women are at higher risk for osteoporosis.

What other factors can increase one's chances of developing osteoporosis?

The older you are, the greater your risk of osteoporosis. Having a family history of the disease can also increase one's risk. Other factors such as diets inadequate in calcium and vitamin D, smoking, ethnicity, and inactivity can also play a role in the development of the disease.

Can taking certain medications increase my chances of developing osteoporosis?

Yes. Some commonly used medicines can result in bone loss and increase your risk of osteoporosis and fracture. These include a type of steroid called glucocorticoids, which are used to control diseases such as arthritis and asthma; some antiseizure drugs; some medicines that treat a common gynecological condition known as endometriosis; and some cancer drugs. Using too much thyroid hormone for an underactive thyroid can also be a problem.

How much calcium and vitamin D do I need each day?

Calcium and vitamin D are important nutrients for bone health. People over fifty should get 1,200 mg of calcium daily. People aged fifty-one to seventy should have 400 IU, or international units, of vitamin D daily and people over seventy should have 600 IU.

How can I be sure I get enough calcium and vitamin D in my diet?

Although foods rich in calcium are believed to be the best source, most American diets do not contain enough calcium. Fortunately, calcium-fortified foods and calcium supplements can help fill the gap, ensuring that you meet your daily calcium requirement.

Milk fortified with vitamin D is a good source of vitamin D. In some cases, supplements may be necessary to meet the daily requirements.

Can I get all the vitamin D I need from sunshine?

Your body makes vitamin D in the skin when it is exposed to sunlight and some people get all the vitamin D they need this way. However, many older people, especially those who are indoors most of the time or live in northern areas, do not get enough vitamin D.

Also, during the winter months, many people do not get enough vitamin D. Many older people will need a dietary supplement to reach recommended levels of vitamin D.

Which exercises are best for bone health?

Exercise can make bones and muscles stronger and help slow the rate of bone loss. It is also a way to stay active and mobile. Weight-bearing exercises, done three to four times a week, are best for preventing osteoporosis. Walking, jogging, playing tennis, and dancing are examples of weight-bearing exercises. Strengthening and balance exercises may help you avoid falls and reduce your chances of breaking a bone.

If I have osteoporosis or low bone mass, what are some tips for safe exercising?

Proper posture and body mechanics are important when doing exercises. Activities that involve twisting your spine or bending forward from the waist, such as conventional sit-ups and toe touches, should be avoided.

Does osteoporosis have any warning signs?

Osteoporosis does not have any symptoms until a fracture occurs. Some people may be unaware that they have already experienced one or more spine fractures. Height loss of one inch or more may be the first sign that someone has experienced spinal fractures due to osteoporosis.

People who have experienced a fracture are at high risk of having another one. A fracture over the age of fifty or several fractures before that age may be a warning sign that a person has already developed osteoporosis. Any fracture in an older person should be followed up for suspicion of osteoporosis.

How is osteoporosis diagnosed?

The test used to diagnose osteoporosis is called a bone density test. This test is a measure of how strong—or dense—your bones are and can help your doctor predict your risk for having a fracture. Bone density tests are painless, safe, and require no preparation on your part.

Are there different types of bone density tests?

Some bone density tests measure the strength of the hip, spine, or wrist, which are the bones that break most often in people with osteoporosis. Other tests measure bone in the heel or hand.

One way to measure bone density is by a dual x-ray absorptiometry (DXA) scan, which estimates what your risk for a fracture is. It could show that you have normal bone density. Or, it could show that you have osteopenia, or even osteoporosis.

Who should get a bone density test?

The United States Preventive Services Task Force recommends that women aged sixty-five and older be screened for osteoporosis, as well as women aged sixty and older who are at increased risk for an osteoporosis-related fracture. However, the decision whether to have a bone density test is best made between a patient and his or her doctor.

Is there a cure for osteoporosis?

Although there is no cure for osteoporosis, it can be treated. The goal of treatment is to prevent fractures. Along with making lifestyle changes, there are several medication options.

What type of doctor specializes in osteoporosis?

If your physician does not specialize in osteoporosis, he or she can refer you to a specialist. There is not one type of doctor who cares for people with osteoporosis. Endocrinologists, rheumatologists, geriatricians, and internists are just a few of the doctors who are likely to specialize in the care of people with osteoporosis.

What treatments are available for osteoporosis?

Several medications are approved by the Food and Drug Administration for the treatment of osteoporosis. Since all medications have side effects, it is important to talk to your doctor about which medication is right for you.

Alendronate, risedronate, and ibandronate are from a class of drugs called bisphosphonates that slow bone loss, reduce fracture risk, and, in some cases, increase bone density.

Estrogen is approved for treating menopausal symptoms and osteoporosis. But because breast cancer, strokes, blood clots, and heart attacks may be increased in some women who take estrogen, women should take the lowest effective dose for the shortest period possible.

Raloxifene is approved for use in postmenopausal women. It is from a class of drugs called SERMs, or selective estrogen receptor modulators. Raloxifene slows bone loss and reduces the risk of fractures in the spine.

Calcitonin is approved for the treatment of osteoporosis in women who are at least five years past menopause. It is a hormone produced in the thyroid gland that slows bone loss and reduces the risk of spine fractures.

Teriparatide, a form of human parathyroid hormone, is approved for use in postmenopausal women and men who are at high risk of fracture. Given daily as an injection, it increases bone density and reduces the risk of spine and other fractures.

None of these medications have been approved for children.

Chapter 41

Prostate Problems

What is the prostate?

The prostate is part of a man's sex organs. It's about the size of a walnut and surrounds the tube called the urethra, located just below the bladder.

The urethra has two jobs: to carry urine from the bladder when you urinate and to carry semen during a sexual climax, or ejaculation. Semen is a combination of sperm plus fluid that the prostate adds.

What are prostate problems?

For men under fifty, the most common prostate problem is prostatitis.

For men over fifty, the most common prostate problem is prostate enlargement. This condition is also called benign prostatic hyperplasia or BPH. Older men are at risk for prostate cancer as well, but this disease is much less common than BPH.

What is prostatitis?

"Prostatitis" means that the prostate is inflamed; it could be swollen, red, and warm. If you have prostatitis, you may have a burning

Reprinted from "What I Need to Know about Prostate Problems," National Institute of Diabetes and Digestive and Kidney Diseases, National Institutes of Health, NIH Publication No. 05-4806, November 2004.

feeling when you urinate, or you may have to urinate more often. You may have a fever or just feel tired.

Inflammation in any part of the body is usually a sign that the body is fighting germs or repairing an injury. Some kinds of prostatitis are caused by germs, or bacteria. If you have bacterial prostatitis, your doctor can look through a microscope and find bacteria in a sample of your urine. Your doctor can then give you an antibiotic medicine to fight the bacteria.

If you keep getting infections, you may have a defect in your prostate that allows bacteria to grow. This defect can usually be corrected by surgery.

Most of the time, doctors don't find any bacteria in men with prostatitis. If you have urinary problems, the doctor will look for other possible causes, such as a kidney stone or cancer.

If no other causes are found, the doctor may decide that you have a condition called nonbacterial prostatitis.

Antibiotics will not help nonbacterial prostatitis. You may have to work with your doctor to find a treatment that's good for you. Changing your diet or taking warm baths may help. Your doctor may give you a medicine called an alpha blocker to relax the muscle tissue in the prostate. No single solution works for everyone with this condition.

What is prostate enlargement, or BPH?

If you're a man over fifty and have started having problems urinating, the reason could be an enlarged prostate, or BPH. As men get older, their prostate keeps growing. As it grows, it squeezes the urethra. Since urine travels from the bladder through the urethra, the pressure from the enlarged prostate may affect bladder control.

If you have BPH, you may have one or more of these problems:

- A frequent and urgent need to urinate. You may get up several times a night to go to the bathroom.

- Trouble starting a urine stream. Even though you feel you have to rush to get to the bathroom, you find it hard to start urinating.

- A weak stream of urine.

- A small amount of urine each time you go.

- The feeling that you still have to go, even when you have just finished urinating.

- Leaking or dribbling.

- Small amounts of blood in your urine.

You may barely notice that you have one or two of these symptoms, or you may feel as though urination problems have taken over your life.

Is BPH a sign of cancer?

No. It's true that some men with prostate cancer also have BPH, but that doesn't mean that the two conditions are always linked. Most men with BPH don't develop prostate cancer. However, because the early symptoms are the same for both conditions, you should see a doctor to evaluate these symptoms.

Is BPH a serious disease?

By itself, BPH is not a serious condition, unless the symptoms are so bothersome that you can't enjoy life. But BPH can lead to serious problems. One problem is urinary tract infections.

If you can't urinate at all, you should get medical help right away. Sometimes this happens suddenly to men after they take an over-the-counter cold or allergy medicine.

In rare cases, BPH and its constant urination problems can lead to kidney damage.

What tests will my doctor order?

Several tests help the doctor identify the problem and decide on the best treatment:

- **Digital rectal exam:** This exam is usually the first test done. The doctor inserts a gloved finger into the rectum and feels the part of the prostate that sits next to it. This exam gives the doctor a general idea of the size and condition of the prostate.

- **Blood test:** The doctor may want to test a sample of your blood to look for prostate-specific antigen, or PSA. If your PSA is high, it may be a sign that you have prostate cancer. But this test isn't perfect. Many men with high PSA scores don't have prostate cancer.

- **Imaging:** The doctor may want to get a picture of your prostate using either x-rays or a sonogram. An IVP, or intravenous pyelogram, is an x-ray of the urinary tract. For an IVP, dye will be injected into a vein. Later, when the dye passes out of your blood into your urine, it will show up on the x-ray. A rectal sonogram uses a probe, inserted into the rectum, to bounce sound waves off the prostate.

- **Urine flow study:** You may be asked to urinate into a special device that measures how quickly the urine is flowing. A reduced flow may mean that you have BPH.

- **Cystoscopy:** Another way to see a problem from the inside is with a cystoscope, which is a thin tube with lenses like a microscope. The tube is inserted into the bladder through the urethra while the doctor looks through the cystoscope.

How is BPH treated?

Several treatments are available. You'll have to work with your doctor to find the one that's best for you:

- **Watchful waiting:** If your symptoms don't bother you too much, you may choose to live with them rather than take pills every day or have surgery. But you should have regular checkups to make sure your condition isn't getting worse. With watchful waiting, you can be ready to choose a treatment as soon as you need it.

- **Medicines:** In recent years, scientists have developed several medicines to shrink or relax the prostate to keep it from blocking the bladder opening.

- **Nonsurgical procedures:** A number of devices have been developed to remove parts of the prostate. These procedures can usually be done in a clinic or hospital without an overnight stay. The procedures are transurethral, which means the doctor reaches the area by going through the urethra. The doctor's devices use thin tubes inserted through the urethra to deliver controlled heat to small areas of the prostate. A gel may be applied to the urethra to prevent pain or discomfort. You won't need general drugs that make you go to sleep. These procedures are called transurethral microwave thermotherapy (TUMT) and transurethral needle ablation (TUNA).

- **Surgical treatment:** Surgery to remove a piece of the prostate can be done through the urethra or in open surgery, which requires cutting through the skin above the base of the penis. Your doctor may recommend open surgery if your prostate is especially large. The most common surgery is called transurethral resection of the prostate, or TURP. In TURP, the surgeon inserts a thin tube up the urethra and cuts away pieces of the prostate with a wire loop under direct vision through a cystoscope. TURP and open surgery both require general anesthesia and a stay in the hospital.

Is TURP the same as removing the prostate?

No. TURP and other procedures for BPH remove only enough tissue to relieve urine blockage. In a few cases, the prostate may continue to grow, and urinary problems return.

You should continue to have your prostate checked once a year even after surgery to make sure that BPH or prostate cancer has not developed.

A prostate removal, or prostatectomy, is usually done only to stop prostate cancer from spreading.

What are the side effects of prostate treatments?

Surgery for BPH may have a temporary effect on sexual function. Most men recover complete sexual function within a year after surgery. The exact length of time depends on how long you had symptoms before surgery was done and on the type of surgery. After TURP, some men will find that semen does not go out of the penis during orgasm. Instead, it goes backward into the bladder. In some cases, this condition can be treated with a drug that helps keep the bladder closed. A doctor who specializes in fertility problems may be able to help if this backward ejaculation causes a problem for a couple trying to get pregnant.

If you have any problems after treatment for a prostate condition, talk with your doctor or nurse. Erection problems and loss of bladder control can be treated, and chances are good that you can be helped.

If your prostate is removed completely to stop cancer, you're more likely to have long-lasting sexual and bladder control problems (leaking or dribbling). Your doctor may be able to use a technique that leaves the nerves around the prostate in place. This makes it easier for you to regain bladder control and sexual function. Not all men can have this technique, but most men can be helped with other medical treatments.

Hope through Research

The National Institute of Diabetes and Digestive and Kidney Diseases (NIDDK) has many research programs aimed at finding treatments for urinary disorders, including prostatitis and BPH. The Medical Therapy of Prostate Symptoms (MTOPS) program is studying the results of medical therapy used to treat thousands of men with

BPH in several research centers throughout the country. MTOPS will provide valuable information about the effectiveness and side effects of drugs being used for BPH.

Research is also under way to evaluate new approaches to surgical treatment of BPH. The Minimally Invasive Surgical Therapies (MIST) treatment group is looking at TUMT, TUNA, and other transurethral treatments for BPH that generally do not require a hospital stay. Studies are planned to assess the effectiveness of saw palmetto and other herbal remedies for this disorder.

Part Six

Menopause

Chapter 42

Understanding Menopause

Chapter Contents

Section 42.1

Perimenopause

Excerpted from "Perimenopause," National Women's Health
Information Center, March 2006.

What is perimenopause?

Perimenopause is the time leading up to menopause when you start
to notice menopause-related changes—plus the year after menopause.
During perimenopause, your ovaries start to shut down, making less
of certain hormones (estrogen and progesterone), and you begin to lose
the ability to become pregnant. This change is a natural part of aging that signals the ending of your reproductive years.

When does perimenopause start?

Women normally go through perimenopause between ages forty-
five and fifty-five, but some women start perimenopause earlier, even
in their thirties. When perimenopause starts, and how long it lasts,
varies from woman to woman. You will likely notice menopause-related
symptoms, such as changes in periods.

What are some of the signs and symptoms?

Menopause affects every woman differently. Your only symptom
may be your period stopping. You may have other symptoms, too. Many
symptoms at this time of life are because of just getting older. But
some are due to approaching menopause. Menopause-related symptoms you might have during perimenopause include the following:

- Changes in pattern of periods (can be shorter or longer, lighter
  or heavier, more or less time between periods)

- Hot flashes (sudden rush of heat in upper body)

- Night sweats (hot flashes that happen while you sleep), often
  followed by a chill

- Trouble sleeping through the night (with or without night sweats)

- Vaginal dryness

- Mood changes, feeling crabby (probably because of lack of sleep)

- Trouble focusing, feeling mixed-up or confused

- Hair loss or thinning on your head, more hair growth on your face

When you visit your doctor, take along a diary about what's happening with your period. For a few months before your visit, record when your period starts and stops each month, and indicate whether it is light or heavy. Also note any other symptoms you have.

Is there any treatment for perimenopause? What can I do?

Some women take oral contraceptives (birth control pills, or "the pill") to ease perimenopausal symptoms—even if they don't need them for birth control. These hormone treatments of combined estrogen and progestin can help keep your periods regular plus ease all the symptoms listed above. Talk with your doctor to see if this option is for you. If you are over thirty-five, you should not take birth control pills if you smoke or have a history of blood clots. You need a prescription to get oral contraceptives.

After a woman reaches menopause, if she still needs treatment for menopause symptoms, she should switch from birth control pills to menopause hormone therapy (HT). HT contains much lower doses of hormones, and thus has less risk for bad side effects.

Making some changes in your life can also help ease your symptoms and keep you healthy:

- **Eat healthy:** A healthy diet is more important now than before because your risks of osteoporosis (extreme bone loss) and heart disease go up at this stage of life. Eat lots of whole-grain foods, vegetables, and fruits. Add calcium-rich foods (milk, cheese, yogurt) or take a calcium supplement to obtain your recommended daily intake. Get adequate vitamin D from sunshine or a supplement. Avoid alcohol or caffeine, which also can trigger hot flashes in some women.

- **Get moving:** Regular exercise helps keep your weight down, helps you sleep better, makes your bones stronger, and boosts your mood. Try to get at least thirty minutes of exercise most days of the week, but let your doctor recommend what's best for you.

- **Find healthy ways to cope with stress:** Try meditation or yoga—both can help you relax, as well as handle your symptoms more easily.

Can I get pregnant while in perimenopause?

Yes, you can get pregnant until you've gone twelve months in a row without a period. Talk to your doctor about your birth control options.

Section 42.2

Menopause: A Summary

Excerpted from "Menopause," National Institute on Aging, National Institutes of Health, May 2005.

What is menopause?

Menopause is a normal part of life, just like puberty. It is the time of your last period, but symptoms can begin several years before that. And these symptoms can last for months or years after. Sometime around forty, you might notice that your period is different—how long it lasts, how much you bleed, or how often it happens may not be the same. Or, without warning, you might find yourself feeling very warm during the day or in the middle of the night. Changing levels of estrogen and progesterone, which are two female hormones made in your ovaries, might lead to these symptoms.

This time of change, called perimenopause by many women and their doctors, often begins several years before your last menstrual period. It lasts for one year after your last period, the point in time known as menopause. A full year without a period is needed before you can say you have been "through menopause." Postmenopause follows menopause and lasts the rest of your life.

Menopause doesn't usually happen before you are forty, but it can happen any time from your thirties to your mid-fifties or later. The average age is fifty-one. Smoking can lead to early menopause. Some types of surgery can bring on menopause. For example, removing your uterus (hysterectomy) before menopause will make your periods stop, but your ovaries will still make hormones. That means you could still have symptoms of menopause like hot flashes when your ovaries start to make less estrogen. But, when both ovaries are also removed (oophorectomy), menopause symptoms can start right away, no matter what your age is, because your body has lost its main supply of estrogen.

What are the signs of menopause?

Women may have different signs or symptoms at menopause. That's because estrogen is used by many parts of your body. So, changes in how much estrogen you have can cause assorted symptoms. But that doesn't mean you will have all, or even most, of them. In fact, some of the signs that happen around the time of menopause may really be a result of growing older, not changes in estrogen.

Changes in your period: This might be what you notice first. Your period may no longer be regular. How much you bleed could change. It could be lighter than normal. Or, you could have a heavier flow. Periods may be shorter or last longer. These are all normal results of changes in your reproductive system as you grow older. But, just to make sure there isn't a problem, see your doctor if:

- Your periods are coming very close together;
- You have heavy bleeding;
- You have spotting;
- Your periods are lasting more than a week.

Hot flashes: These are very common around the time of menopause because they are related to changing estrogen levels. They may last a few years after menopause. A hot flash is a sudden feeling of heat in the upper part or all of your body. Your face and neck become flushed. Red blotches may appear on your chest, back, and arms. Heavy sweating and cold shivering can follow. Flashes can be as mild as a light blush or severe enough to wake you from a sound sleep (called night sweats). Most hot flashes last between thirty seconds and ten minutes.

Problems with the vagina and bladder: Changing estrogen levels can cause your genital area to get drier and thinner. This could make sexual intercourse uncomfortable. You could have more vaginal or urinary infections. You might find it hard to hold urine long enough to get to the bathroom. Sometimes your urine might leak during exercise, sneezing, coughing, laughing, or running.

Sex: Around the time of menopause you may find that your feelings about sex have changed. You could be less interested. Or, you could feel freer and sexier after menopause. You can stop worrying about becoming pregnant after one full year without a period. But, remember you can't ever stop worrying about sexually transmitted diseases (STDs), such as human immunodeficiency virus (HIV)/AIDS or gonorrhea. If you think you might be at risk for an STD, make sure your partner uses a condom each time you have sex.

Sleep problems: You might start having trouble getting a good night's sleep. Maybe you can't fall asleep easily, or you wake too early. Night sweats might wake you up. You might have trouble falling back to sleep if you wake during the night.

Mood changes: You might find yourself more moody, irritable, or depressed around the time of menopause. It's not clear why this happens—is there is a connection between changes in estrogen levels and emotions or not? It's possible that stress, family changes such as growing children or aging parents, or always feeling tired could be causing these mood changes.

Changes in your body: You might think your body is changing. Your waist could get larger. You could lose muscle and gain fat. Your skin could get thinner. You might have memory problems, and your joints and muscles could feel stiff and achy. Are these a result of having less estrogen or just related to growing older? We don't know.

What about my heart and bones?

Two common health problems can start to happen at menopause, and you might not even notice.

Osteoporosis: Day in and day out your body is busy breaking down old bone and replacing it with new healthy bone. Estrogen helps control bone loss. So losing estrogen around the time of menopause causes women to begin to lose more bone than is replaced. In time, bones can become weak and break easily. This condition is called osteoporosis. Talk to your doctor to see if you should have a bone density test to find out if you are at risk for this problem. Your doctor can also suggest ways to prevent or treat osteoporosis.

Heart disease: After menopause, women are more likely to have heart disease. Changes in estrogen levels may be part of the cause. But, so is getting older. As you age, you may develop other problems, like high blood pressure or weight gain, that put you at greater risk for heart disease. Be sure to have your blood pressure and levels of triglycerides, fasting blood glucose, and low-density lipoprotein (LDL), high-density lipoprotein (HDL), and total cholesterol checked regularly. Talk to your healthcare provider to find out what you should do to protect your heart.

How can I stay healthy after menopause?

Staying healthy after menopause may mean making some changes in the way you live.:

- **Don't smoke:** If you do use any type of tobacco, stop—it's never too late to benefit from quitting smoking.

- **Eat a healthy diet:** One low in fat, high in fiber, with plenty of fruits, vegetables, and whole-grain foods, as well as all the important vitamins and minerals.

- **Make sure you get enough calcium and vitamin D:** In your diet or in vitamin/mineral supplements.

- **Keep a healthy weight:** Learn what your healthy weight is, and try to stay there.

- **Exercise:** Do weight-bearing exercise, such as walking, jogging, or dancing, at least three days each week for healthy bones. But try to be physically active in other ways for your general health.

Other things to remember:

- Take medicine to lower your blood pressure if your doctor prescribes it for you.

- Use a water-based vaginal lubricant (not petroleum jelly) or a vaginal estrogen cream or tablet to help with vaginal discomfort.

- Get regular pelvic and breast exams, Pap tests, and mammograms. You should also be checked for colon and rectal cancer and for skin cancer. Contact your doctor right away if you notice a lump in your breast or a mole that has changed.

Are you bothered by hot flashes? Menopause is not a disease that has to be treated. But you might need help with symptoms like hot flashes. Here are some ideas that have helped some women:

- Try to keep track of when hot flashes happen—a diary can help. You might be able to use this information to find out what triggers your flashes and then avoid it.

- When a hot flash starts, go somewhere cool.

- If night sweats wake you, try sleeping in a cool room or with a fan on.

- Dress in layers that you can take off if you get too warm.

- Use sheets and clothing that let your skin "breathe."

- Have a cold drink (water or juice) when a flash is starting.

You could also talk to your doctor about whether there are any medicines to manage hot flashes. Gabapentin, megestrol acetate, and certain antidepressants seem to be helpful to some women.

What about those lost hormones?

These days you hear a lot about whether you should use hormones to help relieve some menopause symptoms. It's hard to know what to do.

During perimenopause, some doctors suggest birth control pills to help with very heavy, frequent, or unpredictable menstrual periods. These pills might also help with symptoms like hot flashes, as well as prevent pregnancy.

As you get closer to menopause, you might be bothered more by symptoms like hot flashes, night sweats, or vaginal dryness. Your doctor might then suggest taking estrogen (as well as progesterone, if you still have a uterus). This is known as menopausal hormone therapy (MHT). Some people still call it hormone replacement therapy or HRT. Taking these hormones will probably help with menopause symptoms and prevent the bone loss that can happen at menopause. However, there is a chance your symptoms will come back when you stop MHT.

Also, menopausal hormone therapy has risks. That is why the U.S. Food and Drug Administration suggests that women who want to try MHT to manage their hot flashes or vaginal dryness use the lowest dose that works for the shortest time it's needed.

Do phytoestrogens help?

Phytoestrogens are estrogen-like substances found in some cereals, vegetables, legumes (beans), and herbs. They might work in the body like a weak form of estrogen. They might relieve some symptoms of menopause, but they could also carry risks like estrogen. We don't know. Be sure to tell your doctor if you decide to try eating a lot more foods that contain phytoestrogens or to try using an herbal supplement. Any food or over-the-counter product that you use for its drug-like effects could change how other prescribed drugs work or cause an overdose.

How do I decide what to do?

Talk to your healthcare provider for help deciding how to best manage menopause. You can see a gynecologist, geriatrician, general practitioner, or internist. Talk about your symptoms and whether they bother you. Make sure the doctor knows your medical history and your family medical history. This includes whether you are at risk for heart disease, osteoporosis, and breast cancer. Remember that your decision is never final. You can—and should—review it with your doctor during a checkup. Your needs may change, and so might what we know about menopause.

A hundred years ago life expectancy was a lot shorter. Reaching menopause then often meant that a woman's life was nearing its end. Not so now. Women are living much longer. Today, a woman turning fifty can expect to live, on average, almost thirty-two more years. You have the time and freedom to make them active, busy years. Follow a healthy lifestyle and plan to make the most of those years ahead of you!

Section 42.3

Stages of Menopause

Reprinted from "Stages of Menopause," National Women's Health Information Center, March 2006.

Menopause is only one of several stages in the reproductive life of a women. The whole menopause transition is divided into the following stages:

1. **Premature menopause:** Menopause that happens before the age of forty, whether it is natural or induced.

2. **Premenopause:** Refers to the entirety of a woman's life from her first to her last regular menstrual period. It is best defined as a time of "normal" reproductive function in a woman.

3. **Perimenopause:** Means "around menopause" and is a transitional stage of two to ten years before complete cessation of the menstrual period and is usually experienced by women from thirty-five to fifty years of age. This stage of menopause is characterized by hormone fluctuations, which cause the typical menopause symptoms, such as hot flashes.

4. **Menopause:** Represents the end stage of a natural transition in a woman's reproductive life. Menopause is the point at which estrogen and progesterone production decreases permanently to very low levels. The ovaries stop producing eggs and a woman is no longer able to get pregnant naturally.

5. **Postmenopause:** Refers to a women's time of life after menopause has occurred. It is generally believed that the postmenopausal phase begins when twelve full months have passed since the last menstrual period. From here a woman will be postmenopausal for the rest of her life.

Male Menopause

Women may not be the only ones who suffer the effects of changing hormones. Some doctors are noticing that their male patients are reporting some of the same symptoms that women experience in menopause.

Section 42.4

Premature Menopause

Reprinted from "Premature Menopause," National Women's Health Information Center, March 2006.

Premature menopause is menopause that happens before the age of forty—whether it is natural or induced. Women who enter menopause early get symptoms similar to those of natural menopause, like hot flashes, emotional problems, vaginal dryness, and decreased sex drive. For some women with early menopause, these symptoms are severe. Also, women who have early menopause tend to get weaker bones faster than women who enter menopause later in life. This raises their chances of getting osteoporosis and breaking a bone. Premature menopause can happen for these reasons:

- **Chromosome defects:** Defects in the chromosomes can cause premature menopause. For example, women with Turner syndrome are born without a second X chromosome or born without part of the chromosome. The ovaries don't form normally, and early menopause results.

- **Genetics:** Women with a family history of premature menopause are more likely to have early menopause themselves.

- **Autoimmune diseases:** The body's immune system, which normally fights off diseases, mistakenly attacks a part of its own reproductive system. This hurts the ovaries and prevents them from making female hormones. Thyroid disease and rheumatoid arthritis are two diseases in which this can happen.

- **Surgery to remove the ovaries:** Surgical removal of both ovaries, also called a bilateral oophorectomy, puts a woman into menopause right away. She will no longer have periods, and hormones decline rapidly. She may have menopausal symptoms right away, like hot flashes and diminished sexual desire. Women who have a hysterectomy, but have their ovaries left in place, will not have induced menopause because their ovaries will continue to make hormones. But because their uterus is removed, they no longer have their periods and cannot get pregnant. They might have hot flashes since the surgery can sometimes disturb the blood supply to the ovaries. Later on, they might have natural menopause a year or two earlier than expected.

• **Chemotherapy or pelvic radiation treatments for cancer:** Cancer chemotherapy or pelvic radiation therapy for reproductive system cancers can cause ovarian damage. Women may stop getting their periods, have fertility problems, or lose their fertility. This can happen right away or take several months. With cancer treatment, the chances of going into menopause depend on the type of chemotherapy used, how much was used, and the age of the woman when she gets treatment. The younger a woman is, the less likely she will go into menopause.

How to Find Out If You Have Premature Menopause

Your doctor will ask you if you've had changes typical of menopause, like hot flashes, irregular periods, sleep problems, and vaginal dryness. Normally, menopause is confirmed when a woman hasn't had her period for twelve months in a row.

However, with certain types of premature menopause, these signs may not be enough for a diagnosis. A blood test that measures follicle-stimulating hormone (FSH) can be done. Your ovaries use this hormone to make estrogen. FSH levels rise when the ovaries stop making estrogen. When FSH levels are higher than normal, you've reached menopause. However, your estrogen levels vary daily, so you may need this test more than once to know for sure.

You may also have a test for levels of estradiol (a type of estrogen) and luteinizing hormone (LH). Estradiol levels fall when the ovaries fail. Levels lower than normal are a sign of menopause. LH is a hormone that triggers ovulation. If you test above normal levels, you've gone through menopause.

Chapter 43

Managing the Symptoms of Menopause

Chapter Contents

Section 43.1

Managing Your Body's Changes during Menopause

Excerpted from "Menopause and Menopause Treatments," National Women's Health Information Center, March 2006. The information in Table 43.1 is reprinted from "Pros and Cons for Treatment of Menopause Symptoms," © 2007 The Hormone Foundation. Reprinted with permission. For additional information, visit www.hormone.org.

What are the symptoms of menopause?

Menopause affects every woman differently. Your only symptom may be your period stopping. You may have other symptoms, too. Many symptoms at this time of life are because of you getting older. But some are due to menopause. Common symptoms of menopause include the following:

- Change in pattern of periods (can be shorter or longer, lighter or heavier, more or less time between periods)

- Hot flashes (sometimes called hot flushes), night sweats (sometimes followed by a chill)

- Trouble sleeping through the night (with or without night sweats)

- Vaginal dryness

- Mood swings, feeling crabby, crying spells (probably because of lack of sleep)

- Trouble focusing, feeling mixed-up or confused

- Hair loss or thinning on your head, more hair growth on your face

Does menopause cause bone loss?

When a woman is young, estrogen helps to keep bone strong. When estrogen levels fall at menopause, bones weaken. When bones weaken a lot, the condition is called osteoporosis. Weak bones can break more easily.

How do I manage menopause? What are my options?

Most women do not need any special treatment for menopause. But some women may have menopause symptoms that need treatment. Several treatments are available. It's a good idea to talk about the treatments with your doctor so you can choose what's best for you.

Hormone therapy (HT): If used properly, hormone therapy (once called hormone replacement therapy or HRT) is one way to deal with the more difficult symptoms of menopause. It's the only therapy that is approved by the government for treating more difficult hot flashes and vaginal dryness. Hormone therapy should *not* be used solely to prevent heart or bone disease, stroke, memory loss, or Alzheimer disease. There are many kinds of hormone therapies, so your doctor can suggest what's best for you. As with all treatments, HT has both possible benefits and possible risks; it is important to talk about these issues with your doctor. If you decide to use HT, use the lowest dose that helps and for the shortest time needed. Check with your doctor every six months to see if you still need HT.

HT can help with menopause by doing the following things:

- Reducing hot flashes
- Treating vaginal dryness
- Slowing bone loss
- Improving sleep (and thus decreasing mood swings)

For some women, HT may increase their chance of the following:

- Blood clots
- Heart attack
- Stroke
- Breast cancer
- Gall bladder disease

Who should **not** *take HT for menopause?*

You should not take HT for menopause if any of the following are true:

- You think you are pregnant.
- You have problems with vaginal bleeding.
- You have had certain kinds of cancers (such as breast or uterine cancer).
- You have had a stroke or heart attack.
- You have had blood clots.
- You have liver disease.
- You have heart disease.

HT can also cause several side effects:

- Vaginal bleeding
- Bloating
- Breast tenderness or swelling
- Headaches
- Mood changes
- Nausea

Be sure to see your doctor if you have any of these side effects while using HT.

What about so-called natural treatments for menopause?

Some women decide to take herbal or other plant-based products to help relieve hot flashes. Some of the most common ones are described here:

- **Soy:** Soy contains phytoestrogens (chemicals that are like estrogen). But, there is no proof that soy—or other sources of phytoestrogens—really do make hot flashes better. And the risks of taking soy—mainly soy pills and powders—are not known. These soy products are more likely to work on mild hot flashes.

- **Other sources of phytoestrogens:** These include herbs such as black cohosh, wild yam, dong quai, and valerian root. Again, there is no proof that these herbs (or pills or creams containing these herbs) help with hot flashes.

Products that come from plants may sound like they are safe, but there is no proof they really are. Make sure to discuss these types of products with your doctor before taking them. You also should tell your doctor about other medicines you are taking, since some plant products can be harmful when combined with other drugs.

What about "bioidentical" hormone therapy?

This term means different things to different people. It's really hormones that are just the same as the hormones the body makes. There are several products with hormone like this that are on the market and are well tested. But some people use this term to mean drugs that are custom-made from a doctor's order. There is no proof that these custom-made products are better or safer than hormone therapy that's on the market.

How much physical activity should I do?

A woman should first talk to her doctor to see what's best for her. The goal is to exercise regularly so you can lower the risk of serious disease (such as heart disease or diabetes), and maintain a healthy weight. This usually takes at least thirty minutes of exercise (such as brisk walking) on most days of the week.

How else can I help my symptoms?

Hot flashes: Some women report that eating or drinking hot or spicy foods, alcohol, or caffeine, feeling stressed, or being in a hot place can bring on hot flashes. Try to avoid any triggers that bring on your hot flashes. Dress in layers, and keep a fan in your home or workplace. Regular exercise might also ease hot flashes, but sometimes exercise can cause a hot flash. If hot flashes continue and HT is not an option, ask your doctor about taking an antidepressant or epilepsy medicine. There is proof that these can relieve hot flashes for some women.

Vaginal dryness: A water-based, over-the-counter vaginal lubricant (like KY® Jelly) can be helpful if sex is painful. A vaginal moisturizer (also over the counter) can provide lubrication and help keep needed moisture in vaginal tissues. Really bad vaginal dryness may need HT. If vaginal dryness is the only reason for considering HT, an estrogen product for the vagina is the best choice. Vaginal estrogen products (creams, tablet, ring) treat only the vagina.

Table 43.1. Pros and Cons of Treating Your Menopausal Symptoms, continued on next page

Symptom/ Treatments	Pros and Cons of Treatment
Hot flashes	
Vitamin E	Pros: May reduce number and severity of hot flashes Cons: No toxicity of vitamin E; some people get headaches; scientific support for its effectiveness is very weak
Megestrol acetate/ Medroxyproges- terone acetate	Pros: Effective progestin treatment for hot flashes Cons: Weight gain; not studied well in women who have had breast cancer
SSRI drugs	Pros: Shown to be effective for hot flashes and also for depression Cons: Causes mood changes; can affect sex drive; paroxetine and sertraline hydrochloride have adverse interactions with tamoxifen
Estrogen*	Pros: Very effective at relieving hot flashes; also helps prevent vaginal thinning; prevents bone loss Cons: Increased risk of breast cancer when combined with a progestin; increased risk of uterine cancer if estrogen is taken without progesterone; increased risk of blood clots
Neurontin	Pros: Effective for relieving hot flashes, particularly at night; aids in getting to sleep Cons: Dizziness and lethargy if used during daytime
Dry vagina and painful intercourse	
Vaginal moisturizers	Pros: Over-the-counter solution Cons: Some people don't like these products, because of consistency or smell; does not thicken the vaginal lining; not as effective as estrogens
Water-soluble lubricants	Pros: Over-the-counter solution (Note: There is difference between lubricant and moisturizer) Cons: Some people don't like these products because of their consistency or smell; does not thicken the vaginal lining
Low dose vaginal estrogen ring	Pros: Helps keep vaginal tissue from thinning; local estrogen believed to have fewer risks compared to systemic estrogen pills taken in higher doses Cons: Some absorption of estrogen into the body occurs but this is small.
Estrogen* (by mouth)	Pros: Helps keep vaginal tissue from thinning; also helps prevent bone loss; very effective against hot flashes Cons: Increased risk of breast cancer if taken with a progestin; increased risk of uterine cancer if estrogen is taken without progesterone; increased risk of blood clots
Bone loss	
Bisphosphonates	Pros: Very effective against bone loss Cons: Common to have gastrointestinal problems when taking these drugs; can cause injury to esophagus unless taken with lots of water while sitting upright or standing; rarely causes jaw necrosis (death cells in the jaw)
Raloxifene	Pros: Very effective against bone loss, lowers risk of breast cancer Cons: Increases risk of blood clots; hot flashes; leg cramps

Table 43.1. Pros and Cons of Treating Your Menopausal Symptoms, continued from previous page

Symptom/ Treatments	Pros and Cons of Treatment
Bone loss, continued	
Calcitonin	Pros: Slows bone breakdown
	Cons: Headaches, dizziness, diarrhea, lack of desire for eating, nose bleeds (with nasal form); much less effective than bisphosphonates
Vitamin D	Pros: Helps body absorb calcium
	Cons: Very large amounts of vitamin D can cause build-up of calcium in blood, which could lead to heart and lung problems and kidney stones
Estrogen*	Pros: Helps prevent vaginal tissue from thinning; also helps prevent bone loss; very effective against hot flashes
	Cons: Increased risk of breast cancer if taken with a progestin; increased risk of uterine cancer if estrogen is taken without progesterone; increased risk of blood clots
Tamoxifen	Pros: Lowers risk of breast cancer; reduces risk of fractures
	Cons: Increases risk of uterine cancer, blood clots; more hot flashes; irregular vaginal bleeding
Depression and mood changes	
Counseling	Pros: Can be empowering; leads to increased insight
	Cons: Can be expensive; may not work as well as medications
SSRI drugs	Pros: Shown to be effective for hot flashes and also for depression
	Cons: Can affect sex drive; some types such as paroxetine or sertraline hydrochloride may interfere with effect of tamoxifen
Estrogen*	Pros: Very effective at preventing bone loss and preventing fractures; very effective at preventing hot flashes; prevents vaginal tissue thinning; may reduce the risk of dementia (in younger menopausal women taking HT for 10 years or more)
	Cons: Increased risk of breast cancer if taken with a progestin; increased risk of uterine cancer if estrogen is taken without progesterone; increased risk of blood clots; increased risk of dementia (in women 65 years and older taking HT for five years or less)

*A note on estrogen: Short-term goals of estrogen treatment are different from the long-term goals. Short-term therapy is designed to relieve symptoms; long-term therapy helps to prevent bone loss. If you take hormones for less than three to five years, the risks are relatively low. If you are concerned about bone loss and are thinking about taking hormone therapy for more than five years, consult with your doctor to see whether hormone therapy or an alternative treatment is best for you.

You should not take estrogen if you have had breast cancer or are at risk for breast cancer. There is an increased risk of breast cancer if taken with progestin, increased risk of uterine cancer if not taken with progesterone and increased risk of blood clots for women taking estrogen.

Table Editors: Nanette Santoro, MD, Director, Division of Reproductive Endocrinology, Dept. of OB/GYN and Women's Health, Albert Einstein College of Medicine; and Richard J. Santen, MD, Professor of Medicine, University of Virginia Health System

Problems sleeping: One of the best ways to get a good night's sleep is to get at least thirty minutes of physical activity on most days of the week. But don't exercise close to bedtime. Also avoid large meals, smoking, and working right before bedtime. Caffeine and alcohol should be avoided after noon. Drinking something warm before bedtime might help you to feel sleepy. Keep your bedroom dark, quiet, and cool, and use your bedroom only for sleeping and sex. Avoid napping during the day, and try to go to bed and get up at the same times every day. If you wake during the night and can't get back to sleep, get up and read until you're sleepy. Don't just lie there. If hot flashes are the cause of sleep problems, treating the hot flashes will usually improve sleep.

Mood swings: Some women report mood swings or "feeling blue" as they reach menopause. Women who had mood swings (premenstrual syndrome, or PMS) before their periods or postpartum depression after giving birth may have more mood swings around menopause. These are women who are sensitive to hormone changes. Often the mood swings will go away with time. If a woman is using HT for hot flashes or another menopause symptom, sometimes her mood swings will get better, too. Also, getting enough sleep and staying physically active will help you to feel your best.

Memory problems: As people age, their memory is not as good as it once was. Some women say they have "fuzzy thinking" as they reach menopause. This may be caused by changing hormones and can improve over time. Getting enough sleep and keeping physically active can help. If memory problems are really bad, talk to your doctor right away. This is not caused by menopause.

Section 43.2

Do Complementary and Alternative Therapies Help Menopausal Symptoms?

Reprinted from the National Center for Complementary and Alternative Medicine, National Institutes of Health, NCCAM Publication No. D297, November 2005.

Menopause is a natural process for women as they age. Menopause can also occur as a result of certain medical treatments that affect a woman's ovaries. Many women and their healthcare providers have become interested in complementary and alternative medicine (CAM) for menopausal symptoms. This information is based on findings from a 2005 National Institutes of Health (NIH) State-of-the-Science (SoS) conference on the management of menopause-related symptoms.

Key Points

Many women have few or no symptoms related to menopause, or feel that their symptoms are not enough of a problem that they need to seek treatment. Some symptoms traditionally seen as menopausal may be related to aging in general.

Menopause should not be viewed as a disease, according to the SoS conference panel.

For many years, menopausal hormone therapy (MHT; in the past, it was called hormone replacement therapy or HRT) was the primary treatment for troubling menopausal symptoms. Recent studies have found increased risks, however, for certain serious health problems from prolonged use of MHT.

Women with severe or long-lasting symptoms of menopause that have not been adequately relieved in other ways should consult their healthcare providers about their personal risks and benefits for using MHT. Certain lifestyle changes can also be helpful.

There is very little high-quality scientific evidence about the effectiveness and long-term safety of CAM therapies for menopausal symptoms. More research is needed.

It is very important for women who are considering or using CAM therapies for any health concern to discuss them with their healthcare provider. This is to help ensure safety and a comprehensive treatment plan.

What is menopause?

Menopause (also called the "change of life") is a normal part of a woman's aging. It is the time when her ability to have children comes to an end. In American women, the transition into menopause usually begins around age forty-seven, with the final menstrual period usually around age fifty-one. However, some women experience it earlier. Menopause occurs over a period of time because the levels of a hormone called estrogen, which is produced by the ovaries, begin to decline slowly. A woman is said to have completed natural menopause when she has not had a period for twelve months in a row. Menopause will occur immediately if a woman has her uterus and/or both ovaries removed surgically (an operation to remove the uterus is called a hysterectomy). This is because at least one ovary and the uterus are needed for a woman to have menstrual periods. Menopause also begins right away if a woman's ovaries are damaged by cancer treatment with radiation therapy or certain anticancer drugs.

What are the most common symptoms that women have during the menopausal transition?

Some symptoms that women experience are related to menopause and decreased activity of the ovaries. Others are related to aging in general. The scientific evidence that certain symptoms are linked to menopause is strongest for the following symptoms:

- Hot flashes, night sweats, or perspiring excessively (these are examples of what are called vasomotor symptoms, because they involve expansion of the blood vessels)

- Sleep difficulties

- Vaginal dryness, which can lead to painful intercourse and sexual problems

It is not certain whether the following symptoms are due to menopause, other factors that can come with aging (such as stress, economic concerns, or changes in personal relationships), or a combination of them:

- Changes in mood, such as depression, anxiety, or irritability

- Problems in thinking or in remembering things

- Urinary incontinence (that is, loss of ability to control urination)

- Painful joints or muscles, or other physical complaints, such as tiredness and stiff joints

The expert panel assembled for the NIH SoS conference noted that menopause is a normal part of women's aging, and advised that menopause not be viewed as a disease (that it be "demedicalized").

What treatment does conventional medicine offer for menopausal symptoms?

For many decades, estrogen (available by prescription with or without another hormone called progestin) has been the main treatment in conventional medicine for menopausal symptoms.[1] For a long time this treatment was called hormone replacement therapy (HRT), but the preferred term now is menopausal hormone therapy (MHT). MHT has been the most effective therapy to date for women who have severe or long-lasting problems related to menopause. It is especially effective against hot flashes and night sweats.

MHT has some other beneficial effects as well. For example, it helps to protect against osteoporosis, an age-related disease in which the bones become brittle and can break more easily. The risk for osteoporosis goes up in both men and women as they age, but it is greater for women after menopause. Drug treatments other than MHT, however, are available for reducing the risk of osteoporosis in both men and women, and certain lifestyle changes also may help.

Why are many people concerned about the effectiveness and safety of MHT?

MHT was widely prescribed until a few years ago. In 2002, findings from a large study called the Women's Health Initiative raised concerns about its safety and side effects. Researchers found increased risks for serious health problems (including heart disease, breast cancer, stroke, and blood clots) in women who had taken a combination of estrogen and progestin for several years. Women who were taking estrogen alone had an increased risk for stroke and blood clots.

469

MHT is being used more cautiously now. The U.S. Food and Drug Administration (FDA) recommends that it be used at the lowest dose for the shortest period of time possible. However, the specific risks and benefits of these low doses, and how long to use them, are not known. The NIH SoS conference panel noted that estrogen may not be an appropriate treatment for some menopausal complaints. This situation is one reason that many women and their healthcare providers have become interested in whether CAM treatments could be helpful for menopausal symptoms.

What should women consider if they are thinking about using CAM for menopausal symptoms?

There is very little scientific evidence to support the effectiveness of CAM therapies for menopausal symptoms. However, it is possible that some CAM therapies, while not as effective as MHT, may provide some relief to women during the menopausal transition. Here are some points to keep in mind about these therapies:

- It is important for women who are considering or using CAM therapies for any health reason to discuss them with their healthcare provider. This is to help ensure safety and a comprehensive treatment plan.

- Botanical and other dietary supplements can interact with prescription and over-the-counter drugs, affecting how the body reacts. Supplements can pose other safety issues as well. Some have been found to be contaminated, contain unlabeled ingredients, or have different amounts of ingredients than are listed on the label. "Natural" does not automatically mean "safe."

- Pharmacists can be a helpful source of information about supplements. However, their advice should not be viewed as a substitute for the advice of a healthcare provider.

- The claims for many CAM therapies can be attractive, ranging from enhancing well-being to producing health results that might seem unbelievable. Check whether such claims are based only on personal stories (testimonials) or on the results of controlled research studies. It is important to know whether scientific research has proven that a therapy works.

- The cost of a CAM therapy may be a concern, as many CAM therapies are not covered by insurance.

About dietary supplements: Dietary supplements were defined in a law passed by Congress in 1994. A dietary supplement must meet all of the following conditions:

- It is a product (other than tobacco) intended to supplement the diet, which contains one or more of the following: vitamins; minerals; herbs or other botanicals; amino acids; or any combination of the above ingredients.

- It is intended to be taken in tablet, capsule, powder, softgel, gelcap, or liquid form.

- It is not represented for use as a conventional food or as a sole item of a meal or the diet.

- It is labeled as being a dietary supplement.

Other important information about dietary supplements:

- They are regulated as foods, not drugs, so there could be quality issues in the manufacturing process.

- Supplements can interact with prescribed or over-the-counter medicines, and other supplements.

- "Natural" does not necessarily mean "safe" or "effective."

- Consult your healthcare provider before starting a supplement, especially if you are pregnant or nursing, or considering giving a supplement to a child.

CAM therapies are not the only alternatives to MHT to consider. Certain lifestyle changes can contribute to healthy aging, including during the menopausal transition. For example, quitting smoking, eating a healthy diet, and exercising regularly have been shown to reduce the risks of heart disease and osteoporosis. Women may want to try one or more of these changes as well.

What are phytoestrogens?

Some botanical products, such as soy and red clover, are called phytoestrogens. Plants rich in phytoestrogens may help relieve some symptoms of menopause. However, it is uncertain whether this relief comes from actual estrogens or from other compounds in the plant. Much remains to be learned about these plant products, including exactly how they work in the human body. Doctors caution that certain women need to be particularly careful before using phytoestrogens:

- Women who have had or are at increased risk for diseases or conditions that are affected by hormones, such as breast, uterine, or ovarian cancer; endometriosis; or uterine fibroids

- Women who are taking drugs that increase estrogen levels in the body, such as birth control pills; MHT; or a type of cancer drug called selective estrogen receptor modulators (SERMs), such as tamoxifen

Which CAM therapies were considered by the NIH SoS conference panel?

The panel discussed the evidence on ten of these therapies:

- Six botanicals—black cohosh, red clover, dong quai root, ginseng, kava, and soy

- DHEA (dehydroepiandrosterone), a dietary supplement

- Exercise

- Paced respiration

- Health education

What is known about the effectiveness and safety of these therapies for menopausal symptoms?

As mentioned in previously, very little well-designed research has been done on CAM therapies for menopausal symptoms. A small number of studies have been published, but they have had limitations (such as the way the research was done or treatment periods that may not have been long enough). As a result, the findings from these studies are not strong enough for scientists to draw any conclusions. Also, many studies of botanicals have not used a standardized (that is, chemically consistent) product. NCCAM is sponsoring a number of studies on botanicals using products that are both well characterized and well standardized (that is, their ingredients have been carefully studied and the dosages are controlled), and on other CAM therapies that have shown possible promise for reducing menopausal symptoms. The aim is to learn more about their safety and effectiveness and how they work in the body.

It is important to know that botanicals and other supplements can have side effects and can interact with herbs, other supplements, or drugs.

Botanicals

Black cohosh (Actaea racemosa, Cimicifuga racemosa): This herb has received more scientific attention for its possible effects on menopausal symptoms than have other botanicals. Studies of its effectiveness in reducing hot flashes have had mixed results. Recent research suggests that black cohosh does not act like estrogen, as once was thought. Black cohosh has had a good safety record over a number of years. Some concerns have been raised about whether it may cause liver problems, but an association has not been proven.

Red clover (Trifolium pratense): The panel reported that five controlled studies found no consistent or conclusive evidence that red clover leaf extract reduces hot flashes. Clinical studies in women report few side effects, and no serious health problems have been discussed in the literature. However, there are some cautions. Animal studies have raised concerns that red clover might have harmful effects on hormone-sensitive tissue (for example, in the breast and uterus).

Dong quai (Angelica sinensis): Only one randomized clinical study of dong quai has been done. The researchers did not find it to be useful in reducing hot flashes. Dong quai is known to interact with, and increase the activity in the body of, the anticoagulant drug warfarin. This can lead to bleeding complications in women who take this medicine.

Ginseng (Panax ginseng or Panax quinquefolius): The panel concluded that ginseng may help with some menopausal symptoms, such as mood symptoms and sleep disturbances, and with one's overall sense of well-being. However, it has not been found helpful for hot flashes.

Kava (Piper methysticum): Kava may decrease anxiety, but there is no evidence that it decreases hot flashes. It is important to note that kava has been associated with liver disease. The FDA has issued a warning to patients and providers about kava because of its potential to damage the liver.

Soy: The scientific literature includes both positive and negative results for soy extracts on hot flashes. When taken as a food or dietary supplement for short periods of time, soy appears to have few if any serious side effects. However, long-term use of soy extracts has been associated with thickening of the lining of the uterus.

Dehydroepiandrosterone (DHEA)

DHEA is a naturally occurring substance that is changed in the body to the hormones estrogen and testosterone. It is also manufactured and sold as a dietary supplement. The only randomized clinical trial of DHEA that has been done so far found no benefit for hot flashes. The NIH SoS conference panel added that a few small, nonrandomized studies have suggested that DHEA might possibly have some benefit for hot flashes and decreased sexual arousal, but this has not been confirmed. The side effects, risks, and benefits of using DHEA for longer than a few months have not been well studied.

Concerns have been raised about whether DHEA is safe and effective. For this reason, NCCAM is providing additional information. DHEA has been used in conventional medicine for a range of health problems other than symptoms of menopause, but there is no good scientific evidence to support these uses. Because levels of natural DHEA in the body decline with age, some people believe that taking DHEA as a supplement can help treat or prevent conditions related to aging. However, there is no good scientific evidence to support this popular notion.

NCCAM does not recommend that consumers use over-the-counter DHEA supplements for any health concerns, including for menopausal symptoms. Little is known about the long-term safety of DHEA, and scientists are not certain whether it might increase the risk for breast or prostate cancer. Therefore, consumers who have questions about whether DHEA could be of benefit for their personal situation should discuss those questions with their healthcare provider.

Other CAM Therapies

The NIH SoS conference panel chose to address the three other therapies following, which they considered CAM "behavioral interventions." They noted that these treatments may be an important area for further research because they cause few, if any, health problems. However, their effectiveness has not yet been proven through large, well-designed studies:

- Exercise has improved the quality of life in women with menopausal symptoms. However, it has not had any effect on vasomotor symptoms or vaginal dryness.

- Paced respiration (also called paced breathing) is a technique of slow, deep breathing. One small study found that it appeared to be helpful for hot flashes.

- Health education involves educating women about what to expect from menopause and what they themselves can do. It has been found to improve women's knowledge, but not to have effects on menopausal symptoms.

Does NCCAM support research on CAM for menopausal symptoms?

NCCAM supports a number of studies on CAM treatments for menopausal symptoms, as do some of the other institutes and centers at NIH. A few recent examples of NCCAM-funded projects include:

- An initiative to improve measures of hot flashes, which is expected to add to the understanding of hot flashes and to aid future clinical studies;

- A study of whether black cohosh can help with the anxiety that may be experienced as a symptom of menopause;

- A study to identify botanicals from Central America that have been used by the native population for menopausal symptoms and to develop and test standardized extracts from these plants;

- Several studies looking at the effect of acupuncture on the recurrence and severity of hot flashes in postmenopausal women and other groups that suffer from hot flashes, such as men being treated for prostate cancer.

Note

1. Conventional medicine is medicine as practiced by holders of M.D. (medical doctor) or D.O. (doctor of osteopathy) degrees and by their allied health professionals such as nurses, physical therapists, and dietitians. CAM is a group of diverse medical and healthcare systems, practices, and products that are not currently considered to be part of conventional medicine. Complementary medicine is used along with conventional medicine. Alternative medicine is used instead of conventional medicine. Some conventional medicine practitioners also practice CAM.

Chapter 44

Hormone Therapy

Chapter Contents

Section 44.1

Hormone Therapy:
Tips to Help You Evaluate Your Options

Excerpted from "Hormones and Menopause: Tips from the National Institute on Aging," National Institute on Aging, National Institutes of Health, July 2006.

A hormone is a chemical substance made by a gland or organ to regulate various body functions. To help control the symptoms of menopause some women can take hormones, called menopausal hormone therapy (MHT). MHT used to be called hormone replacement therapy or HRT. Some women should not use MHT. There are many things to learn about hormones before you make the choice that is right for you.

Which hormones are used for menopause?

During perimenopause, the months or years right before menopause, levels of two female hormones, estrogen and progesterone, in a woman's body go up and down irregularly. This happens as the ovaries struggle to keep up with the body's needs. The symptoms of menopause might result from these changing hormone levels. After menopause, when a woman's ovaries make much less estrogen and progesterone, the symptoms of menopause may continue. Menopausal hormone therapy may help control these symptoms. A woman whose uterus has been removed can use estrogen alone to control her symptoms. But a woman who still has a uterus must take progesterone or a progestin (a synthetic progesterone) along with the estrogen. This will prevent unwanted thickening of the lining of the uterus and also cancer of the uterus, an uncommon but possible result of using estrogen alone.

Why take these hormones? Why not?

Menopause is a normal part of life. It is not a disease that has to be treated. Women may decide to use menopausal hormone therapy because of its benefits, but there are also side effects and risks to consider. Here are two good reasons to think about menopausal hormone therapy:

- Treating some of the bothersome symptoms of menopause

- Preventing or treating osteoporosis

But for some women there are noticeable side effects:

- Breast tenderness

- Spotting or a return of monthly periods

- Cramping

- Bloating

By changing the type or amount of the hormones, the way they are taken, or the timing of the doses, your doctor may be able to control these side effects. Or, over time, they may go away on their own.

For some women there are also serious risks (see Table 44.1). These risks are why you need to think a lot before deciding to use menopausal hormone therapy.

Although the risks are small for any one woman, you need to take them into account. Much of the following table on benefits and risks is based on one important clinical trial, the Women's Health Initiative (WHI). This study looked at estrogen (conjugated equine estrogens) used alone or with a particular progestin (medroxyprogesterone acetate). Some other types of estrogen, progesterone, or progestin may have been tested in smaller clinical trials to see if they have an effect on heart disease, breast cancer, or dementia. Others have not.

Here is what scientists can say right now about the benefits and risks of MHT. Remember—which hormones you use, the way you take them, and the dose might affect these benefits and risks.

Because the average age of women participating in the trial was sixty-three, more than ten years past the average age of menopause, some experts now question whether the WHI results apply to women around the time of menopause. The WHI study found that in every ten thousand women using estrogen plus progestin, there would be seven more heart attacks than in every ten thousand women not using these hormones. Other research has suggested that if MHT is begun around the time of menopause, it might provide protection from heart disease, but not if a woman waits too long. This is a subject for further study.

Table 44.1. Benefits and Risks of Menopausal Hormone Therapy (July 2006)

	Women with a Uterus (Estrogen + Progestin)	Women without a Uterus[a] (Estrogen Only)
Benefits		
Relieves hot flashes/night sweats	Yes	Yes
Relieves vaginal dryness	Yes	Yes
Reduces risk of bone fractures	Yes	Yes
Improves cholesterol levels	Yes	Yes
Reduces risk of colon cancer	Yes	Don't know
Risks		
Increases risk of stroke	Yes	Yes
Increases risk of serious blood clots	Yes	Yes
Increases risk of heart attack	Yes	No
Increases risk of breast cancer	Yes	Possibly
Increases risk of dementia, when begun by women age sixty-five and older	Yes	Yes
Unpleasant side effects, such as bloating and tender breasts	Yes	Yes
Pill form can raise level of triglycerides (a type of fat in the blood)	Yes	Yes

[a]Women who have had a hysterectomy have had their uterus removed.

How would I use the hormones?

Estrogen comes in many forms and dosages. You could use a skin patch or vaginal tablet or cream, take a pill, or get an implant, shot, or vaginal ring insert. Progesterone or progestin is often taken as a pill, sometimes in the same pill as the estrogen. It also comes as a patch, shot, IUD (intrauterine device), vaginal gel, or suppository.

The form your doctor suggests may depend on your symptoms. For example, patches or pills can relieve hot flashes, night sweats, and vaginal dryness. They will also slow or prevent bone loss and help delay osteoporosis while you are using them. Other forms—vaginal creams, tablets, or rings—are used for vaginal dryness. The vaginal ring insert might also help some urinary tract symptoms. But, the dose found in these other forms is probably too low to relieve hot flashes.

What are natural hormones?

The natural hormones used to treat menopause symptoms are estrogen and progesterone made from plants such as soy or yams. Some people also call them bioidentical hormones because they are supposed to be chemically the same as the hormones naturally made by a woman's body. So-called natural hormones are put together (compounded) by a compounding pharmacist. This pharmacist follows a formula decided on by your doctor.

Drug companies also make estrogens and progesterone from plants like soy and yams. Some of these are also chemically identical to the hormones made by your body. You get these from any pharmacy with a prescription from your doctor.

One difference between the natural hormones prepared by a compounding pharmacist and those made by a drug company is that the compounded natural hormones are not regulated and approved by the U.S. Food and Drug Administration (FDA). So, we don't know much about how safe or effective they are or how the quality varies from batch to batch. Hormones made by drug companies are regulated and approved by the FDA.

There are also "natural" treatments for the symptoms of menopause that are available over the counter, without a prescription. Some of these are also made from soy or yams. They are not regulated or approved by the FDA.

What's right for me?

There is no "one size fits all" answer for all women who are trying to decide whether to use menopausal hormone therapy (MHT). You have to look at your own needs and weigh your own risks.

Ask yourself and your doctor these questions:

- How much are you bothered by menopausal symptoms such as hot flashes or vaginal dryness? Your hot flashes or night sweats will likely go away over time, but vaginal dryness may not. MHT can help if your symptoms are troubling you.

- Are you at risk for developing osteoporosis? Estrogen might protect bone mass while you use it. However, there are other drugs that can protect your bones without the same risks as MHT.

- Do you have a history of heart disease? Using estrogen and progestin can increase your risk.

- Do you or others in your family have a history of breast cancer? If you have a family history of breast cancer, check with your doctor about your risk.

- Do you have a history of gall bladder disease or high levels of triglycerides? Some experts think that using a patch will not make your triglyceride (a type of fat in the blood) level go up or increase your chance of gall bladder problems. Using an estrogen pill might.

- Do you have liver disease or a history of stroke or blood clots in your veins? MHT might not be safe for you to use.

- Are you over age sixty-five and thinking about using MHT to prevent dementia? Estrogen and progestin could actually increase your risk of dementia. Estrogen alone might do that also.

Then, talk to your doctor about how best to treat or prevent your symptoms or the diseases for which you are at risk. Ask about your other choices. Remember, these too may have risks and benefits. If you decide to use MHT, the FDA suggests that you use the lowest dose that works for the shortest time needed.

If you are already using menopausal hormone therapy and think you would like to stop, first ask your health care provider how to do that. Some doctors suggest tapering off slowly.

Whatever decision you make now about using MHT is not final. You can start or end the treatment at any time. If you stop, your risks will probably lessen over time, but so will the protection. Discuss your decision about menopausal hormone therapy each year with your doctor at your annual checkup.

Unanswered Questions

Don't forget at your checkup to ask your doctor about any new study results. Research on menopause is ongoing. Scientists are looking for answers to questions such as the following:

- How long can a woman safely use menopausal hormone therapy?

- Are some types of estrogen or progesterone safer than others?

- Is one form of hormone therapy (patch, pill, or cream, for example) better than another?

- Is MHT safer if you start it around the time of menopause instead of when you are older?

For now, we know that each woman is different, and the decision for each one will probably also be different. But almost every study gives women and their doctors more information to answer the question: Is menopausal hormone therapy right for me?

Section 44.2

Menopausal Hormone Use and Cancer: Questions and Answers

Reprinted from the National Cancer Institute, October 4, 2006.

What is menopause?

Menopause is the time in a woman's life when menstruation (having a period) ends. It is part of a biological process that begins, for most women, in their mid-thirties. During this time, the ovaries gradually produce lower levels of natural sex hormones—estrogen and progesterone. Estrogen promotes the normal development of a woman's breasts and uterus, controls the cycle of ovulation (when an ovary releases an egg into a fallopian tube), and affects many aspects of a woman's physical and emotional health. Progesterone controls menstruation and prepares the lining of the uterus to receive the fertilized egg.

"Natural menopause" occurs when a woman has her last menstrual period, or stops menstruating, and is considered complete when menstruation has stopped for one year. This usually occurs between ages forty-five and fifty-five, with variations in timing from woman to woman. Women who undergo surgery to remove both ovaries (an operation called bilateral oophorectomy) experience "surgical menopause"—an immediate end to menstruation caused by lack of hormones produced by the ovaries.

By the time a woman has reached natural menopause, estrogen output has decreased significantly. Even though low levels of this hormone are produced by other organs after menopause, these levels are only about one-tenth of the level found in premenopausal women. Progesterone is nearly absent in menopausal women.

What are menopausal hormones and why are they used?

Doctors may recommend menopausal hormones to counter some of the problems often associated with the onset of menopause (hot flashes, night sweats, sleeplessness, and vaginal dryness) or to prevent some long-term conditions that are more common in postmenopausal women, such as osteoporosis (a condition characterized by a decrease in bone mass and density, causing bones to become fragile). Menopausal hormone use (sometimes referred to as hormone replacement therapy or postmenopausal hormone use) usually involves treatment with either estrogen alone or estrogen in combination with progesterone or progestin, a synthetic hormone with effects similar to those of progesterone. Among women who are prescribed menopausal hormones, women who have undergone a hysterectomy (surgery to remove the uterus and, sometimes, the cervix) are generally given estrogen alone. Women who have not undergone this surgery are given estrogen plus progestin, which is known to have a lower risk of causing endometrial cancer (cancer of the lining of the uterus).

How does medical research determine the benefits and risks of taking menopausal hormones?

Researchers commonly conduct two very different, yet important types of studies with people to examine the benefits and risks of hormone use: clinical trials and observational studies. In clinical trials, the participants are given either hormones or placebos (look-alike pills that do not contain any drug) to determine the effect of the hormones on various conditions and diseases. In observational studies, the investigators do not try to affect the outcome; they compare the health status of women taking hormones to that of women not taking hormones.

What has medical research found out about the risks and benefits of hormone use after menopause?

The most comprehensive evidence about the risks and benefits of taking hormones after menopause to prevent disease comes from the Women's Health Initiative (WHI) Hormone Program, which was sponsored by the National Heart, Lung, and Blood Institute (NHLBI) and the National Cancer Institute (NCI), parts of the National Institutes of Health (NIH). This research program examined the effects of menopausal hormones on women's health. The WHI Hormone Program involved two studies—the use of estrogen plus progestin for women with a uterus (the Estrogen-plus-Progestin Study), and the use of estrogen alone for women without a uterus (the Estrogen-Alone Study). In both hormone therapy studies, women were randomly assigned to receive either the hormone medication being studied or the placebo.

The WHI Estrogen-plus-Progestin Study was stopped in July 2002, when investigators reported that the overall risks of estrogen plus progestin, specifically Prempro™, outweighed the benefits.[1] The researchers found that use of this estrogen plus progestin pill increased the risk of breast cancer, heart disease, stroke, blood clots, and urinary incontinence. However, the risk of colorectal cancer and hip fractures was lower among women using estrogen plus progestin than among those taking the placebo.[1] In addition, the WHI Memory Study showed that estrogen plus progestin doubled the risk for developing dementia (a decline in mental ability in which the patient can no longer function independently on a day-to-day basis) in postmenopausal women age sixty-five and older. The risk increased for all types of dementia, including Alzheimer disease.[2]

The WHI Estrogen-Alone Study, which involved Premarin™, was stopped in February 2004, when the researchers concluded that estrogen alone increased the risk of stroke and blood clots. In contrast with the WHI Estrogen-plus-Progestin Study, the risk of breast cancer was decreased in women using estrogen alone compared with those taking the placebo (see following question). Use of estrogen alone did not increase or decrease the risk of colorectal cancer.[3] Similarly to the results seen in the Estrogen-plus-Progestin Study, women using estrogen alone had an increased risk of urinary incontinence and a decreased risk of hip fractures.

How does menopausal hormone use affect breast cancer risk and survival?

The WHI Estrogen-plus-Progestin Study concluded that estrogen plus progestin increases the risk of invasive breast cancer. After five years of follow-up, women taking these hormones had a 24 percent increase in breast cancer risk compared with women taking the placebo. The increase amounted to an additional eight cases of breast cancer for every ten thousand women taking estrogen plus progestin for one year, compared with ten thousand women taking the placebo.[4]

A detailed analysis of data from the WHI Estrogen-plus-Progestin Study showed that, among women taking estrogen plus progestin, the breast cancers were slightly larger and diagnosed at more advanced stages compared with breast cancers in women taking the placebo. Among women taking estrogen plus progestin, 25.4 percent of the cancers had spread outside the breast to nearby organs or lymph nodes compared with 16.0 percent among nonusers. Women taking estrogen plus progestin also had more abnormal mammograms (breast x-rays that require additional evaluation) than the women taking the placebo.[4]

The WHI Estrogen-Alone Study concluded that taking estrogen did not increase the risk of breast cancer in women with a prior hysterectomy, at least for the seven years of follow-up in the study. Further analysis of data from the study indicated a 20 percent decrease in risk of breast cancer in women taking estrogen alone, although this decrease was seen mainly in the occurrence of early-stage breast cancer and ductal breast cancer (a specific type that begins in the lining of the milk ducts in the breast).[5] The observed reduction amounted to six fewer cases of breast cancer for every ten thousand women taking estrogen for one year, compared with ten thousand nonusers, but this lower incidence was not statistically significant—that is, it was less than what might be expected to happen by chance alone.[5] The Estrogen-Alone Study also showed a substantial increase in the frequency of abnormal mammograms.[5]

A comprehensive review of data from fifty-one epidemiological (population) studies published in the 1980s and 1990s found a statistically significant increase in breast cancer risk among current or recent users of any hormone replacement therapy compared with the risk among nonusers. Most women in the analysis (88 percent) had used estrogen alone, and data for estrogen-plus-progestin users was not analyzed separately. Analysis of the pooled data also showed that the risk of breast cancer increased with increasing duration of hormone use, and this effect was more prominent in women with low body weight or a low body mass index. However, breast cancers in hormone users were less likely to have spread to other parts of the body compared with the breast cancers in nonusers. The increase in breast cancer risk largely, if not completely, disappeared about five years after cessation of hormone use.[6]

What are the effects of hormone use on the risk of endometrial cancer?

Studies have shown that long-term exposure of the uterus to estrogen alone increases a woman's risk of endometrial cancer. The risk associated with estrogen plus progestin appears to be much less, but some data suggest that the risk is still increased compared with the risk for nonusers. The long-term effects of estrogen plus progestin on endometrial cancer risk remain uncertain.[7]

The WHI Estrogen-plus-Progestin Study showed that endometrial cancer rates for women taking estrogen plus progestin daily were the same as or possibly less than those for women taking the placebo pill. Uterine bleeding, however, was a common side effect, leading to more frequent biopsies and ultrasounds for women taking estrogen plus progestin compared with those taking a placebo.[8]

The Million Women Study, which took place in the United Kingdom, confirmed a lower risk of endometrial cancer in women taking estrogen plus progestin compared with those taking estrogen only or tibolone, a synthetic steroid that is not available in the United States.[9]

How does menopausal hormone use affect the risk of ovarian cancer?

Several observational studies have found that the use of estrogen alone is associated with a slightly increased risk of ovarian cancer for women who used this hormone for ten or more years. One observational study that followed 44,241 menopausal women for approximately twenty years concluded that women who used estrogen alone for ten or more years were twice as likely to develop ovarian cancer compared with women who did not use menopausal hormones.[10] Another large observational study also found an association between estrogen use and death due to ovarian cancer. In this study, the increased risk appeared to be limited to women who used estrogen for ten or more years.[11]

Data from the WHI Estrogen-plus-Progestin Study indicate that there may be an increased risk of ovarian cancer with use of estrogen plus progestin.[8] After 5.6 years of follow-up, a 58 percent increased risk of ovarian cancer was reported in women using estrogen plus progestin compared with nonusers, but the increased risk was not statistically significant. One observational study suggested that regimens of estrogen plus progestin do not increase the risk of ovarian cancer if progestin is used for more than fifteen days per month,[12] but this study was too small to draw firm conclusions. More research is needed to clarify the relationship between menopausal hormone use, particularly for estrogen plus progestin, and the risk of ovarian cancer.

How does menopausal hormone use affect the risk of colorectal cancer?

After five years of follow-up of women taking estrogen plus progestin, the WHI Estrogen-plus-Progestin Study reported a 37 percent reduction in colorectal cancer cases compared with women taking the placebo.[1] On average, the researchers found that if a group of ten thousand women takes estrogen plus progestin for a year, six fewer cases of colon cancer will occur than in a group of nonusers. These findings are consistent with observational studies, which have suggested that the use of postmenopausal hormones may reduce the risk of colorectal cancer.[1] The WHI Estrogen-Alone Study concluded that estrogen alone had no significant effect on colorectal cancer risk.[3]

Should women with a history of cancer take menopausal hormones?

One of the roles of naturally occurring estrogen is to promote the normal growth of cells in the breast and uterus. For this reason, it is generally believed that menopausal estrogen use by women who have already been diagnosed with breast cancer may promote further tumor growth. Studies of hormone use to treat menopausal symptoms in breast cancer survivors have produced conflicting results.

In one trial, 434 breast cancer survivors receiving either estrogen alone or estrogen plus progestin were followed for two years before the study was stopped because researchers concluded that even short-term use of hormone replacement therapy posed an unacceptable risk of breast cancer recurrence. Among these study participants, twenty-six women in the group receiving hormone replacement therapy had another occurrence of breast cancer compared with seven women in the group receiving no hormone replacement therapy.[13] In another study, which included 378 women who were followed for four years, eleven women receiving hormone replacement therapy had another occurrence of breast cancer compared with thirteen women receiving no hormone replacement therapy, so the risk of breast cancer recurrence was not increased.[14] A review of fifteen studies comprising a total of 1,416 breast cancer survivors and 1,998 women without a history of breast cancer found no increase in risk of cancer recurrence with hormone replacement therapy use.[15]

There is limited research on the risks associated with menopausal hormone use by women who have had other cancers, particularly gynecological cancers. One review of the published research found that no firm conclusion could be drawn about the safety of hormone use in women with a history of cancer. However, survivors of gastric and bladder cancer and meningioma may be at higher risk of a recurrence. Survivors of gynecological cancers may be at higher risk because these cancers tend to be more hormone-dependent, but more studies are needed.[16]

Does the way in which hormones are administered make a difference?

Most of the data on the long-term health effects of hormones come from studies in which hormones (estrogen alone or estrogen plus progestin) are administered orally in the form of pills. Hormones in the form of transdermal patches or gels are also used to treat menopause-related symptoms. Estrogen-containing vaginal creams and rings can be used specifically for vaginal dryness. Progesterone is also available as a pill or gel. The amount of estrogen that enters the bloodstream from estrogen-containing vaginal creams and rings depends on the types of hormones and the dose. Generally, vaginal administration of hormones results in lower levels of circulating hormones compared with an equivalent oral dose. Because the vaginal epithelium (thin layer of tissue that covers the vagina) responds to very small doses of estrogen, low-dose estrogen-containing creams or gels can be used.

What should women do if they are concerned about taking menopausal hormones?

Although menopausal hormones have short-term benefits such as relief from hot flashes and vaginal dryness, several health concerns are associated with their use. Women should discuss with their health care provider whether to take menopausal hormones and what alternatives may be appropriate for them. The U.S. Food and Drug Administration (FDA) currently advises women to use menopausal hormones for the shortest time and at the lowest dose possible to control symptoms.

What are the alternatives for women who choose not to take menopausal hormones?

To decrease the risk of chronic disease, women can adopt a healthy lifestyle by not smoking, exercising regularly, eating a healthy diet, and limiting the consumption of alcohol. Eating foods rich in calcium and vitamin D or taking dietary supplements containing these nutrients can help prevent osteoporosis. Results from the WHI showed that taking calcium and vitamin D supplements provided some benefit in preserving bone mass and preventing hip fractures, particularly in women age sixty and older. Although generally well tolerated, these supplements were associated with an increased risk of kidney stones. Other drugs, such as alendronate (Fosamax®), raloxifene (Evista®), and risedronate (Actonel®) have been shown to prevent bone loss. In addition, parathyroid hormone (Forteo®) is approved by the FDA for osteoporosis treatment.

Short-term menopause-related problems may go away on their own and frequently require no therapy at all. Some women seek relief from these symptoms with nonprescription complementary and alternative therapies containing estrogen-like compounds. Some sources of these estrogen-like compounds include soy-based products, whole-grain cereal, oilseeds (primarily flaxseed), legumes, and the botanical black cohosh. The benefits and risks of most of these agents are unproven, but remain an active area of research. Local therapy is also available for vaginal dryness and urinary bladder conditions. Women should talk with their doctor about the option best for them.

What research still needs to be done?

Unresolved questions include whether different forms of the hormones, lower doses, different hormones, or different methods of administration are safer or more effective; whether risks or benefits persist after women stop taking hormones; whether women might be able to take hormones safely for a short period of time; and whether certain subgroups of women, including women with a history of cancer, might be at higher or lower risk than the general population.

The WHI continues to evaluate the longer-term effects of calcium and vitamin D supplements on preserving bone mass, preventing hip fractures, and reducing colon cancer risk, and continues long-term follow-up of women in the hormone trials.

Other studies funded by the NIH and other institutions are under way to evaluate the safety and effectiveness of complementary and alternative therapies, such as soy-based products, black cohosh, and red clover, for menopausal symptoms and long-term health after menopause. Several NCI-sponsored studies are evaluating the effectiveness of nonhormonal treatments, such as the botanical St. John's wort and the antidepressant drug citalopram hydrobromide, in reducing hot flashes in women with a history of breast cancer.

Selected References

1. Rossouw JE, Anderson GL, Prentice RL, et al. Risks and benefits of estrogen plus progestin in healthy postmenopausal women: Principal results from the Women's Health Initiative randomized controlled trial. *Journal of the American Medical Association* 2002; 288(3):321–33.

2. Shumaker SA, Legault C, Rapp SR, et al. Estrogen plus progestin and the incidence of dementia and mild cognitive impairment in postmenopausal women: The Women's Health Initiative Memory Study: A randomized controlled trial. *Journal of the American Medical Association* 2003; 289(20):2651–62.

3. Anderson GL, Limacher M, Assaf AR, et al. Effects of conjugated equine estrogen in postmenopausal women with hysterectomy: The Women's Health Initiative randomized controlled trial. *Journal of the American Medical Association* 2004; 291(14):1701–12.

4. Chlebowski RT, Hendrix SL, Langer RD, et al. Influence of estrogen plus progestin on breast cancer and mammography in healthy postmenopausal women: The Women's Health Initiative randomized trial. *Journal of the American Medical Association* 2003; 289(24):3243–53.

5. Stefanick ML, Anderson GL, Margolis KL, et al. Effects of conjugated equine estrogens on breast cancer and mammography screening in postmenopausal women with hysterectomy. *Journal of the American Medical Association* 2006; 295(14):1647–57.

6. Collaborative Group on Hormonal Factors in Breast Cancer. Breast cancer and hormone replacement therapy: Collaborative reanalysis of data from 51 epidemiological studies of 52,705 women with breast cancer and 108,411 women without breast cancer. *Lancet* 1997; 350(9084):1047–59.

7. Grady D, Gebretsadik T, Kerlikowske K, Ernster V, Petitti D. Hormone replacement therapy and endometrial cancer risk: A meta-analysis. *Obstetrics and Gynecology* 1995; 85(2):304–13.

8.   Anderson GL, Judd HL, Kaunitz AM, et al. Effects of estrogen plus progestin on gynecologic cancers and associated diagnostic procedures: The Women's Health Initiative randomized trial. *Journal of the American Medical Association* 2003; 290(13):1739–48.

9.   Beral V, Bull D, Reeves G, Million Women Study Collaborators. Endometrial cancer and hormone-replacement therapy in the Million Women Study. *Lancet* 2005; 365(9470):1543–51.

10. Lacey JV Jr., Mink PJ, Lubin JH, et al. Menopausal hormone replacement therapy and risk of ovarian cancer. *Journal of the American Medical Association* 2002; 288(3):334–41.

11. Rodriguez C, Patel AV, Calle EE, Jacob EJ, Thun MJ. Estrogen replacement therapy and ovarian cancer mortality in a large prospective study of US women. *Journal of the American Medical Association* 2001; 285(11):1460–65.

12. Riman T, Dickman PW, Nilsson S, et al. Hormone replacement therapy and the risk of invasive epithelial ovarian cancer in Swedish women. *Journal of the National Cancer Institute* 2002; 94(7):497–504.

13. Holmberg L, Anderson H. HABITS (hormonal replacement therapy after breast cancer—is it safe?), a randomised comparison: Trial stopped. *Lancet* 2004; 363(9407):453–55.

14. von Schoultz E, Rutqvist LE. Menopausal hormone therapy after breast cancer: The Stockholm randomized trial. *Journal of the National Cancer Institute* 2005; 97(7):533–35.

15. Batur P, Blixen CE, Moore HC, Thacker HL, Xu M. Menopausal hormone therapy (HT) in patients with breast cancer. *Maturitas* 2006; 53(2):123–32.

16. Biglia N, Gadducci A, Ponzone R, Roagna R, Sismondi P. Hormone replacement therapy in cancer survivors. *Maturitas* 2004; 48(4):333–46.

Chapter 45

Medical Problems Accompanying Menopause

Chapter Contents

Section 45.1

Menopause and Osteoporosis

Osteoporosis is a health risk directly linked to menopause. The lack of estrogen causes the cells that build new bone to be less active than cells that remove old bone—your bones are being torn down faster than they are being built up. The excessive loss of bone mass causes osteoporosis, a thinning and weakening of the bones. Osteoporosis increases your risk of a fracture and can lead to a loss of height or a humped back. This disease comes on silently—there are no warning signs and it is usually not detected until a fracture is suffered. It moves quickly with up to 20 percent of expected lifetime bone loss occurring within the first five to seven years after menopause. It is also very common—fifty-one million American women over the age of forty-five are at risk for osteoporosis.

Besides menopause, there are other risk factors that may predispose you to develop osteoporosis:

- Age
- Being Caucasian or Asian
- A thin or small frame
- Family history of osteoporosis

Likewise, there are other risk factors that you can control:

- Alcohol intake
- Exercise or activity
- Cigarette smoking
- Calcium intake

The good news is—osteoporosis is highly preventable and treatable. Although you cannot prevent the estrogen loss that occurs with menopause, there are steps you can take to take care of your bones, and your doctor can help you.

First, if you are under the age of sixty-five and have one or more risk factors for osteoporosis, you should have a bone density test performed. Over the age of sixty-five, a bone density test should be performed whether any of the risk factors appear or not.

Possible Treatments

Hormone replacement therapy (HRT): HRT replaces the estrogen that your body no longer produces, thereby slowing down and even stopping the loss of bone mass.

Calcium intake: Include more calcium-rich foods, such as milk and yogurt, in your diet, or consider taking a daily calcium supplement. Peri- and postmenopausal women taking estrogen need 1,200 mg of calcium per day, and postmenopausal women not on estrogen require about 1,500 mg per day (the average menopausal women gets only about 750 mg per day).

Vitamin D: Vitamin D is activated by the liver and kidneys to boost calcium absorption. Women age fifty-one to seventy require 400 units of vitamin D per day, and women over the age of seventy need 600 units. Vitamin D–fortified milk is one of the best food sources for this nutrient—one eight-ounce glass provides 100 units, or 25 percent, of the daily requirement. Likewise, most vitamin supplements contain 100 percent of the daily requirement.

Exercise: Exercise can't stop bone loss, but the activity, especially walking, can slow down the pace of osteoporosis. In addition, exercise keeps muscles toned and strong, making falls less damaging. Just thirty minutes of brisk walking several days a week is all you need to increase strength and overall fitness.

Medications: Various medications are available that help preserve bone loss. Ask your doctor for further information on these treatments.

Section 45.2

Menopause and Depression

"Menopause," is reprinted with permission from the University of Michigan Depression Center, www.depressioncenter.org. © 2007 Regents of the University of Michigan.

Why am I depressed?

Depression affects twice as many women as men. Midlife is often considered a period of increased risk for depression in women. It is not known why, but it may be related to having a personal or family history of depression, life stressors, and role changes. Menopause is often believed to be a time when women are more likely to become depressed. Studies actually show that depression is more likely to occur in the years during transition to menopause, perimenopause years. This period is associated with gradual declines in estrogen levels. Some studies suggest that changes in estrogen levels are associated with onset of depression.

What are the symptoms of depression during midlife?

The symptoms of depression in menopause or perimenopause are: two or more weeks of depressed mood, decreased interest or pleasure in activities, change in appetite, change in sleep patterns, fatigue or loss of energy, difficulty concentrating, excessive feeling of guilt or worthlessness, thoughts of suicide, extreme restlessness and irritability. Many symptoms of menopause overlap with symptoms of depression, including problems with sleep and physical symptoms such as hot flashes, fatigue, irritability, anxiety, and difficulty concentrating. Some women suffer needlessly because they think these discomforts and problems are a natural part of aging. Depression should not be dismissed as a normal consequence of later life for women.

Depression that goes untreated can lead to more severe episodes of depression and even physical complications. For example, depression is associated with increased risk for heart attacks. A recent study suggests that depression leads to loss of bone mineral density, therefore increasing a women's risk for broken bones.

What can I do about depression in midlife?

You have already taken one of the most important steps in helping your depression—you have come for help. Fortunately, depression is treatable. Believing one's condition is "incurable" is part of the hopelessness that accompanies depression. This way of thinking is a symptom of depression and will improve with treatment. There are many treatment options available to help depression.

Medication: There are many effective, well-tolerated antidepressant medications. Antidepressant medications are an essential part of treatment for women who are moderately to severely depressed.

Hormone replacement therapy: Some clinical studies indicate that estrogen may help with depression in the early stages of menopause. Although the usefulness of estrogen as an antidepressant has not been well established, it may be an important adjunct to other treatments for depression. Be sure to discuss the benefits and risks of hormone replacement therapy with your healthcare provider, including the potential benefits to your mood.

Get a physical examination: A thorough physical examination is important to rule out any physical illnesses that may cause depressive symptoms. As you get older, you may be more likely to develop some of these physical health problems. Certain medications can cause symptoms that mimic depression. Be sure to review all medications that you are taking with your healthcare provider.

Therapy: Therapy involves talking with a trained professional (psychologist, psychiatrist, clinical nurse, or social worker) on a short term (twelve to twenty weeks) or a long-term basis and can take many forms. Two types of therapy are particularly effective for depression. Cognitive behavioral therapy (CBT) targets negative thoughts and behaviors that tend to worsen depressed mood and teaches better ways of thinking and behaving. Interpersonal therapy (IPT) helps a person communicate more effectively with others, therefore decreasing stressors. Some studies suggest that women with depression are more likely to engage in excessive rumination. This increased pondering and brooding causes the length and severity of depression. Therapy can help you address these negative ruminations.

Alternative medicine, herbal remedies, and dietary supplements: There has been rising interest in the use of herbs and dietary supplements for the treatment of depression. St. John's wort (*Hypericum perforatum*) has been the most common of these. However, scientific studies of these alternative forms of treatment have so far been short-term and not well controlled. There is no uniformity of dose or amounts and types of ingredients because the Food and Drug Administration does not regulate them. Be sure to tell your healthcare provider if you are taking an herbal or dietary supplement. Some of them may negatively interact with antidepressant medication or other medications you are taking.

Is there anything else that I can do?

Along with professional treatment, there are several other things that you can do to help yourself feel better.

Support: It is not uncommon for women in midlife to have double caretaking responsibilities—still caring for their own children while also caring for elderly relatives. It is very important that you get support for yourself and communicate your needs to others. Ask for help with housekeeping, preparing meals, and other daily tasks. Don't feel you have to do it all yourself.

Exercise: The benefits of exercise in depression are well documented. Be sure to discuss any changes you make in your exercise routine with your healthcare provider. Exercise helps treat depression by releasing the body's mood-elevating compounds, reducing the depression hormone cortisol, providing perspective on life, providing a feeling of accomplishment, enhancing self-esteem, and increasing levels of serotonin (a neurotransmitter found to be key in the development of depression). It doesn't matter what you do as long as you do something physical for twenty to thirty minutes three times a week or more. Even exercising as little as ten minutes a day has been found to have beneficial effects. Walking is perhaps the most accessible form of exercise because it costs nothing and you can start immediately.

Stress management: Depression can also be made worse by stress. Midlife is identified with stressors and life transitions such as children leaving home, loss of a parent, caring for a parent, occupational problems, marital changes, and even death of a loved one. These life changes, particularly loss and interpersonal role transitions, have been associated with depression in women. Identify stressors that you are putting on yourself (trying to be "perfect," doing too much). Set priorities and let unnecessary tasks wait.

Promote sleep: Inadequate sleep can make depression worse. Take care to keep your sleep cycle regular by going to bed and waking around the same time. Develop relaxing bedtime rituals such as reading or a warm bath. Take time to rest during bedtime hours, even if you aren't asleep.

Dietary changes: Eating a well-balanced diet and regularly scheduled meals is important. Decreasing refined sugar, caffeine, alcohol, and chocolate may help. Use of calcium and B vitamins (B_6) may also decrease symptoms.

Spend time with others: Depressed women often withdraw from others because they mistakenly feel they would not be good company. Being with others is another way to gain perspective, which helps with the symptoms of depression. If you live alone, it is especially important to establish contact with others. Consider joining a support group for others experiencing problems with depression.

Make time to do what you enjoy: Depressed women sometimes temporarily lose the ability to enjoy themselves. Avoiding enjoyable activities only makes this worse. Continue doing pleasurable activities even if you don't feel like it. You will soon find that you have come to enjoy yourself again, at least for short periods.

Give yourself a break: You will feel like yourself again and better able to handle everyday pressures. Be realistic about the demands and expectations you make on yourself.

References

Coyne JC, Pepper C, Flynn HA: The significance of prior history of depression in two populations. *Journal of Consulting and Clinical Psychology* 67(1):76–81, 1999.

Hay AG, Banckroft J, Johnstone EC: Affective symptoms in women attending a menopause clinic. *Br J Psychiatry* 164(4):513–16, 1994.

Rubinow DR, Schmidt PJ, Roca CA: Estrogen-Serotonin Interactions: Implications for Affective Regulation. *Biol Psychiatry* 44:839–50, 1998.

Schmidt PJ, Rubinow DR: Menopause-related affective disorders: A justification for further study. *Am J Psychiatry* 148:844–52, 1994.

Schwingl PJ, Hulka BS, Harlow SD: Risk factors for menopausal hot flashes. *Obst Gyn* 84:29–34, 1994.

Weissman, M.M., Markowitz, J.C., Klerman, G.L. (2000). *Comprehensive Guide to Interpersonal Psychotherapy*. New York: Basic Books.

Section 45.3

Menopause and Bladder Control

Reprinted from the National Institute of Diabetes and Digestive and Kidney Diseases, National Institutes of Health, NIH Publication No. 04-4186, April 2004.

Does menopause affect bladder control?

Yes. Some women have bladder control problems after they stop having periods (menopause or change of life). If you are going through menopause, talk to your healthcare team.

After your periods end, your body stops making the female hormone estrogen. Estrogen controls how your body matures, your monthly periods, and body changes during pregnancy and breast-feeding.

Some scientists believe estrogen may help keep the lining of the bladder and urethra plump and healthy. They think that lack of estrogen could contribute to weakness of the bladder control muscles.

Pressure from coughing, sneezing, or lifting can push urine through the weakened muscle. This kind of leakage is called stress incontinence. It is one of the most common kinds of bladder control problems in older women.

Recent studies have raised doubts about the benefits of taking estrogen after menopause. The studies also point to added risks from taking estrogen for many years. No studies have shown that taking estrogen improves bladder control in women who have gone through menopause. Your doctor can suggest many other possible treatments to improve bladder control.

What else causes bladder control problems in older women?

Sometimes bladder control problems are caused by other medical conditions. These problems include the following:

- Infections

- Nerve damage from diabetes or stroke

- Heart problems

- Medicines
- Feeling depressed
- Difficulty walking or moving

A very common kind of bladder control problem for older women is urge incontinence. This means the bladder muscles squeeze at the wrong time—or all the time—and cause leaks.

If you have this problem, your healthcare team can help you retrain yourself to go to the toilet on a schedule.

What should you do about bladder control after menopause?

Talk to your healthcare team. You may have stress or urge incontinence, but other things could also be happening.

Medicines and exercises can restore bladder control in many cases. Your doctor will give you a checkup first.

What treatments can help you regain bladder control?

It depends on what kind of bladder control problem you have. Your healthcare team may also recommend some of the following:

- Limiting caffeine
- Exercising pelvic muscles
- Training the bladder to hold more urine

If these simple treatments do not work, your healthcare team may have you try something different. These treatments might include the following:

- Biofeedback
- Electrical stimulation of pelvic muscles
- A device inserted in the vagina to hold up the bladder
- A device inserted directly into the urethra to block leakage
- Surgery to lift a sagging bladder into a better position

What professionals can help you with bladder control?

Professionals who can help you with bladder control include the following:

- Your primary care doctor

- A gynecologist: a women's doctor
- A urogynecologist: an expert in women's bladder problems
- urologist: an expert in bladder problems
- A nurse or nurse practitioner
- A physical therapist

Points to Remember

- Some women have bladder control problems after they stop having periods.
- Exercising pelvic muscles can help you maintain or improve bladder control.
- Treatment depends on the type of bladder control problem(s) you have. Talk to your healthcare team to find the treatment that's right for you.

Section 45.4

Menopause and Insomnia

How is sleep affected by perimenopause, menopause, and postmenopause?

Many female patients who come to my office in their late thirties and forties with symptoms of insomnia are actually experiencing the beginning of their transition to menopause, which is called perimenopause. Sleep can be impacted by many things, such as hormonal and lifestyle changes.

Hormonal changes: During the course of perimenopause through menopause, a woman's ovaries gradually decrease production of estrogen and progesterone, a sleep-promoting hormone. The shifting of ratios of hormones can be an unsettling process, sometimes contributing to the inability to fall asleep. Also, waning levels of estrogen may make you more susceptible to environmental and other factors or stressors, which disrupt sleep.

Hot flashes: A hot flash is a surge of adrenaline, awakening your brain from sleep. It often produces sweat and a change of temperature that can often be disruptive to sleep and comfort levels. Unfortunately it may take time for your adrenaline to recede and let you settle down into sleep again.

Depression/mood swings: About 20 percent of women will experience depression during this time frame and some cases have been linked to estrogen loss. However, hormonal changes may not be the only cause. Precipitants such as life stress and a history of menopause are important causes as well.

Coincidental social issues: Aside from the hormonal changes you may be experiencing, this time in life can present many social changes. Whether your children and moving out of the house, retiring, moving to a smaller home or you are just feeling some of the "midlife crisis" stress of getting to a new phase in life, these issues can interfere with your ability to sleep.

Since hormonal and social issues are at play, it is important for you to be in touch with how your sleep is impacted by this transitional period. The perimenopausal period may last from three to ten years. Some women "learn" to have insomnia and adjust their life around it—and as their hormones settle down, they have built a lifestyle of insomnia.

What should you do if menopause is preventing you from getting a good night's sleep? How do you know if you need to talk to your doctor?

If you are finding symptoms of perimenopause keeping you up or waking you up every night or ongoing, see your gynecologist or general practitioner. There are some things you can control (like your sleep habits) and things you can't control (like your hormones, without medication). Using good sleep hygiene, do everything in your power to stack the odds for good sleep and hopefully you can make up for the hot flashes and other natural sleep obstacles.

I stress that women need to be consistent with wake-up times and give themselves time to fall asleep at night. Build a very tight sleep structure and sleep environment by paying attention to your sleep environment:

- Make your room dark quiet and safe.

- Keep your room as cool as you can.

- Skip alcohol and tobacco.

- Keep a cloth in a bucket of ice near your bed so that you can cool yourself quickly.

What treatments are available for women whose sleep is affected by menopausal symptoms?

Hormone replacement therapy (HRT) works by supplementing estrogen hormone that is no longer being made by your body in the same way as it was before perimenopause. Estrogen reduces hot flashes, vaginal symptoms, and difficulty with urination. HRT is recommended for the shortest possible term in the lowest possible dose. HRT has been found to help women. I know many women who have gone back on their HRT simply because they need to sleep. Again, sleep is so vital. One has to weigh the consideration of good sleep when we are discussing whether or not to discontinue HRT.

Another of the things that helps some women is a low-dose birth control pill, which acts to stabilize mild fluctuations of estrogen that may be occurring.

What kinds of treatments are available for a woman who does not want to use hormone replacement therapy (HRT)?

There are some herbal products that have been tried but I don't recommend them. The data shows that they are not effective. I try to avoid those. Relaxation therapy, paced breathing, and exercise may help—burn energy while relaxing. Again, if you can get all your sleep ducks in a row, you can combat the hormonal issues. You can try acupuncture or shiatsu (shiatsu uses pressure areas like acupuncture but without needles—it is based on the Eastern study of body energies and how they flow). I have had good results with shiatsu and yoga. Relaxation and exercise helps you focus on yourself and helps you settle down. Some success has been seen with antidepressants such as the selective serotonin reuptake inhibitors (SSRIs) or anti-epilepsy drugs.

Chapter 46

Male Menopause

Male menopause is a term used to refer to an age-related decline in testosterone levels in men. However, male menopause is a misleading description because it suggests a comparison with the dramatic end of reproductive function in women.

All women experience a profound fall in oestrogen levels at the time of the menopause. However, in men, testosterone levels fall much less and more gradually. This decline may not affect all men.

Other terms used to refer to a decline in testosterone levels include andropause or viropause. These terms have no established medical meaning.

Testosterone Treatment Is Often Not Necessary

Testosterone treatment should not be endorsed, sought or prescribed as a "cure-all" for symptoms of ageing. There is no evidence that testosterone treatment will benefit older men with slight falls in testosterone levels.

Only men with proven testosterone deficiency (also referred to as androgen deficiency) will benefit from testosterone treatment.

Reprinted from "Male Menopause," April 2007. This information was provided by the Better Health Channel, a Victorian Government (Australia) website. Material on the Better Health Channel is regularly updated. For the latest version of this information please visit: www.betterhealth.vic.gov.au.

Diagnosis

Symptoms associated with a low testosterone level may include low energy, fatigue, poor concentration or memory, mood changes, low sex drive or loss of muscle strength. However, these symptoms occur in other conditions and are often not a good guide to a man's testosterone level.

A diagnosis of androgen deficiency may be made only after an appropriate medical examination and blood tests to check hormone levels. Other tests may also be required, either to rule out other medical conditions or to identify causes (other than age) of the low testosterone level.

Illness May Lead to a Drop in Testosterone Levels

Many illnesses that are common in older men can cause a drop in testosterone levels. Illnesses that may cause either a drop in testosterone levels or symptoms similar to testosterone (androgen) deficiency include:

- Cardiovascular disease;
- Some lung diseases;
- Depression.

There is no evidence to support the use of testosterone therapy for these conditions.

Obesity Is a Major Cause of Reduced Testosterone

Obesity is strongly associated with lower testosterone levels. However, this does not mean that obese men with lowered testosterone levels should automatically receive testosterone treatment.

Obese men with low testosterone levels should consult their doctor for a complete review of their health, lifestyle and physical activity levels.

Treatment for Men with Androgen Deficiency

For older men (aged over forty) with proven androgen deficiency, a number of treatment options are available. The treatment prescribed can vary according to cost and what suits the individual person. The options include:

- Injections;
- Implants;
- Capsules;
- Patches;
- Gels;
- Creams.

Men who are treated with testosterone will need to be regularly monitored by their doctor; this will include prostate checks as required according to their age and family history. Cholesterol levels should also be measured.

Where to Get Help

- Your doctor

Things to Remember

- The term male menopause is misleading.
- Testosterone levels gradually fall with age but the effects are variable.
- Symptoms may not be a good guide to testosterone levels.

Part Seven

Other Concerns
That Impact Adult Health

Chapter 47

Work-Related Health Concerns

Chapter Contents

Section 47.1

Protecting Your Back at Work

Back pain is one of the most common medical problems in the United States. The cause is often poor posture and body mechanics in the workplace.

A supervised program of back protection and exercise may be the key to alleviating and even preventing such problems.

Correct posture and body mechanics play a vital role in preventing back pain because pressure on the discs and strain of the muscles, ligaments, and back joints is aggravated by incorrect posture and body mechanics. At the same time, when your posture is good and you move your body correctly, you reduce the strain on your back.

Sitting Down on the Job

Sitting is often the greatest cause of back pain. When sitting either in a relaxed position, driving, or while at work, support your lower back. Use a rolled towel, small pillow, or a specially designed seat support, available at medical supply stores.

Remove this low back support every half hour for five minutes to give your lower back a change of position. Your head should be positioned so that your ear is in a line with your shoulder and your chin is parallel with the floor.

Avoid leaning to one side when you are sitting, and avoid over-stuffed furniture as it does not offer adequate support.

When working at a desk, your chair should be pulled close to the desk. An office chair with short arm rests will allow this. Office chairs should also have adjustable height, back rests, and seats. The back rest spring should be adjusted so that the back rest moves with you. A seat that tilts forward is a particularly useful feature.

Use a swivel chair to enable you to work without twisting your back. Place objects such as adding machines and computers as close to you as possible to minimize the amount of twisting and turning you need to do.

When you lean forward at your desk, bend forward at the hips instead of rounding your lower back. This will allow you to keep your back straight and in good alignment.

Talking on the Phone Can Be a Pain in the Neck

Holding the phone between your ear and shoulder is a common cause of neck pain. Use a clipboard to hold your papers down so that your hands are free. Special phone adapters also are available.

After sitting for a prolonged period, it is helpful to straighten your back to an upright position and, if possible, stand and walk for awhile.

Don't Forget Exercise

Appropriate exercise, done regularly, will provide the strength and flexibility in the muscles of your legs and back that you need to help avoid excessive strain and possible injury.

Some forms of exercise, such as yoga and tai chi, may help relieve or prevent back pain by increasing flexibility and reducing tension. These exercises should not be done, however, if they are uncomfortable or place a strain on the back.

And don't neglect strength training; strong abdominal, back, and leg muscles play a vital role in helping you maintain good posture and body mechanics.

Section 47.2

Ergonomics for Computer Workstations

Reprinted from the Division of Occupational Health and Safety, National Institutes of Health, July 2006.

Monitors

With regard to the monitor, one must take into consideration how the placement and maintenance of the monitor can effect both the eyes and the musculoskeletal system. The following suggestions can help prevent the development of eye strain, neck pain, and shoulder fatigue while using your computer workstation:

- Make sure the surface of the viewing screen is clean.

- Adjust brightness and contrast to optimum comfort.

- Position the monitor directly in front of user to avoid excessive twisting of the neck.

- Position the monitor approximately 20–26 inches (arm's length) from user.

- Tilt top of the monitor back 10 to 20 degrees.

- Position monitors at right angles from windows to reduce glare.

- Position monitors away from direct lighting that creates excessive glare or use a glare filter over the monitor to reduce glare.

- The top of the viewing screen should be at eye level when the user is sitting in an upright position (Note: Bifocal wearers may need to lower monitor a couple of inches).

Adjusting Your Chair

Contrary to popular belief, sitting, which most people believe is relaxing, is hard on the back. Sitting for long periods of time can cause increased pressure on the intervertebral discs—the springy, shock-absorbing part of the spine. Sitting is also hard on the feet and legs.

Gravity tends to pool blood in the legs and feet and create a sluggish return to the heart.

The following recommendations can help increase comfort for computer users:

- "Dynamic sitting": Don't stay in one static position for extended periods of time.

- When performing daily tasks, alternate between sitting and standing.

- Adjust height of backrest to support the natural inward curvature of the lower back:

  - It may be useful to use a rolled towel or lumbar pad to support the low back.

  - The backrest angle should be set so that your hip-torso angle is 90 degrees or greater.

- Adjust height of chair so feet rest flat on floor (use footrest if necessary):

  - Sit upright in the chair with the low back against the backrest and the shoulders touching the backrest.

  - Thighs should be parallel to the floor and knees at about the same level as the hips.

  - Back of knees should not come in direct contact with the edge of the seat pan (there should be two to three inches between the edge of the seat and the back of the knee).

- Don't use armrests to slouch.

- Adjust height and/or width of armrests so they allow the user to rest arms at his or her sides and relax/drop his or her shoulders while keyboarding.

- Where armrests are used, elbows and lower arms should rest lightly so as not to cause circulatory or nerve problems.

Desktops for Computer Workstations

If you are like many computer users, your computer, keyboard, and mouse are resting on your desk or a portable computer workstation. There is no specific height recommended for your desktop; however, the working height of your desk should be approximately elbow height for light duty desk work.

To allow for proper alignment of your arms your keyboard should be approximately one to two inches above your thighs. Most times this requires a desk that is twenty-five to twenty-nine inches in height (depending upon size of individual) or the use of an articulating keyboard tray. The area underneath the desk should always be clean to accommodate the user's legs and allow for stretching.

The desktop should be organized so frequently used objects are close to the user to avoid excessive extended reaching. If a document holder is used, it should be placed at approximately the same height as the monitor and at the same distance from the eyes to prevent frequent eye shifts between the screen and reference materials.

Keyboard and Mouse

Many ergonomic problems associated with computer workstations occur in the forearm, wrist, and hand. Continuous work on the computer exposes soft tissues in these areas to repetition, awkward postures, and forceful exertions.

The following adjustments should be made to your workstation to help prevent the development of an ergonomic problem in the upper extremities:

- Adjust keyboard height so shoulders can relax and allow arms to rest at sides (an articulating keyboard tray is often necessary to accommodate proper height and distance).

- Keyboard should be close to the user to avoid excessive extended reaching.

- Forearms parallel to the floor (approximately 90 degree angle at elbow).

- Mouse should be placed adjacent to keyboard and at the same height as the keyboard (use articulating keyboard tray if necessary).

- Avoid extended and elevated reaching for keyboard and mouse. Wrist should be in neutral position (not excessively flexed or extended).

- Do not rest the hand on the mouse when you are not using it. Rest hands in your lap when not entering data.

Lighting for Computer Workstations

Lighting not suited to working with a video display terminal is a major contributing factor in visual discomforts including eyestrain, burning or itching eyes, and blurred or double vision. Typical office environments have illumination levels of 75 to 100 foot-candles, but according to the American National Standards Institute (ANSI), computer workstations require only 18 to 46 foot-candles.

Use the following recommendations to reduce eyestrain and eye fatigue:

- Close drapes/blinds to reduce glare. Adjust lighting to avoid glare on screen (light source should come at a 90 degree angle, with low watt lights rather than high.) Place monitor at 90 degree angle to windows (where possible). Reduce overhead lighting (where possible). Use indirect or shielded lighting where possible. Walls should be painted medium or dark color and not have reflective finish.

- Use a glare screen to reduce glare (alternatively, place a large manila folder on top of the monitor and let it hang over the monitor two to three inches to reduce glare from overhead lighting).

Eye Exercises and Stretches

Eye Comfort Exercises

1. Blinking (produces tears to help moisten and lubricate the eyes)
2. Yawning (produces tears to help moisten and lubricate the eyes)
3. Expose eyes to natural light

Palming Exercise

1. While seated, brace elbows on the desk and close to the desk edge.
2. Let weight fall forward.
3. Cup hands over eyes.
4. Close eyes.
5. Inhale slowly through nose and hold for four seconds.
6. Continue deep breathing for fifteen to thirty seconds.

Eye Movements

1. Close eyes.

2. Slowly and gently move eyes up to the ceiling, then slowly down to the floor.

3. Repeat three times.

4. Close eyes.

5. Slowly and gently move eyes to the left, then slowly to the right.

6. Repeat three times.

Focus Change

1. Hold one finger a few inches away from the eye.

2. Focus on the finger.

3. Slowly move the finger away.

4. Focus far into the distance and then back to the finger.

5. Slowly bring the finger back to within a few inches of the eye.

6. Focus on something more than eight feet away.

7. Repeat three times.

Musculoskeletal System Exercises and Stretches

Deep Breathing

1. While standing, or in an otherwise relaxed position, place one hand on the abdomen and one on the chest.

2. Inhale slowly through the nose.

3. Hold for four seconds.

4. Exhale slowly through the mouth.

5. Repeat.

Cable Stretch

1. While sitting with chin in, stomach in, shoulders relaxed, hands relaxed in lap, and feet flat on the floor, imagine a cable pulling the head upward.

2. Hold for three seconds and relax.

3. Repeat three times.

Side Bend: Neck Stretch

1. Tilt head to one side (ear toward shoulder).
2. Hold for fifteen seconds.
3. Relax.
4. Repeat three times on each side.

Diagonal Neck Stretch

1. Turn head slightly and then look down as if looking in your pocket.
2. Hold for fifteen seconds.
3. Relax.
4. Repeat three times on each side.

Shoulder Shrug

1. Slowly bring shoulders up to the ears and hold for approximately three seconds.
2. Rotate shoulders back and down.
3. Repeat ten times.

Executive Stretch

1. While sitting, lock hands behind head.
2. Bring elbows back as far as possible.
3. Inhale deeply while leaning back and stretching.
4. Hold for twenty seconds.
5. Exhale and relax.
6. Repeat one time.

Foot Rotation

1. While sitting, slowly rotate each foot from the ankle.
2. Rotate three times in one direction, then three times in the opposite direction.
3. Relax.
4. Repeat one time.

Hand Shake

1. While sitting, drop arms to the side.

2. Shake hands downward gently.

3. Repeat frequently.

Hand Massage (Note: Perform very gently!)

1. Massage the inside and outside of the hand using the thumb and fingers.

2. Repeat frequently (including before beginning work).

Finger Massage (Note: Perform very gently!)

1. Massage fingers of each hand individually, slowly, and gently.

2. Move toward nail gently.

3. Massage space between fingers.

4. Perform daily.

Wrist Stretch

1. Hold arm straight out in front of you.

2. Pull the hand backward with the other hand, then pull downward.

3. Hold for twenty seconds.

4. Relax.

5. Repeat three times each.

Section 47.3

Carpal Tunnel Syndrome

Reprinted from "Carpal Tunnel Syndrome Fact Sheet," National Institute of Neurological Disorders and Stroke, National Institutes of Health, NIH Publication No. 03-4898, August 2, 2006.

You're working at your desk, trying to ignore the tingling or numbness you've had for months in your hand and wrist. Suddenly, a sharp, piercing pain shoots through the wrist and up your arm. Just a passing cramp? More likely you have carpal tunnel syndrome, a painful progressive condition caused by compression of a key nerve in the wrist.

What is carpal tunnel syndrome?

Carpal tunnel syndrome occurs when the median nerve, which runs from the forearm into the hand, becomes pressed or squeezed at the wrist. The median nerve controls sensations to the palm side of the thumb and fingers (although not the little finger), as well as impulses to some small muscles in the hand that allow the fingers and thumb to move. The carpal tunnel—a narrow, rigid passageway of ligament and bones at the base of the hand—houses the median nerve and tendons. Sometimes, thickening from irritated tendons or other swelling narrows the tunnel and causes the median nerve to be compressed. The result may be pain, weakness, or numbness in the hand and wrist, radiating up the arm. Although painful sensations may indicate other conditions, carpal tunnel syndrome is the most common and widely known of the entrapment neuropathies in which the body's peripheral nerves are compressed or traumatized.

What are the symptoms of carpal tunnel syndrome?

Symptoms usually start gradually, with frequent burning, tingling, or itching numbness in the palm of the hand and the fingers, especially the thumb and the index and middle fingers. Some carpal tunnel sufferers say their fingers feel useless and swollen, even though little or no swelling is apparent. The symptoms often first appear in one or both hands during the night, since many people sleep with flexed wrists. A person with carpal tunnel syndrome may wake up feeling the need to "shake out" the hand or wrist. As symptoms worsen, people might feel tingling during the day. Decreased grip strength may make it difficult to form a fist, grasp small objects, or perform other manual tasks. In chronic or untreated cases, the muscles at the base of the thumb may waste away. Some people are unable to tell between hot and cold by touch.

What are the causes of carpal tunnel syndrome?

Carpal tunnel syndrome is often the result of a combination of factors that increase pressure on the median nerve and tendons in the carpal tunnel, rather than a problem with the nerve itself. Most likely the disorder is due to a congenital predisposition—the carpal tunnel is simply smaller in some people than in others. Other contributing factors include trauma or injury to the wrist that cause swelling, such as sprain or fracture; overactivity of the pituitary gland; hypothyroidism; rheumatoid arthritis; mechanical problems in the wrist joint; work stress; repeated use of vibrating hand tools; fluid retention during pregnancy or menopause; or the development of a cyst or tumor in the canal. In some cases no cause can be identified.

There is little clinical data to prove whether repetitive and forceful movements of the hand and wrist during work or leisure activities can cause carpal tunnel syndrome. Repeated motions performed in the course of normal work or other daily activities can result in repetitive motion disorders such as bursitis and tendonitis. Writer's cramp—a condition in which a lack of fine motor skill coordination and ache and pressure in the fingers, wrist, or forearm is brought on by repetitive activity—is not a symptom of carpal tunnel syndrome.

Who is at risk of developing carpal tunnel syndrome?

Women are three times more likely than men to develop carpal tunnel syndrome, perhaps because the carpal tunnel itself may be smaller in women than in men. The dominant hand is usually affected first and produces the most severe pain. Persons with diabetes or other metabolic disorders that directly affect the body's nerves and make them more susceptible to compression are also at high risk. Carpal tunnel syndrome usually occurs only in adults.

The risk of developing carpal tunnel syndrome is not confined to people in a single industry or job, but is especially common in those performing assembly line work—manufacturing, sewing, finishing, cleaning, and meat, poultry, or fish packing. In fact, carpal tunnel syndrome is three times more common among assemblers than among data-entry personnel. A 2001 study by the Mayo Clinic found heavy computer use (up to seven hours a day) did not increase a person's risk of developing carpal tunnel syndrome.

During 1998, an estimated three of every ten thousand workers lost time from work because of carpal tunnel syndrome. Half of these workers missed more than ten days of work. The average lifetime cost of carpal tunnel syndrome, including medical bills and lost time from work, is estimated to be about $30,000 for each injured worker.

How is carpal tunnel syndrome diagnosed?

Early diagnosis and treatment are important to avoid permanent damage to the median nerve. A physical examination of the hands, arms, shoulders, and neck can help determine if the patient's complaints are related to daily activities or to an underlying disorder, and can rule out other painful conditions that mimic carpal tunnel syndrome. The wrist is examined for tenderness, swelling, warmth, and discoloration. Each finger should be tested for sensation, and the muscles at the base of the hand should be examined for strength and signs of atrophy. Routine laboratory tests and x-rays can reveal diabetes, arthritis, and fractures.

Physicians can use specific tests to try to produce the symptoms of carpal tunnel syndrome. In the Tinel test, the doctor taps on or presses on the median nerve in the patient's wrist. The test is positive when tingling in the fingers or a resultant shock-like sensation occurs. The Phalen, or wrist-flexion, test involves having the patient hold his or her forearms upright by pointing the fingers down and pressing the backs of the hands together. The presence of carpal tunnel syndrome is suggested if one or more symptoms, such as tingling or increasing numbness, is felt in the fingers within one minute. Doctors may also ask patients to try to make a movement that brings on symptoms.

Often it is necessary to confirm the diagnosis by use of electrodiagnostic tests. In a nerve conduction study, electrodes are placed on the hand and wrist. Small electric shocks are applied and the speed with which nerves transmit impulses is measured. In electromyography, a fine needle is inserted into a muscle; electrical activity viewed on a screen can determine the severity of damage to the median nerve. Ultrasound imaging can show impaired movement of the median nerve. Magnetic resonance imaging (MRI) can show the anatomy of the wrist but to date has not been especially useful in diagnosing carpal tunnel syndrome.

How is carpal tunnel syndrome treated?

Treatments for carpal tunnel syndrome should begin as early as possible, under a doctor's direction. Underlying causes such as diabetes or arthritis should be treated first. Initial treatment generally involves resting the affected hand and wrist for at least two weeks, avoiding activities that may worsen symptoms, and immobilizing the wrist in a splint to avoid further damage from twisting or bending. If there is inflammation, applying cool packs can help reduce swelling.

Nonsurgical Treatments

Drugs: In special circumstances, various drugs can ease the pain and swelling associated with carpal tunnel syndrome. Nonsteroidal anti-inflammatory drugs, such as aspirin, ibuprofen, and other nonprescription pain relievers, may ease symptoms that have been present for a short time or have been caused by strenuous activity. Orally administered diuretics ("water pills") can decrease swelling. Corticosteroids (such as prednisone) or the drug lidocaine can be injected directly into the wrist or taken by mouth (in the case of prednisone) to relieve pressure on the median nerve and provide immediate, temporary relief to persons with mild or intermittent symptoms. (Caution: persons with diabetes and those who may be predisposed to diabetes should note that prolonged use of corticosteroids can make it difficult to regulate insulin levels. Corticosteroids should not be taken without a doctor's prescription.) Additionally, some studies show that vitamin B_6 (pyridoxine) supplements may ease the symptoms of carpal tunnel syndrome.

Exercise: Stretching and strengthening exercises can be helpful in people whose symptoms have abated. These exercises may be supervised by a physical therapist, who is trained to use exercises to treat physical impairments, or an occupational therapist, who is trained in evaluating people with physical impairments and helping them build skills to improve their health and well-being.

Alternative therapies: Acupuncture and chiropractic care have benefited some patients but their effectiveness remains unproved. An exception is yoga, which has been shown to reduce pain and improve grip strength among patients with carpal tunnel syndrome.

Surgery

Carpal tunnel release is one of the most common surgical procedures in the United States. Generally recommended if symptoms last for six months, surgery involves severing the band of tissue around the wrist to reduce pressure on the median nerve. Surgery is done under local anesthesia and does not require an overnight hospital stay. Many patients require surgery on both hands. The following are types of carpal tunnel release surgery.

Open release surgery: The traditional procedure used to correct carpal tunnel syndrome, this procedure consists of making an incision up to two inches long in the wrist and then cutting the carpal ligament to enlarge the carpal tunnel. The procedure is generally done under local anesthesia on an outpatient basis, unless there are unusual medical considerations.

Endoscopic surgery: This may allow faster functional recovery and less postoperative discomfort than traditional open release surgery. The surgeon makes two incisions (about one-half inch each) in the wrist and palm, inserts a camera attached to a tube, observes the tissue on a screen, and cuts the carpal ligament (the tissue that holds joints together). This two-portal endoscopic surgery, generally performed under local anesthesia, is effective and minimizes scarring and scar tenderness, if any. One-portal endoscopic surgery for carpal tunnel syndrome is also available.

Although symptoms may be relieved immediately after surgery, full recovery from carpal tunnel surgery can take months. Some patients may have infection, nerve damage, stiffness, and pain at the scar. Occasionally the wrist loses strength because the carpal ligament is cut. Patients should undergo physical therapy after surgery to restore wrist strength. Some patients may need to adjust job duties or even change jobs after recovery from surgery.

Recurrence of carpal tunnel syndrome following treatment is rare. The majority of patients recover completely.

How can carpal tunnel syndrome be prevented?

At the workplace, workers can do on-the-job conditioning, perform stretching exercises, take frequent rest breaks, wear splints to keep wrists straight, and use correct posture and wrist position. Wearing fingerless gloves can help keep hands warm and flexible. Workstations, tools and tool handles, and tasks can be redesigned to enable the worker's wrist to maintain a natural position during work. Jobs can be rotated among workers. Employers can develop programs in ergonomics, the process of adapting workplace conditions and job demands to the capabilities of workers. However, research has not conclusively shown that these workplace changes prevent the occurrence of carpal tunnel syndrome.

What research is being done?

The National Institute of Neurological Disorders and Stroke (NINDS), a part of the National Institutes of Health, is the federal government's leading supporter of biomedical research on neuropathy, including carpal tunnel syndrome. Scientists are studying the chronology of events that occur with carpal tunnel syndrome in order to better understand, treat, and prevent this ailment. By determining distinct biomechanical factors related to pain, such as specific joint angles, motions, force, and progression over time, researchers are finding new ways to limit or prevent carpal tunnel syndrome in the workplace and decrease other costly and disabling occupational illnesses.

Randomized clinical trials are being designed to evaluate the effectiveness of educational interventions in reducing the incidence of carpal tunnel syndrome and upper extremity cumulative trauma disorders. Data to be collected from a NINDS-sponsored clinical study of carpal tunnel syndrome among construction apprentices will provide a better understanding of the specific work factors associated with the disorder, furnish pilot data for planning future projects to study its natural history, and assist in developing strategies to prevent its occurrence among construction and other workers. Other research will discern differences between the relatively new carpal compression test (in which the examiner applies moderate pressure with both thumbs directly on the carpal tunnel and underlying median nerve at the transverse carpal ligament) and the pressure provocative test (in which a cuff placed at the anterior of the carpal tunnel is inflated, followed by direct pressure on the median nerve) in predicting carpal tunnel syndrome. Scientists are also investigating the use of alternative therapies, such as acupuncture, to prevent and treat this disorder.

Section 47.4

Noise-Induced Hearing Loss

Reprinted from the National Institute on Deafness and Other Communication Disorders, National Institutes of Health, NIH Publication No. 97-4233, September 2002. Reviewed by David A. Cooke, M.D., July 2007.

Every day we experience sound in our environment such as the television, radio, washing machine, automobiles, buses, and trucks. But when an individual is exposed to harmful sounds—sounds that are too loud or loud sounds over a long time—sensitive structures of the inner ear can be damaged, causing noise-induced hearing loss (NIHL).

How do we hear?

Hearing is a series of events in which the ear converts sound waves into electrical signals that are sent to the brain and interpreted as sound. The ear has three main parts: the outer, middle, and inner ear. Sound waves enter through the outer ear and reach the middle ear, where they cause the eardrum to vibrate.

The vibrations are transmitted through three tiny bones in the middle ear, called the ossicles. These three bones are named the malleus, incus, and stapes (and are also known as the hammer, anvil, and stirrup). The eardrum and ossicles amplify the vibrations and carry them to the inner ear. The stirrup transmits the amplified vibrations through the oval window and into the fluid that fills the inner ear. The vibrations move through fluid in the snail-shaped hearing part of the inner ear (cochlea) that contains the hair cells. The fluid in the cochlea moves the top portion of the hair cells, called the hair bundle, which initiates the changes that lead to the production of nerve impulses. These nerve impulses are carried to the brain, where they are interpreted as sound. Different sounds move the hair bundles in different ways, thus allowing the brain to distinguish one sound from another, such as vowels from consonants.

What sounds cause NIHL?

NIHL can be caused by a one-time exposure to loud sound as well as by repeated exposure to sounds at various loudness levels over an extended period of time. The loudness of sound is measured in units called decibels. For example, normal conversation is approximately 60 decibels, the humming of a refrigerator is 40 decibels, and city traffic noise can be 80 decibels. Examples of sources of loud noises that cause NIHL are motorcycles, firecrackers, and firearms, all emitting sounds from 120 to 140 decibels. Sounds of less than 80 decibels, even after long exposure, are unlikely to cause hearing loss.

Exposure to harmful sounds causes damage to the sensitive hair cells of the inner ear as well as the hearing nerve. These structures can be injured by two kinds of noise: loud impulse noise, such as an explosion, or loud continuous noise, such as that generated in a woodworking shop.

What are the effects of NIHL?

Impulse sound can result in immediate hearing loss that may be permanent. The structures of the inner ear may be severely damaged. This kind of hearing loss may be accompanied by tinnitus, a ringing, buzzing, or roaring in the ears or head, which may subside over time. Hearing loss and tinnitus may be experienced in one or both ears, and tinnitus may continue constantly or occasionally throughout a lifetime.

Continuous exposure to loud noise also can damage the structure of the hair cells, resulting in hearing loss and tinnitus. Exposure to impulse and continuous noise may cause only a temporary hearing loss. If the hearing recovers, the temporary hearing loss is called a temporary threshold shift. The temporary threshold shift largely disappears sixteen to forty-eight hours after exposure to loud noise.

Both forms of NIHL can be prevented by the regular use of hearing protectors such as earplugs or earmuffs.

What are the symptoms of NIHL?

The symptoms of NIHL increase gradually over a period of continuous exposure. Sounds may become distorted or muffled, and it may be difficult for the person to understand speech. The individual may not be aware of the loss, but it can be detected with a hearing test.

Who is affected by NIHL?

More than thirty million Americans are exposed to hazardous sound levels on a regular basis. Individuals of all ages, including children, adolescents, young adults, and older people, can develop NIHL. Exposure occurs in the workplace, in recreational settings, and at home. Noisy recreational activities include target shooting and hunting, snowmobiling, riding go-carts, woodworking and other noisy hobbies, and playing with power horns, cap guns, and model airplanes. Harmful noises at home include vacuum cleaners, garbage disposals, gas-powered lawn mowers, leaf blowers, and shop tools. And it makes no difference where a person lives—both urban and rural settings offer their own brands of noisy devices on a daily basis. Of the twenty-eight million Americans who have some degree of hearing loss, about one-third can attribute their hearing loss, at least in part, to noise.

Can NIHL be prevented?

NIHL is preventable. All individuals should understand the hazards of noise and how to practice good health in everyday life.

- Know which noises can cause damage (those above 90 decibels).

- Wear earplugs or other hearing protective devices when involved in a loud activity (special earplugs and earmuffs are available at hardware stores and sporting good stores).

- Be alert to hazardous noise in the environment.

- Protect children who are too young to protect themselves.

- Make family, friends, and colleagues aware of the hazards of noise.

- Have a medical examination by an otolaryngologist, a physician who specializes in diseases of the ears, nose, throat, head, and neck, and a hearing test by an audiologist, a health professional trained to identify and measure hearing loss and to rehabilitate persons with hearing impairments.

What research is being done for NIHL?

Scientists are studying the internal workings of the ear and the mechanisms that cause NIHL so that better prevention and treatment strategies can be developed. For example, scientists have discovered that damage to the structure of the hair bundle is related to temporary and permanent loss of hearing. When the hair bundle is exposed to prolonged periods of damaging sound, the basic structure of the hair bundle is destroyed and the important connections among hair cells are disrupted. These structural changes lead directly to hearing loss.

Recent NIDCD Research

Recent findings by NIDCD researchers show that hair bundles are capable of rebuilding their structure from top to bottom over a forty-eight-hour period (the common duration of temporary hearing loss). Researchers suggest that permanent hearing loss may occur when damage is so severe that it overwhelms the self-repair mechanism.[1]

Drug Therapies

Other studies involve potential drug therapies for NIHL. For example, scientists are studying how changes in blood flow in the cochlea affect hair cells. When a person is exposed to loud noise, blood flow in the cochlea drops. However, a drug that is used to treat peripheral vascular disease (any abnormal condition in blood vessels outside the heart) maintains circulation in the cochlea during exposure to noise. These findings may lead to the development of treatment strategies to reduce NIHL.

Continuing efforts will provide opportunities that can aid research on NIHL as well as other diseases and disorders that cause hearing loss.

Notes

1. Schneider M.E., Belyantseva I.A., Azevedo R.B., Kachar B. Rapid renewal of auditory hair bundles. *Nature.* 22 Aug 2002. 418(6900): 837–38.

Section 47.5

Managing Job Stress

"Managing Job Stress" by Robin Jacobs. From Career and Employment Guide for Job Seekers and Employees, Office of Students with Disabilities, Portland Community College, © 2003.

Does this sound familiar? Christmas crowds fill the aisles, and your cash register breaks down. You're short-staffed at the restaurant, and a busload of tourists stream through the door. You're giving a presentation to your biggest client company in an hour, and your materials and lost luggage are heading for Europe!

No matter where you work or what you do, you'll undoubtedly face stress on the job. In fact, research surveys and studies reveal:

- Forty percent of workers report their job is "very or extremely stressful" (Northwestern National Life).

- Twenty-six percent of workers report they are "often or very often burned out or stressed by their work" (The Families and Work Institute).

- Twenty-nine percent of workers report they feel "quite a bit or extremely stressed at work" (Yale University).

- Three-fourths of employees believe the worker has more on-the-job stress than a generation ago (Princeton Survey Research Associates).

- Problems at work are more strongly associated with health complaints than are any other life stressor—more so than even financial problems or family problems (St. Paul Fire and Marine Insurance Company).

What is job stress?

According to the National Institute for Occupational Safety and Health, job stress can be defined as the harmful physical and emotional responses that occur when the requirements of the job do not match the capabilities, resources, or needs of the worker.

531

Job stress is often linked or equated with challenge, but the two are very different. Challenge motivates and energizes us psychologically and physically to learn new skills and master given tasks. When a challenge is met, we feel a great sense of accomplishment. We feel relaxed and satisfied. Challenge is beneficial in the work environment, as it helps increase productivity. This is what people are referring to when they say "a little bit of stress is good for you." It might be more accurate to say "a little challenge is good for you."

Stress, on the other hand, is when job demands can't be met, relaxation has turned to exhaustion, and a sense of satisfaction has turned into feelings of tension. In short, the worker feels overly taxed both psychologically and physically, and the stage is set for illness, injury, and job failure.

What are the causes of job stress?

Quite simply, job stress results from the interaction of the worker and the conditions of the work. Views differ on the importance of worker characteristics versus working conditions as the primary cause of job stress.

Some view differences in individual characteristics, such as personality and coping style, as most important in predicting whether certain job conditions will result in stress. What may be stressful for one person may not be a problem for someone else. This viewpoint leads to prevention strategies that focus on workers and ways to help them cope with demanding job conditions.

Although individual differences can't be ignored, research studies indicate certain working conditions are stressful to most people. This scientific evidence places greater emphasis on working conditions as the key source of job stress, and job redesign as the primary prevention strategy. Excessive workload demands and conflicting expectations, for example, are key sources of job stress.

Other sources may include:

- Infrequent rest breaks;

- Long work hours and demanding work shifts;

- Hectic and routine tasks that have little inherent meaning, do not utilize a worker's skills, and provide little sense of control;

- Management styles: A lack of participation by workers in decision making, poor communication in the organization, lack of family-friendly policies;

- Interpersonal relationships: Poor social environment, lack of support or help from co-workers and supervisors;

- Work roles: Conflicting or uncertain job expectations, too much responsibility, too many "hats to wear";

- Career concerns: Job insecurity, lack of growth opportunity, rapid changes for which workers are unprepared;

- Environmental conditions: Unpleasant physical conditions such as crowding, noise, air pollution; ergonomic problems;

- Work conditions that pose risk to health and safety.

Short-lived episodes of stress pose little risk. But if stressful situations go unresolved, the body can suffer from wear and tear, and the ability of a person's body to repair and defend itself can become seriously compromised.

What are the warning signs of job stress?

The following may indicate signs of stress:

- Headaches
- Sleep disturbances
- Difficulty concentrating
- Short temper
- Upset stomach
- Job dissatisfaction
- Low morale

Signs of stress may also be associated with increased absenteeism, tardiness, and intentions of workers to quit their jobs.

What can be done about job stress?

Job stress may need to be approached in two ways. The two approaches would include:

- Stress management to improve a worker's ability to cope with difficult work situations. Companies sometimes offer stress management training or offer assistance through an Employee Assistance Program.

533

- Organizational change by the company upon identifying stressful aspects of work and designing strategies and improving work conditions to reduce or eliminate the identified stressors.

Be aware that management is often uncomfortable with the "organizational change" approach because it can involve changes in workloads, work routines, work schedules, work production, or organizational structure. As a general rule, however, it takes organizational change to improve working conditions, and it takes improved working conditions to reduce job stress. And it takes reduced to job stress to boost morale and retain workers.

What organizational changes can help reduce job stress?

Helpful organizational changes may include:

- Ensuring the workload is in line with workers' capabilities and resources;

- Designing jobs to provide meaning, stimulation, and opportunities for workers to use their skills;

- Clearly defining workers' roles and responsibilities;

- Giving workers opportunities to participate in decisions and actions affecting their jobs;

- Improving communications;

- Providing opportunities for social interaction among workers;

- Establishing work schedules that are compatible with demands and responsibilities outside the job.

What worker characteristics can cause job stress?

Worker characteristics that can cause job stress may include:

- **A need to be in control:** The worker feels a need to be in control at all times; the worker views lack of control as a sign of weakness; the worker has difficulty delegating assignments to others; the worker avoids showing signs of weakness or nervousness.

- **A lack or perceived lack of competence:** The worker feels his or her work is inferior compared to others; the worker feels he or she makes poor judgments; the worker feels a lack of common sense; the worker feels doubts about his or her competence and ability to do the job.

- **A desire to please people:** The worker relies on favorable opinions and input from others as a basis for building self-esteem; the worker fears he or she may disappoint others; the worker cares more about others' needs than his or her own; the worker avoids communications and actions that would displease others.

- **A need to be perfect (perfectionism):** The worker feels under pressure to achieve; the worker is highly self-critical; the worker feels a job well done could have been done even better; the worker sacrifices pleasure in order to excel and achieve.

What can workers with these characteristics do to relieve job stress?

If one of the above profiles rings true for you, the following suggestions may help.

Mentally reframe: Identify situations that are stressful for you. At what times, and under what circumstances, do you feel job stress? Make note.

Gauge your thinking. During those stressful times, do your thoughts turn negative and self-defeating? Do your thoughts only add more pressure?

Consider these examples:

- Negative thoughts: "People can tell I'm nervous"; "I'm always making mistakes;" "I can't do anything right"; "That was a stupid thing I did"; "I'll never meet the deadline"; "My performance was awful."

- Pressure thoughts: "I can't show I'm nervous or people will think I'm weak"; "I can't make a mistake or people will think poorly of me"; "If I don't do this right, everyone will see I'm not very skilled"; "The manager must not like me as she never returns my greeting."

Change your thinking. If during stressful times you find yourself thinking negative or pressure thoughts, stop those self-defeaters in their tracks and reframe your thinking!

Using the above examples, let's reframe.

Negative Thoughts

- Stress producing: "People can tell I'm nervous."
- Stress reducing: "People seem interested in what I have to say."

- Stress producing: "I'm always making mistakes."
- Stress reducing: "I made a mistake, but it's okay. Next time I'll know what to do."

- Stress producing: "I can't do anything right."
- Stress reducing: "I do most things well. Some things just take practice, then I get it."

- Stress producing: "That was a stupid thing I did."
- Stress reducing: "I made a wrong judgment, but that's okay. Next time I'll know to do it differently."

- Stress producing: "I'll never meet the deadline."
- Stress reducing: "I'll get it done. I'll just start by making a list of what I need to do."

- Stress producing: "My performance was awful."
- Stress reducing: "I did many things well, but there are a few things I'd like to improve."

Pressure Thoughts

- Stress producing: "I can't show I'm nervous or people will think I'm weak."
- Stress reducing: "I'm well-prepared and confident I'll do a good job."

- Stress producing: "I can't make a mistake or people will think poorly of me."
- Stress reducing: "No one's perfect. If I make a mistake, it's okay. I'll just show I'm like everyone else!"

- Stress producing: "If I don't do this right, everyone will see I'm not very skilled."
- Stress reducing: "I have many good skills, and I can learn and improve with time."

- Stress producing: "The manager must not like me as she never returns my greeting."
- Stress reducing: "The manager must have a lot on her mind."

Replacing self-defeating thoughts with positive ones takes practice, but the results are worth the effort.

What other strategies may help reduce job stress?

The following strategies are also helpful for reducing job stress.

Organize your time: Use a schedule planner and schedule tasks. Stick to the schedule! Be sure to schedule in time you need to meet deadlines, make phone calls, send correspondence, write reports, and so on.

Follow your bio-clock: Try to schedule the hardest tasks during your hours of peak performance and concentration.

Make "To Do" lists: List everything you need to do in order of priority. As you finish a task, check it off and go to the next one.

Throw it away: Don't let things accumulate! Sort mail and toss what you don't need. Sort e-mails and delete what you don't need to read. Sort files and toss what's out-of-date.

Organize your work space: Organize papers, files, or items so that you know where everything is, and things can be found quickly.

Don't procrastinate: Don't wait. Do it now. You'll be happy you got it done!

Think in steps: Take a large project and break it down into small steps. Then do the project one small step at a time.

Take breaks: Avoid working around the clock. Go get a cup a coffee. Eat lunch away from your desk or work area. Try to go home on time.

Share a problem: If you encounter an unusually challenging work problem, talk with co-workers. They may not have a solution, but it helps to talk through issues. Sometimes just by talking through a problem, you can recognize a solution.

Sleep: Make sure you get enough sleep. Lack of sleep impairs concentration, which can add pressure and anxiety.

Target ideas: Each time you feel stress, write down a list of targeted things you need to do to reduce the stress for that event.

Take a real vacation: When you take time off, avoid thinking about work. Focus on things you enjoy. This applies to your time off on weekends as well.

Transition: Between work and home, do something to get your mind off work. Listen to the car radio, stop for a coffee, drop by the library, stop at the store.

Leave work at work: Take home as little work as possible.

Practice relaxation techniques: During times of stress, try deep breathing, muscle relaxation techniques, exercising, taking a walk, mentally rehearsing by mentally walking through an upcoming event, talking with a friend, listening to relaxing music, meditating, or engaging in an activity you enjoy to divert your attention.

These are just a few suggestions that will hopefully help should you encounter stress in the workplace.

Chapter 48

Travel-Related Health Concerns

Chapter Contents

Section 48.1

Healthy Travel: What You Should Know

"Tips for Safe and Healthy Travel" is excerpted from "Traveling This Summer? Here Are Tips for Safe and Healthy Travel," Centers for Disease Control and Prevention, June 21, 2006. "Travelers' Health Kit" is reprinted from Centers for Disease Control and Prevention, 2006.

Tips for Safe and Healthy Travel

Each year millions of Americans travel abroad for vacation, business, or to visit friends and family. Unfortunately, about half of these international travelers get sick or injured during their trip.

The good news is that most travel-related sickness and injury can be prevented. You are likely to be a traveler who has an enjoyable trip free from illness or injury when you follow these tips:

1. **Be informed:** Learn about travel health risks and what to do to avoid them before your trip.

2. **Be ready:** Get any vaccinations (shots) or medicines that you will need before your trip.

3. **Be smart while you travel:** Make sure you follow travel safety tips while you are on your trip.

Be Informed

Find out what you need to know about staying healthy and safe in the area where you are traveling.

Be Ready

If you will need any vaccinations (shots) or medicines, go to your healthcare provider or a travel medicine clinic at least four to six weeks before your trip. This will give your shots time to work so that you will be protected during your trip. If it is less than four weeks before you leave, you should still see your doctor. It might not be too late to get your shots, medications, and other useful information.

Some countries require you to present a certificate that says you have had a yellow fever vaccination before you can enter. Only authorized healthcare providers can give the yellow fever vaccine. The vaccine should be given at least ten days before travel and a stamped vaccine certificate will be issued to you by the immunization center.

Prepare a traveler's health kit so you have all the medications and supplies you may need before you go.

Be Smart while You Travel

- Wash your hands often with soap and water. If soap and water are not available and your hands are not visibly dirty, use alcohol-based hand gel (with at least 60 percent alcohol) to clean your hands.

- Drink only bottled or boiled water or carbonated (bubbly) drinks from sources you trust. Do not drink tap water or fountain drinks, or eat ice cubes.

- Only eat food that has been fully cooked or fruits and vegetables that have been washed and peeled by you. Remember: boil it, cook it, peel it, or forget it.

- If visiting an area where you might get malaria, make sure to take your malaria prevention medication before, during, and after your trip, as directed.

- If you might be bitten by insects (like mosquitoes or ticks) use insect repellent (bug spray) with 30-50 percent DEET (N,N-diethylmetatoluamide). The label on the container will tell you the DEET content.

- Make sure you know how to protect yourself from injury while you travel. Motor vehicle accidents are a leading cause of injury and deaths in travelers. Swimming-related accidents are also a major cause of injury among travelers.

- Avoid poultry farms, bird markets, and other places where live poultry is raised or kept.

- Do not handle animals, especially monkeys, dogs, and cats, to avoid bites and serious diseases (including rabies and plague).

Follow the tips and recommendations your health-care provider and the Centers for Disease Control and Prevention (CDC) offer, and you are more likely to remain healthy and safe, so you can enjoy your time away from home.

Travelers' Health Kit

The purpose of a travel kit is twofold: to allow the traveler to take care of minor health problems as they occur and to treat exacerbations of preexisting medical conditions. A variety of health kits are available commercially and may even be purchased over the internet; however, similar kits can be assembled at home. The specific contents of the health kit are based on destination, duration of travel, type of travel, and the traveler's preexisting medical conditions. Basic items that should be included are listed below.

Medications

- Personal prescription medications (copies of all prescriptions, including the generic names for medications, and a note from the prescribing physician on letterhead stationary for controlled substances and injectable medications should be carried)

- Antimalarial medications, if applicable

- Antidiarrheal medication (e.g., bismuth subsalicylate, loperamide)

- Antibiotic for self-treatment of moderate to severe diarrhea

- Antihistamine

- Decongestant, alone or in combination with antihistamine

- Anti–motion sickness medication

- Acetaminophen, aspirin, ibuprofen, or other medication for pain or fever

- Mild laxative

- Cough suppressant/expectorant

- Throat lozenges

- Antacid

- Antifungal and antibacterial ointments or creams

- One percent hydrocortisone cream

- Epinephrine auto-injector (e.g., EpiPen), especially if history of severe allergic reaction. Also available in smaller-dose package for children.

Other Important Items

- Insect repellent containing DEET (up to 50 percent)
- Sunscreen (preferably SPF 15 or greater)
- Aloe gel for sunburns
- Digital thermometer
- Oral rehydration solution packets
- Basic first-aid items (adhesive bandages, gauze, ace wrap, antiseptic, tweezers, scissors, cotton-tipped applicators)
- Antibacterial hand wipes or alcohol-based hand sanitizer
- Moleskin for blisters
- Lubricating eye drops (e.g., Natural Tears)
- First aid quick reference card

Other Items That May Be Useful in Certain Circumstances

- Mild sedative (e.g., zolpidem) or other sleep aid
- Anti-anxiety medication
- High-altitude preventive medication
- Water purification tablets
- Commercial suture/syringe kits (to be used by local healthcare provider. These items will also require a letter from the prescribing physician on letterhead stationary)
- Latex condoms
- Address and phone numbers of area hospitals or clinics

Commercial medical kits are available for a wide range of circumstances, from basic first aid to advanced emergency life support. Many outdoor sporting goods stores sell their own basic first aid kits. For more adventurous travelers, a number of companies produce advanced medical kits and will even customize kits based on specific travel needs. In addition, specialty kits are available for managing diabetes, dealing with dental emergencies, and handling aquatic environments. If travelers choose to purchase a health kit rather than assemble their own, they should be certain to review the contents of the kit carefully to ensure that it has everything needed; supplementation with additional items for comfort may be necessary.

A final reminder: a health kit is useful only if it is available. It should be carried with the traveler at all times (e.g., in carry-on baggage and on excursions). All medications, especially prescription medications, should be stored in carry-on baggage, in their original containers with clear labels. With heightened airline security, sharp objects will have to remain in checked luggage.

Section 48.2

What You Need to Know about Vaccinations and Travel

Reprinted from "What You Need to Know about Vaccinations and Travel: A Checklist," Centers for Disease Control and Prevention, January 12, 2006.

Have you scheduled a visit to your doctor or a travel medicine provider?

Ideally, set up one up four to six weeks before your trip.

Most vaccines take time to become effective in your body and some vaccines must be given in a series over a period of days or sometimes weeks.

If it is less than four weeks before you leave, you should still see your doctor. You might still benefit from shots or medications and other information about how to protect yourself from illness and injury while traveling.

Are you aware of which types of vaccinations you or those traveling with you may need?

CDC divides vaccines for travel into three categories: routine, recommended, and required. While your doctor will tell you which ones you should have, it's best to be aware of them ahead of time.

Routine vaccinations: Be sure that you and your family are up to date on your routine vaccinations. These vaccines are necessary for protection from diseases that are still common in many parts of the world even though they rarely occur in the United States.

Recommended vaccinations: These vaccines are recommended to protect travelers from illnesses present in other parts of the world and to prevent the importation of infectious diseases across international borders. Which vaccinations you need depends on a number of factors, including your destination, whether you will be spending time in rural areas, the season of the year you are traveling, your age, health status, and previous immunizations.

Required vaccinations: The only vaccine required by International Health Regulations is yellow fever vaccination for travel to certain countries in sub-Saharan Africa and tropical South America. Meningococcal vaccination is required by the government of Saudi Arabia for annual travel during the Hajj.

Section 48.3

Cruising with Confidence

Reprinted from *FDA Consumer Magazine*, U.S. Food and Drug Administration, May–June 2003.

Shaking hands may be the conventional greeting for landlubbers, but on the high seas, the "forearm tap" has become popular. This greeting of knocking elbows together instead of shaking hands was encouraged by a number of cruise lines to raise awareness of the importance of personal hygiene onboard ship, according to a representative for Carnival Cruise Lines.

Poor personal hygiene is the likely cause of gastrointestinal illness (gastroenteritis) on cruise ships, according to the Centers for Disease Control and Prevention (CDC). The CDC investigated twenty-two reports of gastroenteritis outbreaks aboard eighteen cruise ships from January 1, 2002, through December 31, 2002. Of the twenty-two outbreaks, three were blamed on bacteria and seven could not be traced with certainty, but the remaining twelve were confirmed to be associated with noroviruses—a group of viruses that cause gastroenteritis, also known as Norwalk-like viruses.

Symptoms of norovirus infection include nausea, vomiting, diarrhea, and stomach cramping that can last from twelve to sixty hours. The symptoms usually begin twenty-four to forty-eight hours after a virus is ingested. Although people may feel very ill and vomit frequently, norovirus infections are not considered serious in most individuals. But they may become serious in the very young, in older people, and in those with weakened immune systems.

Noroviruses are found in the stool or vomit of infected people, and infection can spread in several ways:

- Eating food or drinking liquids that are contaminated with the virus

- Touching contaminated surfaces or objects and then placing your hands in or near your mouth

- Having direct contact with another person who is infected and showing symptoms (for example, sharing foods or eating utensils)

Viruses aren't the vacationer's only cause of gastrointestinal illness. "Travelers can also get diarrhea from bacterial infections," says Renata Albrecht, M.D., the director of the Food and Drug Administration's Division of Special Pathogen and Immunologic Drug Products. Bacterial infections usually go away over time without treatment, but doctors may prescribe antibiotics to treat some and shorten the duration of the diarrhea, says Albrecht. No medications are approved for preventing bacterial infection, nor are there medications that prevent or treat noroviruses.

Advice for Travelers

Frequent and thorough hand washing with warm, soapy water is the best prevention against gastroenteritis, says LeeAnne Jackson, Ph.D., a health science policy adviser in the FDA's Center for Food Safety and Applied Nutrition. Travelers who don't have ready access to soap and water may want to carry along a hand gel sanitizer, found in most supermarkets and drugstores.

Jackson also advises travelers to choose foods and beverages carefully. Foods should be thoroughly cooked and served hot. Poor sanitation in some countries may lead to contaminated food and drink, which are the major sources of stomach or intestinal illness while traveling, according to the CDC. Just about any food can become contaminated if handled improperly, but items of particular concern include raw meat, raw seafood, green salads, and raw sprouts. "In some countries, it's wise to steer clear of street food vendors, especially if they serve fresh-cut fruits," says Jackson, who advocates purchasing fruits whole, peeling them, and cutting them up yourself.

Travelers should avoid unpasteurized milk or products made with unpasteurized milk, unpasteurized juices, and ciders, says Jackson. Beverages that may be safer than tap water in some countries are hot beverages, such as coffee or tea made with boiled water, canned or bottled carbonated beverages, and beer and wine. Avoid ice made with tap water. Water on the surface of a beverage can or bottle may be contaminated, so wipe clean and dry the area of the container that will touch your mouth.

The Cruise Ship Connection

CDC investigators believe that most of the recent norovirus infections on cruise ships were spread person-to-person through hand-to-mouth activity. "We suspect that people are probably coming onboard with the virus," says Dave Forney, chief of the CDC's Vessel Sanitation Program. "On a cruise ship, people are out and about in very public areas, and so we have this depositing of the virus on various surfaces that then would be easily picked up by others."

Forney advises cruisers who are ill to avoid contact with other individuals and to report to the ship's medical facility. Unfortunately, many of them don't want to be told to stay in their cabins, adds Forney, so passengers spreading the virus around the ship are contributing to the ongoing problem.

Outbreaks on cruise ships have gained media attention, but an estimated 60 to 80 percent of all outbreaks of severe gastroenteritis occur on land, says the CDC. Norovirus infection is the most common cause of nonbacterial gastrointestinal illness in the United States; about twenty-three million cases of severe gastroenteritis a year are due to noroviruses. Noroviruses may be found in areas where people congregate together for days at a time, such as in schools, hotels, camps, nursing homes, and hospitals. Gastroenteritis is not a reportable illness in the United States except on cruise ships, so the public may be more aware of the shipboard incidences, says Forney.

By law, cruise ships that enter a U.S. port from a foreign port are required to report to the CDC, twenty-four hours prior to arrival, the number of passengers and crew onboard who go to the ship's medical facility with gastrointestinal illness, even if the number is zero, says Forney. Having 3 percent or more of either passengers or crew reported with a gastrointestinal illness is considered an outbreak and cause for investigation.

Travelers shouldn't shun cruises, says Forney. "It is perfectly safe to go on cruise ships. The standard by which they are held for sanitation is the highest in the world." Extensive cleaning and disinfecting were carried out on ships immediately following reports of illness, Forney adds. And cruise lines continue to scrub and sanitize public areas of their ships, especially frequently touched surfaces such as handrails, elevator buttons, and even poker chips.

The Importance of Hand Washing

Healthcare specialists generally cite hand washing as the single most effective way to prevent the spread of disease, according to the Centers for Disease Control and Prevention. If you do not wash your hands frequently, you can pick up germs and then infect yourself when you touch your eyes, nose, or mouth. Wash your hands before eating, after using the bathroom, and after changing diapers or playing with a pet.

For best results, use warm water to moisten your hands and then apply soap. Rub your hands together vigorously for at least twenty seconds. It is the soap combined with the scrubbing action that helps loosen and remove the germs on your hands.

Section 48.4

Jet Lag

Basics

Anyone who has ever flown is likely to have experienced some degree of time zone change disorder, commonly known as jet lag. Until recently, jet lag was not treated as a medical condition. It is now included as one of the eighty-four known or suspected sleep disorders and affects millions of people each year.

Jet lag occurs when the body's biological clock is out of sync with local time. When traveling to a new time zone, our bodies are slow to adjust and remain on their original biological schedule for several days. The result is that we feel excessively sleepy during the day or wide awake at night.

People may experience jet lag in varying degrees. In general, the severity of jet lag symptoms is directly related to the number of time zones crossed by a flight. Jet lag symptoms typically last longer following eastward flights. Flying east usually results in difficulty initiating sleep, whereas flying west results in early morning awakenings. All age groups are susceptible, but individuals over the age of fifty are more likely to develop jet lag than those under the age of thirty. Also, individual susceptibility tends to vary considerably and it is possible that preexisting sleep deprivation will intensify jet lag.

Symptoms

Symptoms of jet lag include the following:

- Daytime sleepiness
- Nighttime alertness (insomnia)
- Loss of appetite and other gastrointestinal dysfunction
- Mood disturbances
- Difficulty concentrating or focusing

Treatment

Researchers believe that gradually adjusting your bedtime to coincide with the time zone of your destination in the days before travel may prevent or reduce jet lag. On average, it takes about a day for each hour of time zone change to recover from jet lag.

In addition to adjusting your sleep schedule, prescription sleep aids may help reduce the amount of sleep lost as a result of jet lag. Over-the-counter sleep aids and alcohol should be avoided. Nonprescription sleep aids can cause sleepiness long after the intended sleep time and exacerbate the sleepiness associated with jet lag. Alcohol can disrupt sleep. Daytime sleepiness can be treated with caffeine, as long as it is not taken in the few hours before bedtime.

Melatonin, a naturally secreted hormone that regulates the body's internal clock, is used by some people to initiate sleep when traveling. Currently, melatonin is largely available only in health food stores and is not regulated. Therefore, melatonin is, at present, an experimental approach to sleep problems and travelers should consult their physicians before using it. Pregnant or breastfeeding women and children should not take melatonin for jet lag. Melatonin (0.5 mg) is probably of use only when traveling east. Travelers can take it a few days before, during, or after traveling east and should take it five to seven hours before their usual bedtime in their old time zone. Melatonin can induce sleepiness, so people should not drive or operate heavy machinery for several hours after ingestion.

Coping

The following are additional steps you can take to minimize jet lag:

- Shift your sleep times before you travel. In the few days before traveling west, go to bed and wake up one hour later each day. In the few days before traveling east, go to bed and wake up one hour earlier each day.

- Regulate your light exposure before you travel. In the few days before traveling west, seek evening light and avoid morning light. In the few days before traveling east, seek morning light and avoid evening light. People can use a bright light box to get light, although people who experience migraines or mood disorders or have eye diseases should first consult with their physician before using one.

- Regulate your light exposure in your new time zone. If you traveled west, on arrival, seek morning light and avoid afternoon light. If you traveled east, on arrival seek evening light and avoid morning light. Weather conditions permitting, people can seek light by going outdoors and wearing only lightly tinted sunglasses. Do not look directly at the sun. Light can be avoided by staying indoors away from windows, wearing very dark sunglasses when outside, and sleeping.

- Avoid alcohol and caffeine for at least three to six hours before bedtime.

- Avoid heavy exercise close to bedtime.

- Bring earplugs and blindfolds to reduce noise and light while sleeping.

Section 48.5

Motion Sickness

Reprinted from "What's Motion Sickness?" This information was provided by KidsHealth, one of the largest resources online for medically reviewed health information written for parents, kids, and teens. For more articles like this one, visit www.KidsHealth.org, or www.TeensHealth.org. © 2004 The Nemours Foundation.

If you've ever been sick to your stomach while riding in a car, train, airplane, or boat, you know exactly what motion sickness feels like. It's no fun.

To understand motion sickness, it helps to understand a few parts of your body and how they affect the way you feel movement:

- **Inner ears:** The liquid in here sloshes around, helping you sense if you're moving, and, if you are, which way you're moving—up, down, side to side, round and round, forward, or backward.

- **Eyes:** What you see also lets your body know whether you're moving and in which direction.

- **Skin receptors:** These receptors tell your brain which parts of your body are touching the ground.

- **Muscles and joint sensory receptors:** These sensing receptors tell your brain if you're moving your muscles and which position your body is in.

The brain gets an instant report from these different parts of your body and tries to put together a total picture about what you are doing just at that moment. But if any of the pieces of this picture don't match, you can get motion sickness.

For example, if you're riding in a car and reading a book, your inner ears and skin receptors will detect that you are moving forward. However, your eyes are looking at a book that isn't moving, and your muscle receptors are telling your brain that you're sitting still. So the brain gets a little confused. Things may begin to feel a little scrambled inside your head at that point.

When this happens, you might feel really tired, dizzy, or sick to your stomach. Sometimes you might even throw up. And if you're feeling scared or anxious, your motion sickness might get even worse.

Avoiding Motion Sickness

To avoid motion sickness:

- **Put your best face forward:** Always sit facing forward. Don't face backward in your seat or sit in a seat that faces backward. Sitting forward helps keep the motion sensed by your eyes and ears the same.

- **Examine the great outdoors:** Look outside. From inside a car, look at stuff far away, like the barn up ahead or a mountain. If you're seasick on a boat, go to the top deck (in the middle of the boat) and look far out into the horizon—where the sea and sky meet. On an airplane, try looking out the window. This way, your eyes won't be fooled into thinking you're not moving when you actually are.

- **Get to the middle of things:** Whatever you're riding in, find the place with the least amount of movement. This means sitting closer to the center of a plane (in the aisle seats over the wings) or in the middle of a boat—rather than at the sides or the front, where you're more likely to feel seasick.

If you feel this way easily during any kind of movement, it's a good idea to go to the doctor. He or she will want to make sure there's nothing wrong with your inner ears or any of the other body parts that sense movement.

But for typical motion sickness, you may be able to take some medicine before you travel. For some, it may help to wear pressure bracelets that can be bought at the pharmacy or drugstore.

If you feel yourself getting sick while you're traveling in a car, it might help if the driver finds a safe spot, where you can get out and walk around a little bit. If you can't pull over, make sure you have a plastic bag in the car—just in case!

Section 48.6

Travelers' Diarrhea

Excerpted from "Travelers' Diarrhea," Centers for Disease Control and Prevention, November 21, 2006.

Who gets travelers' diarrhea?

Travelers' diarrhea (TD) is the most common illness affecting travelers. Each year between 20 and 50 percent of international travelers, an estimated ten million persons, develop diarrhea. The onset of TD usually occurs within the first week of travel but may occur at any time while traveling, and even after returning home. The most important determinant of risk is the traveler's destination. High-risk destinations are the developing countries of Latin America, Africa, the Middle East, and Asia. Persons at particularly high-risk include young adults, immunosuppressed persons, persons with inflammatory bowel disease or diabetes, and persons taking H2 (Histamine-2) blockers or antacids. Attack rates are similar for men and women. The primary source of infection is ingestion of fecally contaminated food or water.

What are common symptoms of travelers' diarrhea?

Most TD cases begin abruptly. The illness usually results in increased frequency, volume, and weight of stool. Altered stool consistency also is common. Typically, a traveler experiences four to five loose or watery bowel movements each day. Other commonly associated symptoms are nausea, vomiting, diarrhea, abdominal cramping, bloating, fever, urgency, and malaise. Most cases are benign and resolve in one to two days without treatment. TD is rarely life threatening.

What causes travelers' diarrhea?

Infectious agents are the primary cause of TD. Bacterial enteropathogens cause approximately 80 percent of TD cases. The most common causative agent isolated in countries surveyed has been enterotoxigenic *Escherichia coli* (ETEC). ETEC produce watery diarrhea with associated cramps and low-grade or no fever. Besides ETEC and other bacterial pathogens, a variety of viral and parasitic enteric pathogens also are potential causative agents.

What preventive measures are effective for travelers' diarrhea?

Travelers can minimize their risk for TD by practicing the following effective preventive measures:

- Avoid eating foods or drinking beverages purchased from street vendors or other establishments where unhygienic conditions are present.

- Avoid eating raw or undercooked meat and seafood.

- Avoid eating raw fruits (e.g., oranges, bananas, avocados) and vegetables unless the traveler peels them.

If handled properly, well-cooked and packaged foods usually are safe. Tap water, ice, unpasteurized milk, and dairy products are associated with increased risk for TD. Safe beverages include bottled carbonated beverages, hot tea or coffee, beer, wine, and water boiled or appropriately treated with iodine or chlorine.

Is prophylaxis of travelers' diarrhea recommended?

The Centers for Disease Control and Prevention (CDC) does not recommend antimicrobial drugs to prevent TD. Studies show a decrease in the incidence of TD with use of bismuth subsalicylate and with use of antimicrobial chemoprophylaxis. Several studies show that bismuth subsalicylate taken as either two tablets four times daily or two fluid ounces four times daily reduces the incidence of travelers' diarrhea. Use of bismuth subsalicylate should be avoided by persons who are allergic to aspirin, during pregnancy, and by persons taking certain other medications (e.g., anticoagulants, probenecid, or methotrexate). In addition, persons should be informed about potential side effects, in particular about temporary blackening of the tongue and stool, and rarely ringing in the ears. Because of potential adverse side effects, prophylactic bismuth subsalicylate should not be used for more than three weeks.

Some antibiotics administered in a once-a-day dose are 90 percent effective at preventing travelers' diarrhea; however, antibiotics are not recommended as prophylaxis. Routine antimicrobial prophylaxis increases the traveler's risk for adverse reactions and for infections with resistant organisms. Because antimicrobials can increase a traveler 's susceptibility to resistant bacterial pathogens and provide no protection against either viral or parasitic pathogens, they can give travelers a false sense of security. As a result, strict adherence to preventive measures is encouraged, and bismuth subsalicylate should be used as an adjunct if prophylaxis is needed.

What treatment measures are effective for travelers' diarrhea?

TD usually is a self-limited disorder and often resolves without specific treatment; however, oral rehydration is often beneficial to replace lost fluids and electrolytes. Clear liquids are routinely recommended for adults. Travelers who develop three or more loose stools in an eight-hour period—especially if associated with nausea, vomiting, abdominal cramps, fever, or blood in stools—may benefit from antimicrobial therapy. Antibiotics usually are given for three to five days. If diarrhea persists despite therapy, travelers should be evaluated by a doctor and treated for possible parasitic infection.

When should antimotility agents not be used to treat travelers' diarrhea?

Antimotility agents primarily reduce diarrhea by slowing transit time in the gut, and, thus, allow more time for absorption. Some persons believe diarrhea is the body's defense mechanism to minimize contact time between gut pathogens and intestinal mucosa. In several studies, antimotility agents have been useful in treating travelers' diarrhea by decreasing the duration of diarrhea. However, these agents should not be used by travelers with fever or bloody diarrhea, because they can increase the severity of disease by delaying clearance of causative organisms. Because antimotility agents are now available over the counter, their injudicious use is of concern. Adverse complications (toxic megacolon, sepsis, and disseminated intravascular coagulation) have been reported as a result of using these medications to treat diarrhea.

Chapter 49

Caring for Aging Parents

Chapter Contents

Section 49.1

Caregiving: Tips for Daily Life

Excerpted from "Because We Care: A Guide for People Who Care—Living Day to Day," National Family Caregiver Support Program, Administration on Aging, September 9, 2004.

Hands-On Caregiving

If your older relative or friend needs considerable help, a well-planned routine can make the more demanding parts of your caregiving day go more smoothly and take less time and help to ensure that your care receiver does not develop problems which could be prevented.

Make a list of all the things you need for morning and bedtime routines, buy several of these items, and have them close at hand, such as bathing items, medications, and clothing. This saves time and keeps you from having to search or leave the room for them when you are helping your older family member. If you use items in several different places, have duplicate items stored in these rooms, such as the bathroom and bedroom.

If possible, have someone help you with the morning and bedtime routines, if your older relative needs a lot of assistance, since getting up and going to bed often are the most challenging times of the day.

Practice good oral hygiene that includes tooth brushing, denture cleaning, and cleaning around the gums, preferably after every meal. Good oral hygiene helps to prevent tooth decay, tooth loss, and gum diseases, as well as secondary infections that can result from poor dental care. Persons with disabilities or medical problems may need special care in addition to daily hygiene routines.

If your older family member is disabled, has poor eyesight, or has cognitive impairments, you may need to remind him or her about personal hygiene or assist him or her. If your care receiver is incontinent, it is especially important to ensure that he or she is clean at all times, to use protective (barrier) creams, and to change incontinence aids and clothing as often as needed. Poor hygiene can result in diaper rash and blistering of the skin. Poor hygiene also can contribute to the development of decubitus ulcers (pressure sores) and other problems that cause pain, discomfort, and serious, even life-threatening infections. In older women, tight-fitting clothing and diapers can lead to yeast infections.

There are new commercial products that make incontinence much less of a problem than it once was because they keep clothes and bed linens clean and dry. You also can discuss ways in which your care receiver's incontinence may be corrected with your healthcare provider, including exercises and surgical procedures.

Older persons with limited movement should be turned in bed on a regular basis to prevent pressure sores. Correct bedding, such as sheepskin or egg carton bed coverings or an air mattress, helps to prevent pressure sores. It is important to move older persons with disabilities at least once an hour, even if it is just to reposition them, to do range of motion exercises, and to have them sit in various chairs that offer sufficient support.

Make lists of:

- Morning and bedtime routines;
- Medical personnel with their area of expertise, addresses, and telephone numbers;
- Home health agencies;
- Other people who can help or fill in, if you need additional help;
- Lawyers and financial advisors;
- Where needed items are kept, such as thermometers and blood pressure monitors;
- Medications, when they are to be taken, and where they are stored;
- Exercise schedules and directions;
- Emergency contacts in addition to 911.

These lists and other needed information can be put into a clearly marked notebook and kept where others can easily find them in your older relative's room. This book should be complete enough so that someone filling in for you will know exactly what is needed and what to do.

Tips on Safety

Quick, easy, and readily available ways to communicate with others that can help in an emergency are a must for you and your older family member or friend. You can get:

- A cordless speaker phone with memory so that you can simply hit one button in an emergency and get help without compromising the safety of your care receiver;

- A cellular phone, if you and your care receiver travel;

- A signal system that will summon help with the push of a button, if you leave your care receiver alone at times;

- A specially equipped telephone with speed dialing, a large digital display for easy reading, and ring and voice enhancer, if your care receiver has hearing problems;

- An intercom that will alert you if your care receiver is having problems when you are in another room;

- Smoke detectors on each floor, which should be periodically checked to ensure that they are operating properly.

If your family member is disabled, you will want to ensure the following:

- He or she has a clear path through each room, that there are no rugs or raised room dividers to trip over, and no slippery floors. You can carpet the bathroom with all weather carpeting to help prevent falls. This can be pulled up in sections, if it is wet.

- He or she uses a cane or walker, if needed.

- He or she is secure in his or her wheelchair. If your older relative is weak, a tray that attaches to the wheelchair can prevent falls and gives your care receiver a place for drinks, magazines, etc. It is important to ensure that the wheels are securely locked when doing transfers, or if the older person's chair is on an incline.

- He or she cannot fall out of bed. If the bed does not have guardrails, you can place the wheelchair or other guards next to the bed, and position your older relative in the middle of the bed so that she or he can turn over without fear of falling.

Meals

As people age, they sometimes experience problems with chewing and swallowing, but there are ways to minimize these problems. The need for certain nutrients in older person's diets may also change.

Avoid foods that are high in:

- Saturated fats;

- Salts, chemical preservatives, and additives;

- Sugar and calories that do not enhance nutrition, but may add to excessive weight gain.

There are numerous ways to obtain pre-prepared and easy to prepare meals that are nutritious time savers.

For older people who are homebound, meal times can be pleasant social events, when you can be together and talk. If your relative or friend is confined to bed, you can sit and talk while he or she eats and bring a tray in for yourself. There are a host of eating utensils and accessories that make eating easier for persons with disabilities.

Caring for Your Home

Use an attractive plastic tablecloth or placemats that are easy to clean and an attractive towel, apron, or other covering for your care receiver's clothes, if there is a tendency to spill food. Be sure that it is large and long enough to cover his or her lap and fold it inward before taking it off to avoid spillage on the floor. Consider having a vase of flowers (even if they are artificial) on the table or next to the bed, if your older relative is confined to bed, and open the curtains and let the sun shine in.

Use lightweight, plastic, easy-grip glasses, or cups with handles. If there is a lot of spillage, try a drink holder with a lid and plastic straw insert.

If clothes are wrinkled, you can put them in the dryer with a wet towel or sponge on a warm setting. This often saves a lot of time ironing.

If your care receiver is incontinent, you can use the following:

- washable or disposable pads on the bed above the sheet

- rubberized sheets underneath the bed sheet

- a stain- and water-resistant mattress pad

If the mattress does become soiled, it will need to be thoroughly cleaned and aired after being sprayed with a safe (always read the label) antibacterial cleaning agent. You can ask your doctor or pharmacist for recommendations.

You can use water-resistant pads or heavy towels on the wheelchair or furniture that your care receiver uses. If you travel, keep pads in the car for use on the car seat and when visiting other places.

When buying towel sets, you may want to purchase extra wash-cloths since these are used more frequently and wear out faster. Thermal blankets also are useful because they are warm, lightweight, and easy to wash.

Exercise

In consultation with your care receiver's physician and physical therapist, you can plan a routine of exercises. Exercises even for bed- and wheelchair-bound older persons help to improve circulation, lung and heart function, posture, and mental alertness and help to prevent diabetes, pressure sores, osteoporosis, heart disease, and stroke.

If appropriate, encourage your relative to do a little more physical activity each week. Vary the exercises and challenge him or her to do better. Exercise with your relative. If he or she is confined to a bed or wheelchair, try to get him or her to exercise at least five minutes every hour, and again, regularly change his or her position to prevent pressure sores.

Clothing

Regardless of our age or physical condition, we want to look and feel our best. Today's clothing options make that a much easier goal to reach. When buying clothing, consider the following:

- Clothing that is washable and wrinkle-free saves on dry cleaning bills and ironing time.

- Slacks and skirts that have elasticized waistbands or tie waistbands are easier to get on and off and are more comfortable.

- Clothing with snaps or zippers and some that button down the front are easier to manipulate.

- Shoes should not slip off easily, and should have a nonskid tread.

- Interchangeable and color-coordinated clothing (e.g., slacks and tops that can go with several others) make dressing easier.

Entertainment, Entertaining, and Travel

Boredom can sap our intellect and spirit, but you can change this by creating activities that you and your care receiver look forward to and by sharing these with others. There are many activities that frail and disabled older people can enjoy:

- Check the TV listings and choose your favorite programs to watch each day rather than having the TV going nonstop.

- Get large-print and talking books from the library and read together.

- Check for special events that are low-cost or free. Invite a friend or family member to join you, preferably one who can drive or help you if your care receiver has a disability.

- Go out to lunch or take advantage of the early-bird specials at restaurants.

- Visit an art-hobby store and see what is available in the way of arts or crafts projects that you and your care receiver can enjoy.

- Invite family or friends over for dinner or lunch. If you have limited funds to entertain or do not have time to prepare food have them over for dessert or snacks, ask each of them to bring something, or ask them to chip in on a carryout meal.

- Plan day trips to local places of interest. Again, invite a friend or family member to join you.

- If you can afford to do so, go on a vacation. You can share the adventure and expense with other family members or friends. Many places offer senior discounts. Make sure that they can accommodate your needs, especially if your care receiver is disabled. Large hotel and motel chains now go out of their way to help, if you make your needs known to them. In addition, there are companies and organizations that plan trips for persons with limitations in their mobility. Many travel books have special sections on accommodations, travel, and activities for those with limited mobility.

- If you have the room, invite friends or family members to come and stay with you for a while in your home.

- Check colleges, religious organizations, and community centers for free courses and other activities.

- Visit museums, galleries, botanical and zoological parks, or a petting zoo.

- If appropriate, get a pet. Your local shelter or humane society has many nice pets available for adoption.

- Get a computer with internet access so that you can e-mail friends, join in chat rooms, learn about things that are of interest to you, and enjoy computer games.

- Ask your local Area Agency on Aging about friendly visitor, volunteer, and telephone reassurance programs.

- Many fraternal, religious, and social organizations have activities specifically for older people. This can be a great way to extend your circle of friends and supportive network.

Section 49.2

Managing Caregiver Stress

Reprinted from "Caregiver Stress," National Women's Health Information Center, January 2006.

What is a caregiver?

Caregivers are people who take care of other adults, most often parents or spouses, who are ill or disabled. The people who receive care usually need help with basic daily tasks. Caregivers help with many things:

- Grocery shopping
- House cleaning
- Cooking
- Shopping
- Paying bills
- Giving medicine
- Toileting

- Bathing

- Dressing

- Eating

Usually caregivers take care of elderly people. Less often, caregivers are grandparents who are raising their grandchildren. The terms "informal caregiver" and "family caregiver" refer to people who are not paid to provide care. As the American population ages, the number of caregivers and the demands placed on them will grow.

Who are our nation's caregivers?

About one in four American families, or 22.4 million households, care for someone over the age of fifty. The number of American households involved in caregiving may reach 39 million by 2007.

About 75 percent of caregivers are women.

Two-thirds of caregivers in the United States have jobs in addition to caring for another person.

Most caregivers are middle-aged: thirty-five to sixty-four years old.

What is caregiver stress?

Caregiver stress is the emotional strain of caregiving. Studies show that caregiving takes a toll on physical and emotional health. Caregivers are more likely to suffer from depression than their peers. Limited research suggests that caregivers may also be more likely to have health problems like diabetes and heart disease than non-caregivers.

Caring for another person takes a lot of time, effort, and work. Plus, most caregivers juggle caregiving with full-time jobs and parenting. In the process, caregivers put their own needs aside. Caregivers often report that it is difficult to look after their own health in terms of exercise, nutrition, and doctor's visits. So, caregivers often end up feeling angry, anxious, isolated, and sad.

Caregivers for people with Alzheimer disease (AD) or other kinds of dementia are particularly vulnerable to burnout. Research shows that most dementia caregivers suffer from depression and stress. Also, studies show that the more hours spent on caregiving, the greater the risk of anxiety and depression.

Women caregivers are particularly prone to feeling stress and overwhelmed. Studies show that female caregivers have more emotional and physical health problems, employment-related problems, and financial strain than male caregivers. Other research shows that people who care for their spouses are more prone to caregiving-related stress than those who care for other family members.

It is important to note that caring for another person can also create positive emotional change. Aside from feeling stress, many caregivers say their role has had many positive effects on their lives. For example, caregivers report that caregiving has given them a sense of purpose. They say that their role makes them feel useful and capable and that they are making a difference in the life of a loved one.

How can I tell if caregiving is putting too much stress on me?

If you have any of the following symptoms, caregiving may be putting too much strain on you:

- Sleeping problems—sleeping too much or too little

- Change in eating habits resulting in weight gain or loss

- Feeling tired or without energy most of the time

- Loss of interest in activities you used to enjoy, such as going out with friends, walking, or reading

- Easily irritated, angered, or saddened

- Frequent headaches, stomach aches, or other physical problems

What can I do to prevent or relieve stress?

Take care of yourself. In the process, you'll become a better caregiver. Take the following steps to make your health a priority:

- Find out about community caregiving resources.

- Ask for and accept help.

- Stay in touch with friends and family. Social activities can help you feel connected and may reduce stress.

- Find time for exercise most days of the week.

- Prioritize, make lists, and establish a daily routine.

- Look to faith-based groups for support and help.

- Join a support group for caregivers in your situation (like caring for a person with dementia). Many support groups can be found in the community or on the internet.

- See your doctor for a checkup. Talk to him or her about symptoms of depression or sickness you may be having.

- Try to get enough sleep and rest.

- Eat a healthy diet rich in fruits, vegetables, and whole grains and low in saturated fat.

- Ask your doctor about taking a multivitamin.

- Take one day at a time.

Caregivers who work outside the home should consider taking some time off. If you are feeling overwhelmed, taking a break from your job may help you get back on track. Employees covered under the federal Family and Medical Leave Act may be able to take up to twelve weeks of unpaid leave per year to care for relatives. Ask your human resources office about options for unpaid leave.

What is respite care?

The term "respite care" means care that gives the regular caregiver some time off. Respite care gives family caregivers a much-needed break. In the process, respite care reduces caregiver stress.

Respite care may be provided by any of the following:

- Home healthcare workers

- Adult day-care centers

- Short-term nursing homes

- Assisted living homes

Respite care is essential to family caregivers. Studies show that respite care helps caregivers keep their loved ones at home for longer periods of time.

What is the National Family Caregiver Support Program (NFCSP)?

The National Family Caregiver Support Program (NFCSP) is a federally funded program through the Older Americans Act. The NFCSP helps states provide services that assist family caregivers. To be eligible for the NFCSP, caregivers must:

- Care for adults aged sixty years and older, or

- Be grandparents or relatives caring for a child under the age of eighteen.

Each state offers different amounts and types of services. These include the following:

- Information about available services
- Help accessing support services
- Individual counseling and organization of support groups
- Caregiver training
- Respite care
- Limited supplemental services to complement the care provided by caregivers

How can I find out about caregiving resources in my community?

A number of resources can help direct you to the caregiver services you need. These agencies will be able to tell you:

- What kind of services are available in your community;
- If these services are right for you;
- If you are eligible for these services;
- Whom to contact and hours of operation.

People who need help caring for an older person should contact their local Area Agency on Aging (AAA). AAAs are usually listed in the government sections of the telephone directory under "Aging" or "Social Services."

What kind of caregiver services can I find in my community?

There are many kinds of community care services:

- Transportation
- Meals
- Adult day care
- Home care
- Cleaning and yard work services

- Home modification

- Senior centers

- Hospice care

- Support groups

- Legal and financial counseling

What kind of home care help is available?

There are two kinds of home care: home health care and nonmedical home care services. Both types help sick and disabled people live independently in their homes for as long as possible. Caregivers and doctors decide what services are necessary and most helpful.

Home health care includes health-related services such as the following:

- Medicine assistance

- Nursing services

- Physical therapy

Nonmedical home care services include the following:

- Housekeeping

- Cooking

- Companionship

How will I pay for home health care?

Medicare, Medicaid, and some private insurance companies will cover the cost of limited home care. Coverage varies from state to state. Other times, you will have to pay out of pocket for these services.

The cost of home care depends on what types of services are used. Nonmedical workers like housekeepers are much less expensive than nurses or physical therapists. Also, some home care agencies are cheaper than others.

Who is eligible for Medicare home health care services?

To get Medicare home health care, a person must meet all of the following four conditions:

- A doctor must decide that the person needs medical care in the home and make a plan for home care.

- The person must need at least one of the following: sporadic (and not full time) skilled nursing care, physical therapy, or speech language pathology services, or continue to need occupational therapy.

- The person must be homebound. This means that he or she is normally unable to leave home. When the person leaves home, it must be infrequent, for a short time, to get medical care, or to attend religious services.

- The home health agency caring for the person must be approved by the Medicare program.

Will Medicaid help pay for home health care?

To qualify for Medicaid, a person must have a low income and few other assets. Medicaid coverage differs from state to state. In all states, Medicaid pays for basic home health care and medical equipment. In some cases, Medicaid will pay for a homemaker, personal care, and other services not covered by Medicare.

Section 49.3

Balancing Work, Family, and Caregiving

From "Balancing Work and Caregiving: Tips for Employees" by Carolyn S. Wilken, © 2006 University of Florida Institute of Food and Agricultural Sciences. Reprinted with permission.

Providing care for older family members has become a way of life for millions of Americans. In fact, nearly one in ten American workers is a caregiver. By 2007, 15.6 million Americans will be trying to balance working and caregiving responsibilities.

Nearly half of caregivers are employed full-time. Another 11 percent are employed part-time. Employed caregivers struggle to balance their time and energy between work and caregiving. Caregivers are often exhausted, burdened, and stressed.

Employed caregivers often find it necessary to turn down training opportunities or promotions. They may take early retirement or simply quit their jobs altogether. Lost work opportunities take a financial and emotional toll.

Caregivers not only lose current income and benefits. They also face reduced retirement income. Over a lifetime, the average caregiver gives up nearly $700,000 in "wage wealth." Wage wealth includes lost wages, lost Social Security income, and lost pension benefits. Caregivers who enjoy their jobs and who are friends with their co-workers may also become depressed and lonely after quitting.

Men and women seem to have different caregiving responsibilities. Male caregivers are more likely to work full-time. They also spend less time providing care. As caregiving gets harder and takes up more time, women pick up more of the responsibility. As a result, female caregivers are more likely to cut back their working hours or to quit work completely to provide care.

What Can Employed Caregivers Do?

- Openly and honestly describe the situation before it becomes a problem.

- Let your employers know that you are committed to your job. Make sure they know that you don't want to let them down.

- Be honest about the fact that you need your job and your benefits, but that you want to be a dependable and valuable employee.

- Focus on what your employer needs. Think about how you can work together during this hard time.

- Remain professional. Know what you need before you meet with your supervisor. Try to come up with solutions that are creative but practical.

- Be realistic. If your position involves meeting with clients, asking to work evenings is not realistic. On the other hand, if you are making sales calls by phone, you may be able to telecommute from a home office.

Learn What Help Is Available

Contact your company's human resources department for assistance. Ask to speak to someone who knows about caregiving and aging issues.

If you think you will need to leave work temporarily to provide full-time care, learn about the Family Medical Leave Act (FMLA). FMLA provides job protection for employees who must leave their jobs for family medical concerns, such as providing care for a critically ill family member.

Take Steps to Help Yourself

Employed caregivers can take steps to make caregiving less stressful.

Manage Phone Calls

Care receivers may get into the habit of calling for any little thing, or simply because they are lonely. Long, involved phone calls are especially stressful.

Set limits on phone calls. Schedule regular times when you will call and check in.

Support Your Support System

Give your support system time to work. Women are often guilty of the "It's easier if I just do it myself" syndrome. After a while, other people quit offering to help, either because you never let them, or because you've sent the message that you'd just as soon "do it yourself." (This suggests that you don't trust anyone else.) Don't jump in and take over because something doesn't happen as quickly as you think it should.

Avoid Teaching Helplessness

When you are pressed for time, waiting for your mother to brush her hair and put on a sweater seems to take forever. Brushing her hair and putting her sweater on for her is much faster. Over time, though, she will begin to believe that she is helpless and to need more and more help.

"Learned helplessness" occurs when we always do things for or make decisions for people, instead of letting them do it themselves. Over time, people come to believe that they are not capable of doing anything for themselves.

Sometimes, of course, it is faster to "do it for" someone than to wait for that person to do it him- or herself. People with disabilities do need certain kinds of help, but teaching people to be helpless costs the caregiver and the care receiver in the long run.

Set Priorities at Home and Work

What are your priorities? What is most important, and what can you let go? Are home-cooked meals a priority in your life? Is being a caregiver your highest priority? Is spending time with your spouse or children your highest priority? Is your job your most important priority? These are often difficult decisions to make, but sometimes circumstances dictate priorities.

What if you were to lose your job because you missed so much time providing care? What would that mean for you and your family? If keeping your job has to come first, you will need to ask someone else to help. For instance, you may need someone else to take your care receiver to the doctor for you. At some point, you may need to place your care receiver in adult day care or a nursing facility. These are very difficult decisions.

Compartmentalize Your Life

Try to "work when you work," "give care when you are caregiving," and "play when you play." Schedule separate times to be with your children and your care receiver. Everyone will feel more satisfied if they get your complete attention for even a short time, instead of sharing you.

You may have to take the kids with you to check on grandma. But when this happens, neither the children nor grandma feels like they've really had special time with you. Maybe you can stop and check on your mother before you pick the kids up from daycare. Maybe you and your kids can stop for ice cream or at the park before you go to your mother's.

Ask for and Accept Help

No matter where you live, there are resources available to help you as a caregiver. Contact agencies for help.

Check with your employer. Is there an Employee Assistance Program (EAP)? Can Human Resources (HR) help?

Phone 2-1-1 for help locating services.

Communicate Honestly and Often

Make time to communicate clearly with the following people:

- Your employer
- Your family
- Your friends
- Your care receiver
- Your co-workers
- Your spiritual leader
- Yourself

References

Caregiving in the U.S. (2004). National Alliance for Caregiving/AARP. Retrieved July 17, 2005, from http://www.caregiving.org/data/04finalreport.pdf

Older Americans 2000: Key Indicators of Well-Being. Federal Interagency Forum on Aging-related Statistics. Retrieved July 17, 2005, from http://agingstats.gov

Employed Caregivers. (2003). U.S. Department of Health and Human Services, Administration on Aging, Washington D.C. Retrieved October 30, 2006, from http://www.aoa.gov/press/nfc_month/2003/nfcm_factsheets/3%20employed%20caregivers.pdf

Section 49.4

Long-Distance Caregiving

It was the dilemma experienced by many people who live far from their aging parents. Sara, on a business trip as a buyer for her company, stopped in Chicago to visit her eighty-year old mother. During her stay, she observed her mother had become more frail and forgetful since her last visit. She had neglected paying bills, and after seeing her refrigerator, Sara suspected her mother was not eating properly. Sara's suggestion that her mother move in with her was met with an indignant refusal. Sara wanted to provide support to her mother while respecting her autonomy.

How to manage long-distance caregiving? Here are some suggestions that might apply to your situation as well as Sara's:

- **Consider all the options before moving your relative:** In-home services may permit your loved one to remain in his or her home, close to neighbors and friends.

- **If you haven't visited recently, do so as soon as feasible:** Take note of possible problem areas such as nutrition, safety, driving ability, medications, finances, and physical or emotional illness.

- **Make sure legal and financial affairs are in place and up to date:** Make sure that you also know where to locate critical documents and papers.

- **Set up a system of support if necessary for your family member's safety:** For example, ask a friend or relative to check in with your parent on a regular basis. If that is not adequate, you may need to hire someone to help your family member with meals and personal care.

- **Recognize and acknowledge your own limits:** As your relative requires increasing levels of care, you may become overwhelmed. Consider hiring a geriatric care manager to coordinate your family member's care.

- **Plan ahead to have family leave or personal days available in case you need to make an unexpected visit to your relative:** Put aside money in a special fund to pay for such trips.

Section 49.5

Relocating Your Parents

"Relocating Your Parents," reprinted with permission from the Family Caregiver Alliance, http://www.caregiver.org. © 2003 Family Caregiver Alliance. All rights reserved.

As you've watched your parents age, perhaps you have struggled with situations such as these:

You've traveled to visit your mother for the holidays, and found her refrigerator nearly empty, her checkbook misplaced, and her finances in complete disarray.

Or a neighbor calls you to report that your father was wandering in the street, unable to find the home he's lived in for thirty years.

Or your mother has neglected to take her diabetes medications, severely compromising her health.

If there is a decline in cognitive abilities as a result of Alzheimer disease or a related dementia, or a shift in a medical condition that requires increased care, there is clear cause to be concerned about your parent's welfare. The need to relocate your parent to a safer environment may become apparent.

But where should he or she live? Often your first inclination is to move Mom or Dad into your home—but this major life change deserves thoughtful examination, and there are many alternatives to explore. This section offers helpful advice and summarizes the issues to consider before making the important and challenging decisions regarding relocating your parent.

Open Discussions

Open and honest discussion with your parent and other family members becomes an essential first step when you are trying to decide whether relocating your parent is the right thing to do. Family meetings with your parent, spouse, children, siblings, and other key people will help everyone share their views and will help you decide how best to proceed. Active communication among all family members is the building block to a strong support system for an older parent and all family members involved.

Although some of these discussions may be very difficult and emotional, several topics require attention. Together, the family, including your parent, will need to talk about all possible residential options, each person's role in the transition, the type of care to be provided, changes in lifestyle, finances, and the physical setting of the new home. Clear expectations must be defined. The following topics can help guide your discussions.

Level of Care Needed

As your parent gets older, his or her care needs will change, and in most cases become more challenging. Consider what you will and will not be able to do for your parent. Developing a strategy for how the care will be provided is essential and requires practicality and planning:

- Evaluate whether your parent needs constant supervision or assistance throughout the day and consider how this will be provided.

- Determine which activities of daily living (eating, bathing, toileting) your parent can perform independently.

- Determine your comfort level for providing personal care such as bathing or changing an adult diaper.

- Evaluate your health and physical abilities and decide if you are able to provide care for your parent.

- Expect changes in your parent's medical or cognitive condition.

- Explore the availability of services such as a friendly visitor, in-home care, or adult day services.

- Investigate backup long-term arrangements and options if living with your parent does not work or is not your choice.

- Determine the type of medical care that will be needed for your parent, and whether appropriate physicians and services are available in your community.

Family Dynamics

Families are rich in historical experiences, and many of your positive and negative feelings about your parents and other family members will play a role in your decision to relocate or live with a parent. Be honest with yourself and do not allow unresolved conflicts or feelings of guilt or obligation pressure you into taking on more than you can manage:

- Be honest with yourself and others about the significant life changes that relocating your parent will mean for you, your parent, your siblings, your spouse, and children.

- Try to come to terms with past disagreements between you and your parent.

- When deciding whether to relocate or move your parent into your home, consider the opinions of your spouse, children, siblings, and other family members.

- Come to an agreement with your siblings regarding how much and what kind of help you will receive from them.

Consider Various Living Arrangements

Moving your parent into your home is one option, but you and your family should take some time to consider other living arrangements as well. The type of housing and living arrangement will largely depend on your parent's care needs, finances, and available options. Also, when deciding where a parent should live, family members need to discuss, understand, and accept the benefits and drawbacks of living close to one relative versus another.

Often, the choice of location can cause conflict between family members because those living near the parent bear most of the responsibility for the parent's care, and may feel that those living further away do not help enough. On the other hand, family members who live far away can feel frustrated that they do not have the opportunity to participate more in providing care. An open dialogue and an agreement on how to share local and long-distance caregiving is essential.

The following list outlines different types of living arrangements that may be appropriate for your parent. Each community offers different choices. Remember that Medicare does not usually cover these expenses:

- **A nearby apartment, house, or retirement community:** Your parent may still function happily and safely in his or her own independent environment with a little assistance. In this case, renting a nearby apartment or small home will allow your parent to maintain his or her independence and enable family members to provide consistent monitoring and support. Independent retirement communities may offer individual units with group meals and social activities. Sharing an apartment or house with a friend or relative may be another option. There are also agencies in some cities that arrange for shared living situations.

- **Assisted living facility:** Individuals who are fairly independent but require some daily supervision and assistance with house chores and personal care may consider an assisted living facility. Assisted living facilities may offer rooms or apartment-style accommodations and, often, social activities. Meals are provided. Staff is also available to assist with different care needs, such as bathing, grooming, eating, or using the toilet, and care is arranged as needed by the individual. The monthly charge for assisted living is determined by how much care a person requires.

- **Residential care facility:** These facilities are small group homes that provide constant supervision, meals, and care for people who cannot be left alone but do not require skilled nursing care. Residential care facilities provide assistance with bathing, grooming, eating, using the toilet, and walking, and they also provide socialization and recreational activities.

- **Intermediate care facility:** This type of facility provides round-the-clock care for those who require help with bathing, grooming, going to the toilet, and walking. Individuals in these facilities cannot live independently and require nursing care, although the nursing care is not offered twenty-four hours a day.

- **Skilled nursing facility:** Skilled nursing facilities provide continuous nursing services and are designed to provide high levels of personal care and medical care, such as administration of injections, monitoring of blood pressure, managing ventilators, and providing intravenous feedings to individuals who cannot function independently. People in skilled nursing facilities usually require help with the majority of their self-care needs, and such individuals would probably not be able to live in a home environment.

When Your Parent Moves in with You

Change of family roles: Living with a parent will lead to a change in family roles. A once-authoritative parent may no longer act like a "parent"—you may become the guardian who gives direction and controls many aspects of your parent's life. You may need your child/children to help with more household responsibilities and with a grandparent. These role changes are hard adjustments for everyone:

- Determine your ease with becoming the decision maker and the person with authority.

- Be prepared for resistance from your parent if they feel that they can no longer set the rules or control their situation or fear losing independence.

- When possible, allow some negotiation in decision-making activities so that you can have a win-win situation.

- Decide on what you expect from your parent in terms of completion of chores or financial contributions.

- Think about your spouse's and children's readiness to help with caregiving.

Lifestyle changes: You and your parent probably have very different lifestyles. Sleeping cycles, eating patterns, social calendars, and daily activities may need adjustments in order to guarantee a smooth transition:

- Talk about and plan how to accommodate bed times, nap schedules, and sleeping habits of all family members in the house. Discuss what types of food you eat, when meals are prepared, and if special diets are required and how they will be accommodated.

- Assess whether smoking/nonsmoking or drinking/nondrinking practices are compatible.

- Consider how you can support your parent's continued participation in social networks such as visiting friends and attending a place of worship and how transportation to these and other activities will be managed.

- Encourage your parent to keep enjoyable and safe hobbies.

- Consider whether your parent will be fully integrated into your family's activities or whether he or she will maintain an independent social life.

- Consider how the household noise level and general activity pattern will affect your parent.

The Loss of Time

Caregiving requires a significant amount of time and is very likely to impact your work, family time, personal time, and sleep:

- Determine the amount of time you can devote to your parent's care needs. When will you make phone calls for appointments or to set up needed services? When will you be able to take your parent to medical appointments?

- Evaluate whether you will need to make adjustments to your current work schedule.

- If you will reduce your work hours, determine the implications for your financial picture, career advancement, health insurance, and retirement benefits.

- Consider whether you will have time for your spouse, children, and friends.

- If your parent requires full-time supervision, who will provide it while you are at work?

- Consider the reduced amount of private time you will have to pursue your own interests or hobbies or what your need is for time alone on a daily basis.

- Expect that you will, at times, become exhausted and will need to find a way to rest.

- Investigate how to arrange for some time off from caregiving duties ("respite") and enlist the help of your family members, close friends, or an aide.

Your Home

Physical living arrangements must be adequate if your parent is to move in. There must be enough room and a layout that is adaptable to an older adult who may have mobility or vision problems. A home may require special adaptations to make it safe. Many of these changes are inexpensive but need time and planning to implement:

- Evaluate the amount of available space and whether there is enough privacy.

- Think about where your parent will sleep. How will a child feel if he or she has to give up a room for a grandparent?

- If possible, locate your parent on the first floor in order to avoid stairs.

- Consider major changes that may be needed in order to accommodate any disabilities or mobility problems (e.g., wheelchair-accessible bathroom, shower, etc.).

- Determine what assistive devices may be needed such as grab bars in the bathroom, raised toilet seats, handrails, and a ramp.

- If your parent wanders, consider special locks, door chimes, and other devices that will help keep doors and windows safely secured.

- Look through your home for hazards such as dangling cords, toxins, slippery surfaces, unsteady chairs, throw rugs.

- Install bright nonglare lights above all walkways, and low-cost adhesive strips on steps and in other potentially slippery areas such as bathrooms and showers.

- Adjust temperature controls so that the house is not too hot or too cold. Be aware that older people often like their environment warmer and this may affect both your comfort and your utility bills.

- Discuss how you might incorporate your parent's furniture into your home.

- Review how existing or new pets will be integrated into the new home situation.

Financial Arrangements

Individual financial information is not usually shared among family members. However, if you are caring for a parent it may become necessary for you to become more involved in his or her personal finances, including paying bills, monitoring accounts, and managing investments. This could create problems with your parent or siblings, who may question how you are handling your parent's money:

- Agree upon how much, if any, financial payment your parent will provide toward his or her living expenses. Will he or she pay for rent, food, and other costs?

- Your siblings may be resentful of any money you might receive. Openly discuss financial arrangements with siblings to keep them updated on new expenditures and apprised of accounts.

- Come to an agreement between your parent and siblings regarding payment of out-of-pocket expenses.

- Investigate the option of automatic payment of recurring bills.

- Look into free or low-cost services that assist with Medicare paperwork for older adults.

Difficulties with the Move

It is likely that your parent has lived in his or her current home for many years and has developed strong ties to community, family, friends, healthcare providers, social life, and daily routine. Packing and moving out of a house is a significant chore for anybody, but for the older adult who has decades' worth of memories and possessions, moving can represent a tremendous emotional challenge. Moving away from this familiar and comfortable setting is difficult and can cause great sadness. Furthermore, leaving one's own house represents a decrease in independence and signals a new life stage.

In some communities, there are specialized companies that will help organize a senior's move to a new location. But for most families, the adult children perform that task. Again, open communication will help ease the way.

While you help your parent pack, talk through the difficult feelings, acknowledge the loss that your parent is experiencing, and reassure him or her that you are all making the best decision possible.

Allow time and opportunity to reminisce. Your parent will need time to adjust to his or her new living environment and role with your family. Your patience and support will help make this transition smoother. An outside counselor may also be helpful.

Rewards

Despite the challenges, many adult children find that providing support and care for their parents is one of the most rewarding experiences they have ever had. Parents can contribute to the family through sharing their past and become an integral part of your household. Grandchildren have the unique opportunity to learn and absorb family history. Caregiving carries with it the extraordinary opportunity to give back what your parent once provided to you.

Section 49.6

Evaluating and Choosing Housing Options for Elders

Reprinted from "Because We Care: A Guide for People Who Care—Evaluating and Choosing Housing Options for Elders," National Family Caregiver Support Program, Administration on Aging, September 9, 2004.

There are many times when it is not possible for a caregiver and care receiver to live together:

- The level of care that your spouse, relative, or friend needs may require highly skilled healthcare personnel on a regular basis. In this case, an extended care facility, such as assisted living or a nursing home, may be a better care alternative.

- Your relative or friend may live in another town and not want to move.

- There may not be room in your home, or family members, including your relative, may not want to live together.

Whatever the reasons, living in different housing does not mean that you cannot be a good caregiver. You and your relative will, however, need to make arrangements for additional help or services as needed—either in his or her present home or in a new housing arrangement.

Points to Consider when Choosing Housing and Living Arrangements

When providing services to older persons who have limitations in their mobility and multiple needs, the type of housing and living arrangements you choose become critical keys in assuring that they get the care they need. Housing and care in this instance go hand in hand. There are many types of housing arrangements available for older persons, and they often overlap in the types of care and services they provide.

Before making a housing choice, you and your older relative should assess present needs and envision, as well as possible, how these needs may change in the future.

What options will be open to you if the need for more supportive housing and living arrangements arises?

- Will your family member need to move to another care arrangement?

- Are these facilities available in the community, and how much will they cost?

- How are you going to pay for housing and services now and in the future?

- If you enter into housing that requires a substantial deposit at the time of admission, will some of the money be returned if your relative decides to leave?

- What guarantees do you have that the facility is financially secure?

You and your older relative will want to ask these questions before making a decision about moving into a new housing arrangement. If this arrangement involves a large entrance fee or deposit or the signing of a contract, you also will want to consult a lawyer before making the commitment.

Guidelines for Choosing Housing Options

Regardless of what the facility is called, check it out thoroughly before making a decision. The types of facilities listed below range from informal home-share arrangements to commercial enterprises, government-sponsored facilities, and housing options administered by nonprofit organizations. Some are licensed or accredited, while others are not.

Accreditation is an evaluation of a facility's operation against a set of standards. The Continuing Care Accreditation Commission—a membership organization of continuing care communities—is one such organization.

Licensing is an evaluation of a facility's operation in accordance with government regulations. About half of the states currently regulate assisted living facilities.

Many skilled and intermediate care nursing facilities are accredited to accept patients under the Medicare or Medicaid programs, which means that they must meet certain standards and provide certain services.

Regardless of these considerations, you are responsible, in large part, for ensuring that the facility is the right one for your spouse, relative, or friend.

Even if you are not thinking about housing options in the foreseeable future, it is wise to have several in mind in case an emergency arises and you need temporarily care for your relative. Home care agencies often do not have staff available to fill in on short notice, and you may need the services of a long-term care facility.

Here are some things you can do:

- Start your preliminary search by phone.

- Visit those facilities that have the services your care receiver wants and needs.

- Take your older relative to see the facility. Better yet, visit several and let your relative make the final choice, if at all possible.

If your relative is able to make sound decisions, and does not like any of the housing options or does not want to move into a facility after visiting several, keep looking or further explore the possibility of home care in his or her home or yours. Use a checklist (this checklist can be used as a general guide for all types of housing) to ensure that the housing arrangement is the right one for your relative.

Types of Housing and Living Arrangements

Listed below are types of housing and living arrangements, what they generally offer, and for whom they are intended. Added to these considerations are those of costs. While some housing options are modestly priced, others, especially those that are for-profit, tend to be expensive:

- Retirement communities are planned towns with a range of housing, services, and care options.

- Continuing care communities offer varying levels of care in the same building or on the same campus. When selecting a continuing care retirement community or retirement community, remember they may encompass everything from housing for independent living to assisted living and skilled nursing home care. Therefore it may be difficult to identify what is offered simply because a facility has a certain name. These communities are usually designed for older persons with substantial financial resources.

- ECHO housing is a self-contained housing unit temporarily placed on a relative's lot that is suitable for older persons who are largely self-sufficient.

- Accessory apartments are self-contained apartments in the care receiver's home, your home, or the home of another caregiver. They are designed for older persons who may be largely self-sufficient or need help with housekeeping, cooking, and personal care—commonly referred to as activities of daily living (ADLs).

- Shared housing can be in the home of the older person or in someone else's home. Common areas, such as kitchens and dining rooms, are shared. This type of housing offers the older homeowner added income or the older renter an inexpensive place to live. It may offer companionship, and the possibility of having someone else around, at least part of the time, to help out with chores or in case of emergencies, but this depends on the persons sharing the house. This type of arrangement can work well for those elderly who are independent, but who would welcome a little extra income or help. It is important, however, to check the person's references carefully before making a decision.

- Congregate senior housing usually offers small apartments. Some offer group meals and social activities. They are designed for persons who are largely independent and do not need personal care or help with activities of daily living.

- Adult foster care is usually provided in private homes—often by the owner of the residence. The home usually provides meals, housekeeping, and sometimes personal care and assistance with ADLs.

- Senior group homes are located in residential neighborhoods and offer meals, housekeeping, and usually some personal care and assistance with ADLs. Usually a caregiver is on site, with medical personnel making periodic visits. Both adult foster care and group homes may be referred to as board and care homes or residential care facilities.

- Assisted living may provide everything, including skilled nursing care. Others provide only personal care, assistance with ADLs, or social activities. These may also be called retirement homes or residential care facilities, to name a few.

- Nursing homes provide an array of services including twenty-four-hour skilled medical care for total care patients; custodial care; therapy for patients convalescing from hospitalizations; and personal care and help with activities of daily living for persons with dementia, chronic health, or mobility problems.

Part Eight

Additional Help and Information

Chapter 50

Glossary of Terms Related to Adult Health Concerns

adipose tissue: fat tissue in the body.[1]

adjuvants: substances sometimes included in a vaccine formulation to enhance the immune-stimulating properties of a vaccine.[2]

analgesics: drugs that relieve pain. There are two main types: non-narcotic analgesics for mild pain, and narcotic analgesics for severe pain.[3]

angiogram: exam of your blood vessels using x-rays. The doctor inserts a small tube into the blood vessel and injects dye to see the vessels on the x-ray.[4]

antacids: drugs that relieve indigestion and heartburn by neutralizing stomach acid.[3]

antianxiety drugs: drugs that suppress anxiety and relax muscles (sometimes called anxiolytics, sedatives, or minor tranquilizers).[3]

The terms in this glossary were excerpted from "Obesity, Physical Activity, and Weight-Control Glossary," National Institute of Diabetes and Digestive and Kidney Diseases, National Institutes of Health, January 2002 [marked 1]; "Understanding Vaccines," National Institute of Allergy and Infectious Diseases, National Institutes of Health, NIH Publication No. 03-4219, July 2003 [marked 2]; "General Drug Categories," U.S. Food and Drug Administration, March 1998, updated by David A. Cooke M.D., May 2007 [marked 3]; and "Common Screening and Diagnostic Tests," National Women's Health Information Center, October 2006 [marked 4].

antiarrhythmics: drugs used to control irregularities of heartbeat.[3]

antibacterials: drugs used to treat infections.[3]

antibiotics: drugs made from naturally occurring and synthetic substances that combat bacterial infection. Some antibiotics are effective only against limited types of bacteria. Others, known as broad-spectrum antibiotics, are effective against a wide range of bacteria.[3]

antibodies: molecules produced by a B cell in response to an antigen. When an antibody attaches to an antigen, it helps destroy the microbe bearing the antigen.[2]

anticoagulants: drugs that prevent blood from clotting.[3]

anticonvulsants: drugs that prevent epileptic seizures.[3]

antidepressants: there are multiple classes of these medications, which all tend to improve mood and reduce anxiety. The most widely used classes are serotonin-specific reuptake inhibitors (SSRIs) and serotonin-norepinephrine reuptake inhibitors (SNRIs). There are several additional commonly used drugs which fit into neither of these classes. Tricyclics and monoamine oxidase inhibitors are two older drug classes that are prescribed less commonly, but remain in use.[3]

antidiarrheals: drugs used for the relief of diarrhea. Two main types of antidiarrheal preparations are simple adsorbent substances and drugs that slow down the contractions of the bowel muscles so that the contents are propelled more slowly.[3]

antiemetics: drugs used to treat nausea and vomiting.[3]

antifungals: drugs used to treat fungal infections.[3]

antigen: a molecule on a microbe that identifies it as foreign to the immune system and stimulates the immune system to attack it.[2]

antihistamines: drugs used primarily to counteract the effects of histamine, one of the chemicals involved in allergic reactions. These may be further subdivided into first-generation (sedating) antihistamines and second-generation (nonsedating) antihistamines.[3]

antihypertensives: drugs that lower blood pressure. The types of antihypertensives currently marketed include diuretics, beta-blockers, calcium channel blockers, angiotensin-converting enzyme (ACE) inhibitors, angiotensin II receptor blockers (ARBs), renin inhibitors, centrally acting antihypertensives, and sympatholytics.[3]

anti-inflammatories: drugs used to reduce inflammation—the redness, heat, swelling, and increased blood flow found in infections and in many chronic noninfective diseases. These may be subdivided into traditional nonsteroidal anti-inflammatory drugs (NSAIDs, or nonselective COX inhibitors) and COX-2 inhibitors.[3]

antineoplastics: drugs used to treat cancer.[3]

antipsychotics: drugs used to treat symptoms of severe psychiatric disorders. These drugs are sometimes called major tranquilizers. These may be subdivided into first-generation (or typical) antipsychotics and second-generation (or atypical) antipsychotics.[3]

antipyretics: drugs that reduce fever.[3]

antivirals: drugs used to treat viral infections or to provide temporary protection against infections such as influenza.[3]

artificially acquired immunity: immunity provided by vaccines, as opposed to naturally acquired immunity, which is acquired from exposure to a disease-causing organism.[2]

attenuation: the weakening of a microbe so that it can be used in a live vaccine.[2]

B cells: white blood cells crucial to the immune defenses. Also known as B lymphocytes, they come from bone marrow and develop into blood cells called plasma cells, which are the source of antibodies.[2]

bariatric surgery: surgery on the stomach and/or intestines to help the patient with extreme obesity lose weight.[1]

barium enema: a lubricated enema tube is gently inserted into your rectum. Barium flows into your colon. An x-ray is taken of the large intestine.[4]

beta-blockers: beta-adrenergic blocking agents, or beta-blockers for short, reduce the oxygen needs of the heart by reducing heartbeat rate.[3]

biopsy: a test that removes cells or tissues for examination by a pathologist to diagnose for disease.[4]

blood test: blood is taken from a vein in the inside elbow or back of the hand to test for a health problem.[4]

body mass index (BMI): A measure of body weight relative to height. BMI can be used to determine if people are at a healthy weight, overweight, or obese.[1]

bone mineral density test (BMD): special x-rays of your bones are used to test if you have osteoporosis, or a weakening of the bones.[4]

booster shots: supplementary doses of a vaccine, usually smaller than the first dose, that are given to maintain immunity.[2]

bronchodilators: drugs that open up the bronchial tubes within the lungs when the tubes have become narrowed by muscle spasm. Bronchodilators ease breathing in diseases such as asthma.[3]

bronchoscopy: exam of the lungs. A bronchoscope, or flexible tube, is put through the nose or mouth and into your windpipe (trachea).[4]

calorie: a unit of energy in food.[1]

cholesterol: A fat-like substance that is made by the body and is found naturally in animal foods such as meat, fish, poultry, eggs, and dairy products.[1]

clinical breast exam (CBE): a doctor, nurse, or other health professional uses his or her hands to examine your breasts and underarm areas to find lumps or other problems.[4]

clinical trial: an experiment that tests the safety and effectiveness of a vaccine or drug in humans.[2]

colonoscopy: an examination of the inside of the colon using a colonoscope, inserted into the rectum. A colonoscope is a thin, tube-like instrument with a light and lens for viewing. It may also have a tool to remove tissue to be checked under a microscope for disease.[4]

computed tomographic (CT or CAT) scan: the patient lies on a table and x-rays of the body are taken from different angles. Sometimes, a fluid is used to highlight parts of the body in the scan.[4]

conjugate vaccine: a vaccine in which proteins that are easily recognizable to the immune system are linked to the molecules that form the outer coat of disease-causing bacteria to promote an immune response. Conjugate vaccines are designed primarily for very young children because their immune systems cannot recognize the outer coats of certain bacteria.[2]

corticosteroids: these hormonal preparations are used primarily as anti-inflammatories in arthritis or asthma or as immunosuppressives, but they are also useful for treating some malignancies or compensating for a deficiency of natural hormones.[3]

cough suppressants: simple cough medicines, which contain substances such as honey, glycerin, or menthol, soothe throat irritation but do not actually suppress coughing.[3]

cytotoxic T cells (also called killer T cells): a subset of T cells that destroy body cells infected by viruses or bacteria.[2]

cytotoxics: drugs that kill or damage cells. Cytotoxics are used as antineoplastics (drugs used to treat cancer) and also as immunosuppressives.[3]

decongestants: drugs that reduce swelling of the mucous membranes that line the nose by constricting blood vessels, thus relieving nasal stuffiness.[3]

diuretics: drugs that increase the quantity of urine produced by the kidneys and passed out of the body, thus ridding the body of excess fluid. Diuretics reduce waterlogging of the tissues caused by fluid retention in disorders of the heart, kidneys, and liver. They are useful in treating mild cases of high blood pressure.[3]

DNA vaccine (also called naked DNA vaccine): a vaccine that uses a microbe's genetic material, rather than the whole organism or its parts, to simulate an immune response.[2]

echocardiogram: an instrument (that looks like a microphone) is placed on the chest. It uses sound waves to create a moving picture of the heart. A picture appears on a TV monitor, and the heart can be seen in different ways.[4]

electrocardiogram (EKG or ECG): records the electrical activity of the heart, using electrodes placed on the arms, legs, and chest.[4]

electroencephalogram (EEG): measures the electrical activity of the brain, using electrodes that are put on the patient's scalp.[4]

energy expenditure: the amount of energy, measured in calories, that a person uses.[3]

exercise stress test: electrodes are placed on the chest, arms, and legs to record the heart's activity. A blood pressure cuff is placed around the arm and is inflated every few minutes. Heart rate and blood pressure are taken before exercise starts. The patient walks on a treadmill or pedals a stationary bicycle. The pace of the treadmill is increased. The response of the heart is monitored. The test continues until target heart rate is reached. Monitoring continues after exercise for ten to fifteen minutes or until the heart rate returns to normal.[4]

expectorants: drugs that stimulate the flow of saliva and promote coughing to eliminate phlegm from the respiratory tract.[3]

fecal occult blood test (FOBT): detects hidden blood in a bowel movement. There are two types: the smear test and flushable reagent pads.[4]

formalin: a solution of water and formaldehyde, used in toxoid vaccines to inactivate bacterial toxins.[2]

glucose: a building block for most carbohydrates. Digestion causes carbohydrates to break down into glucose. After digestion, glucose is carried in the blood and goes to body cells where it is used for energy or stored.[1]

helper T cells: a subset of T cells that function as messengers. They are essential for turning on antibody production, activating cytotoxic T cells, and initiating many other immune functions.[2]

high blood pressure: Another word for "hypertension." Blood pressure rises and falls throughout the day. An optimal blood pressure is less than 120/80 mmHg.[1]

high-density lipoprotein (HDL): a form of cholesterol that circulates in the blood. Commonly called "good" cholesterol. High HDL lowers the risk of heart disease.[1]

hypoglycemics (oral): drugs that lower the level of glucose in the blood. Oral hypoglycemic drugs may be used in diabetes mellitus if it cannot be controlled by diet alone, with or without insulin injections.[3]

immune: having a high degree of resistance to or protection from a disease.[2]

immune system: a collection of specialized cells and organs that protect the body against infectious diseases.[2]

immunosuppressives: drugs that prevent or reduce the body's normal reaction to invasion by disease or by foreign tissues. Immunosuppressives are used to treat autoimmune diseases (in which the body's defenses work abnormally and attack its own tissues) and to help prevent rejection of organ transplants.[3]

inactivated vaccine: a vaccine made from a whole viruses or bacteria that has been inactivated with chemicals or heat.[2]

insulin: a hormone in the body that helps move glucose (sugar) from the blood to muscles and other tissues. Insulin controls blood sugar levels.[1]

laparoscopy: a small tube with a camera is inserted into the abdomen through a small cut in or just below the belly button to see inside the abdomen and pelvis. Other instruments can be inserted in the small cut as well. It is used for both diagnosing and treating problems inside the abdomen.[4]

laxatives: drugs that increase the frequency and ease of bowel movements, either by stimulating the bowel wall (stimulant laxative), by increasing the bulk of bowel contents (bulk laxative), increasing fluid movement into the bowel (osmotic laxatives), or by lubricating them (stool softeners, or bowel movement softeners).[3]

lipoprotein: compounds of protein that carry fats and fat-like substances, such as cholesterol, in the blood.[1]

live, attenuated vaccine: a vaccine made from microbes that have been weakened in the laboratory so that they can't cause disease.[2]

low-density lipoprotein (LDL): a form of cholesterol that circulates in the blood. Commonly called "bad" cholesterol. High LDL increases the risk of heart disease.[1]

metabolism: all of the processes that occur in the body that turn the food you eat into energy your body can use.[1]

lymph nodes: small bean-shaped organs of the immune system, distributed widely throughout the body and linked by lymphatic vessels. Lymph nodes are gathering sites of B, T, and other immune cells.[2]

lymphocytes: white blood cells that are central to the immune system's response to foreign microbes. B cells and T cells are lymphocytes.[2]

macrophages: large and versatile immune cells that devour and kill invading microbes and other intruders. Macrophages stimulate other immune cells by presenting them with small pieces of the invaders.[2]

magnetic resonance imaging (MRI): a test that uses powerful magnets and radio waves to create a picture of the inside of your body without surgery. The patient lies on a table that slides onto a large tunnel-like tube, which is surrounded by a scanner. Small coils may be placed around your head, arm, leg, or other areas.[4]

mammogram: x-rays of the breast taken by resting one breast at a time on a flat surface that contains an x-ray plate. A device presses firmly against the breast. An x-ray is taken to show a picture of the breast.[4]

memory cells: a subset of T cells and B cells that have been exposed to antigens and can then respond more readily and rapidly when the immune system encounters the same antigens again.[2]

muscle relaxants: drugs that relieve muscle spasm in disorders such as backache.[3]

naturally acquired immunity: immunity produced by antibodies passed from mother to fetus (passive), or by the body's own antibody and cellular immune response to a disease-causing organism (active).[2]

obesity: having a high amount of body fat. A person is considered obese if he or she has a body mass index (BMI) of 30 kg/m2 or greater.[1]

overweight: being too heavy for one's height. It is defined as a body mass index (BMI) of 25 up to 30 kg/m2. Body weight comes from fat, muscle, bone, and body water. Overweight does not always mean over fat.[1]

Pap test: the nurse or doctor uses a small brush to take cells from the cervix (opening of the uterus) to look at under a microscope in a lab.[4]

pelvic exam: a doctor or nurse asks about the patient's health and looks at the vaginal area. The doctor or nurse checks the fallopian tubes, ovaries, and uterus by putting two gloved fingers inside the vagina. With the other hand, the doctor or nurse will feel from the outside for any lumps or tenderness.[4]

physical exam: the doctor or nurse will test for diseases, assess your risk of future medical problems, encourage a healthy lifestyle, and update your vaccinations.[4]

polysaccharides: long, chain-like molecules made up of linked sugar molecules. The outer coats of some bacteria are made of polysaccharides.[2]

polyunsaturated fat: a highly unsaturated fat that is liquid at room temperature.[1]

positron emission tomography (PET) scan: the patient is injected with a radioactive substance, such as glucose. A scanner detects any cancerous areas in the body. Cancerous tissue absorbs more of the substance and looks brighter in images than normal tissue.[4]

preclinical testing: required laboratory testing of a vaccine before it can be given to people in clinical trials. Preclinical testing is done in cell cultures and in animals.[2]

protein: one of the three nutrients that provides calories to the body. Protein is an essential nutrient that helps build many parts of the body, including muscle, bone, skin, and blood.[1]

recombinant DNA technology: the technique by which genetic material from one organism is inserted into a foreign cell or another organism in order to mass-produce the protein encoded by the inserted genes.[2]

recombinant subunit vaccines: vaccines made using recombinant DNA technology to engineer the antigen molecules of the particular microbe.[2]

recombinant vector vaccines: vaccines that use modified viruses or bacteria to deliver genes that code for microbial antigens to cells of the body.[2]

saturated fat: a fat that is solid at room temperature.[1]

sigmoidoscopy: the sigmoidoscope is a small camera attached to a flexible tube. This tube, about 20 inches long, is gently inserted into the colon. As the tube is slowly removed, the lining of the bowel is examined.[4]

sleeping drugs: the main groups of drugs that are used to induce sleep are benzodiazepines, non-benzodiazepine hypnotics, and barbiturates. All such drugs have a sedative effect in low doses and are effective sleeping medications in higher doses.[3]

spirometry: the patient breathes into a mouthpiece that is connected to an instrument called a spirometer. The spirometer records the amount and the rate of air that is breathed in and out over a specified time. It measures how well the lungs exhale.[4]

subunit vaccine: a vaccine that uses one or more components of a disease-causing organism, rather than the whole, to stimulate an immune response.[2]

T cells: white blood cells (also known as T lymphocytes) that direct or participate in immune defenses.[2]

thrombolytics: drugs that help dissolve and disperse blood clots and may be prescribed for patients with recent arterial or venous thrombosis.[3]

toxin: agent produced by plants and bacteria, normally very damaging to cells.[2]

toxoid vaccine: a vaccine containing a toxoid, used to protect against toxins produced by certain bacteria.[2]

toxoids (also called inactivated toxins): toxins, such as those produced by certain bacteria, that have been treated by chemical means, heat, or irradiation and are no longer capable of causing disease.[2]

tranquilizer: This is a term commonly used to describe any drug that has a calming or sedative effect. However, the drugs that are sometimes called minor tranquilizers should be called antianxiety drugs, and the drugs that are sometimes called major tranquilizers should be called antipsychotics.[3]

trans fatty acids: a fat that is produced when liquid fat (oil) is turned into solid fat through a chemical process called hydrogenation.[1]

ultrasound: a clear gel is put onto the skin over the area being examined. An instrument is then moved over that area. The machine sends out sound waves, which reflect off the body. A computer receives these waves and uses them to create pictures of the body.[4]

unsaturated fat: a fat that is liquid at room temperature. Vegetable oils are unsaturated fats. Unsaturated fats include polyunsaturated fats, and monounsaturated fats.[1]

virulent: toxic, causing disease.[2]

viruses: very small microbes that do not consist of cells but are made up of a small amount of genetic material surrounded by a membrane or protein shell. Viruses cannot reproduce by themselves. In order to reproduce, viruses must infect a cell and use the cell's resources and molecular machinery to make more viruses.[2]

vitamins: chemicals essential in small quantities for normal health, which the body cannot produce itself (or in adequate quantities). A normal diet contains adequate amounts of vitamins for most individuals. However, people whose diets are inadequate or who have digestive tract or liver disorders may need to take supplementary vitamins.[3]

Chapter 51

Directory of Adult Health Resources

General

Agency for Healthcare Research and Quality
U.S. Department of Health and Human Services
P.O. Box 8547
Silver Spring, MD 20907-8547
Toll-Free: 800-358-9295
Website: http://www.ahrq.gov

Centers for Disease Control and Prevention
U.S. Department of Health and Human Services
1600 Clifton Road
Atlanta, GA 30333
Toll-Free: 800-311-3435
Phone: 404-639-3311
Website: www.cdc.gov
E-mail: cdcinfo@cdc.gov

Food and Drug Administration
5600 Fishers Lane
Rockville, Maryland 20857
Toll-Free: 888-INFO-FDA
(888-463-6332)
Website: http://www.fda.gov

healthfinder®
P.O. Box 1133
Washington, DC 20013-1133
Toll-Free: 800-336-4797
Phone: 301-565-4167
Fax: 301-984-4256
Website: www.healthfinder.gov
E-mail: healthfinder@nhic.org

The information in this chapter was compiled from various sources deemed accurate. All contact information was verified and updated in July 2007. Inclusion does not imply endorsement. This list is intended to serve as a starting point for information gathering; it is not comprehensive.

National Center for Complementary and Alternative Medicine
National Institutes of Health
P.O. Box 7923
Gaithersburg, MD 20898-7923
Toll Free: 888-644-6226
Phone: 301-519-3153
Fax: 866-464-3616
TTY: 866-464-3615 (for hearing impaired)
Website: nccam.nih.gov
E-mail: info@nccam.nih.gov

National Heart, Lung, and Blood Institute
NHLBI Health Information Center
P.O. Box 30105
Bethesda, MD 20824-0105
Phone: 301-592-8573
Fax: 240-629-3246
TTY: 240-629-3255
Website: http://www.nhlbi.nih.gov
E-mail: nhlbiinfo@nhlbi.nih.gov

National Institute of Arthritis and Musculoskeletal and Skin Diseases
Information Clearinghouse
National Institutes of Health
1 AMS Circle
Bethesda, MD 20892-3675
Toll-Free: 877-22-NIAMS
Phone: 301-495-4484
Fax: 301-718-6366
TTY: 301-565-2966
Website: http://www.niams.nih.gov
E-mail: niamsinfo@mail.nih.gov

National Institute of Neurological Disorders and Stroke
P.O. Box 5801
Bethesda, MD 20824
Toll-Free: 800-352-9424
Phone: 301-496-5751
TTY: 301-468-5981
Website: http://www.ninds.nih.gov
E-mail: braininfo@ninds.nih.gov

National Institute on Aging
P.O. Box 8057
Gaithersburg, MD 20898
Toll-Free: 800-222-2225
Website: http://www.nih.gov/nia

National Jewish Medical and Research Center
1400 Jackson Street
Denver, CO 80206
Toll-Free: 800-222-LUNG (222-5864)
Phone: 303-388-4461
Website: http://www.njc.org

National Women's Health Information Center
U.S. Department of Health and Human Services
8270 Willow Oaks Corporate Dr.
Fairfax, VA 22031
Toll-Free: 800-994-9662
Toll-Free TDD: 888-220-5446
Website: http://www.4women.gov

Osteoporosis and Related Bone Diseases National Resource Center
National Institutes of Health
2 AMS Circle
Bethesda, MD 20892-3676
Toll-Free: 800-624-BONE (2663)
Phone: 202-223-0344
Fax: 202-293-2356
Website: http://www.niams.nih.gov/bone
E-mail: NIAMSBoneInfo@mail.nih.gov

Alcohol and Drug Abuse

National Clearinghouse for Alcohol and Drug Information
Substance Abuse and Mental Health Services Administration
U.S. Department of Health and Human Services
P.O. Box 2345
Rockville, MD 20847-2345
Toll-Free: 800-729-6686
Website: www.ncadi.samhsa.gov

National Institute on Alcohol Abuse and Alcoholism
National Institutes of Health
U.S. Department of Health and Human Services
5635 Fishers Lane, MSC 9304
Bethesda, MD 20892-9304
Phone: 301-443-3860
Website: http://www.niaaa.nih.gov

National Institute on Drug Abuse
National Institutes of Health
U.S. Department of Health and Human Services
6001 Executive Boulevard, Room 5213
Bethesda, MD 20892-9561
Phone: 301-443-1124
Website: http://www.drugabuse.gov

Arthritis

American Academy of Orthopaedic Surgeons
6300 North River Road
Rosemont, Illinois 60018-4262
Phone: 847-823-7186
Fax: 847-823-8125
Website: www.aaos.org
E-mail: custserv@aaos.org

American Chronic Pain Association
P.O. Box 850
Rocklin, CA 95677
Phone: 916-632-0922
Fax: 916-632-3208
Website: www.theacpa.org

American College of Rheumatology
1800 Century Place, Suite 250
Atlanta, GA 30345
Phone: 404-633-3777
Fax: 404-633-1870
Website: www.rheumatology.org

American Pain Society
4700 West Lake Avenue
Glenview, IL 60025-1485
Phone: 847-375-4715
Website: www.ampainsoc.org

American Physical Therapy Association
1111 North Fairfax Street
Alexandria, VA 22314-1488
Toll-Free: 800-999-2782
Phone: 703-684-2782
Website: http://www.apta.org

Arthritis Foundation
P.O. Box 932915
Atlanta, GA 31193-2195
Toll-Free: 800-283-7800
Phone: 404-872-7100
Website: www.arthritis.org
E-mail: help@arthritis.org

National Institute of Arthritis and Musculoskeletal and Skin Diseases Information Clearinghouse (NAMSIC)
National Institutes of Health
1 AMS Circle
Bethesda, MD 20892-3675
Toll-Free: 877-22-NIAMS (226-4267)
Phone: 301-495-4484
Fax: 301-718-6366
TTY: 301-565-2966
Website: www.nih.gov/niams

Cancer Screening

National Cancer Institute
NCI Public Inquiries Office
6116 Executive Boulevard
Room 3036A
Bethesda, MD 20892-8322
Toll-Free: 800-4-CANCER (422-6237)
TTY: 800-332-8615
Website: http://www.cancer.gov

Prostate Cancer Foundation
1250 Fourth Street
Santa Monica, CA 90401
Toll-Free: 800-757-CURE (2873)
Phone: 310-570-4700
Fax: 310-570-4701
Website: http://www.prostatecancerfoundation.org
E-mail: info@prostatecancerfoundation.org

Caregiver Concerns

Administration on Aging
Department of Health and Human Services
Washington, DC 20201
Phone: 202-619-0724
Fax: 202-357-3555
Website: http://www.aoa.gov
E-mail: aoainfo@aoa.hhs.gov

AGS Foundation for Health in Aging
Empire State Building
350 Fifth Avenue, Suite 801
New York, NY 10118
Toll-Free: 800-563-4916
Phone: 212-755-6810
Fax: 212-832-8646
Website: http://
www.healthinaging.org

Family Caregiver Alliance
180 Montgomery Street
Suite 1100
San Francisco, CA 94104
Toll-Free: 800-445-8106
Phone: 415-434-3388
Website: http://
www.caregiver.org
E-mail: info@caregiver.org

National Adult Day Services Association, Inc.
2519 Connecticut Ave. NW
Washington, DC 20008
Toll-Free: 800-558-5301
Fax: 202-783-2255
Website: http://www.nadsa.org
E-mail: info@nadsa.org

National Association of Area Agencies on Aging
1730 Rhode Island Ave., NW
Suite 1200
Washington, DC 20036
Phone: 202-872-0888
Website: http://www.n4a.org

National Family Caregivers Association
10400 Connecticut Avenue
Suite 500
Kensington, MD 20895-3944
Toll-Free: 800-896-3650
Phone: 301-942-6430
Fax: 301-942-2302
Website: http://
www.nfcacares.org
E-mail:
info@thefamilycaregiver.org

National Family Caregivers Support Program
Administration on Aging
Washington, DC 20201
Phone: 202-619-0724
Fax: 202-357-3555
Website: http://www.aoa.gov/prof/
aoaprog/caregiver/caregiver.asp
E-mail: aoainfo@aoa.hhs.gov

Chronic Obstructive Pulmonary Disease and Emphysema

American Lung Association
61 Broadway, 6th Floor
New York, NY 10006
Toll-Free: 800-LUNGUSA
Website: http://www.lungusa.org

COPD Foundation, Inc.
2937 SW 27th Avenue, Suite 302
Miami, FL 33133
Toll-Free: 866-731-2673
Website: http://
www.copdfoundation.org
E-mail:
mmcguire@COPDFoundation.org

National Emphysema Foundation
128 East Avenue
Norwalk, CT 06851
Phone: 203-866-5000
Fax: 203-286 1105
Website: http://www.emphysema foundation.org

National Lung Health Education Program
American Association for Respiratory Care
9425 MacArthur Boulevard
Irving, TX 75063
Phone: 972-910-8555
Fax: 972-484-2720
Website: http://www.nlhep.org
E-mail: NLHEP@aarc.org

Dental Health

American Academy of Periodontology
737 N. Michigan Ave., Suite 800
Chicago, IL 60611
Toll-Free: 800-356-7736
Website: http://www.perio.org

American Dental Association
211 East Chicago Ave.
Chicago, IL 60611-2678
Phone: 312-440-2500
Website: http://www.ada.org

National Institute of Dental and Craniofacial Research
National Institutes of Health
Public Information and Liaison Branch
Bethesda, MD 20892
Phone: 301-496-4261
Website: http://www.nidcr.nih.gov

Depression

American Psychiatric Association
1000 Wilson Boulevard
Suite 1825
Arlington, VA 22209-3901
Toll-Free: 888-35-PSYCH
(888-357-7924)
Phone: 703-907-7300
Fax: 703-907-1085
Website: http://www.psych.org
E-mail: apa@psych.org

American Psychological Association
750 First Street, NE
Washington, DC 20002-4242
Toll-Free: 800-374-2721
Phone: 202-336-5500
TDD/TTY: 202-336-6123
Website: http://www.apa.org

Depression and Bipolar Support Alliance
730 N. Franklin St., Suite 501
Chicago, IL 60610-7204
Toll-Free: 800-826-3632
Fax: 312-642-7243
Website: http://www.dbsalliance.org
E-mail:
questions@dbsalliance.org

Mental Health America

2000 N. Beauregard Street
6th Floor
Alexandria, VA 22314
Toll-Free: 800-969-6642
Fax: 703-684-5968
Website: http://
www.mentalhealthamerican.net

National Alliance on Mental Illness

Colonial Place Three
2107 Wilson Blvd., Suite 300
Arlington, VA 22201-3042
Toll-Free: 800-950-NAMI (6264)
Phone: 703-524-7600
Fax: 703-524-9094
TDD: 703-516-7227
Website: http://www.nami.org

National Institute of Mental Health

Public Information and
Communications Branch
6001 Executive Boulevard,
Room 8184, MSC 9663
Bethesda, MD 20892-9663
Toll-Free: 866-615-6464
Phone: 301-443-4513
Fax: 301-443-4279
TTY: 866-415-8051
Website: http://www.nimh.nih.gov
E-mail: nimhinfo@nih.gov

Postpartum Education for Parents

P.O. Box 6154
Santa Barbara, CA 93130
Phone: (805) 564-3888
Website: http://www.sbpep.org
E-mail: pepboard@gmail.com

Postpartum Support International

927 N. Kellogg
Santa Barbara, CA 93111
Phone: 805-967-7636
Fax: 805-967-0608
Website: http://
www.postpartum.net

Diabetes

American Diabetes Association

ATTN: National Call Center
1701 North Beauregard Street
Alexandria, VA 22311
Toll-Free: 800-DIABETES
(800-342-2383)
Website: http://www.diabetes.org
E-mail: AskADA@diabetes.org

Lower Extremity Amputation Prevention Program (LEAP)

Bureau of Primary Health Care
Health Resources and Services
Administration
U.S. Department of Health and
Human Services
1770 Physicians Park Drive
Baton Rouge, Louisiana 70816
Toll-Free: 888-275-4772
Website: http://
www.bphc.hrsa.gov/leap

National Diabetes Information Clearinghouse
1 Information Way
Bethesda, MD 20892–3560
Phone: 301-654-3327
Fax: 703-738-4929
Website: http://
diabetes.niddk.nih.gov
E-mail: ndic@info.niddk.nih.gov

National Institute of Diabetes and Digestive and Kidney Diseases
National Institutes of Health
U.S. Department of Health and Human Services
Building 31, Rm. 9A06
31 Center Drive, MSC 2560
Bethesda, MD 20892-2560
Toll-Free: 800-891-5390
Phone: 301-496-3583
Website: http://www.niddk.nih.gov
E-mail:
dwebmaster@extra.niddk.nih.gov

Endometriosis

American College of Obstetricians and Gynecologists
409 12th Street, SW
Washington, DC 20024
PO Box 96920
Washington, DC 20090
Phone: 202-863-2487 or 202-638-5577
Fax: 202-484-3917
Toll-Free: 800-762-2264
Website: http://www.acog.org
E-mail: adolhlth@acog.org

Endometriosis Association
8585 N. 76th Place
Milwaukee, WI 53223
Phone: 414-355-2200
Fax: 414-355-6065
Website: http://
www.endometriosisassn.org

Food and Nutrition

American Dietetic Association
120 South Riverside Plaza
Suite 2000
Chicago, IL 60606-6995
Toll-Free: 800-877-1600
Website: www.eatright.org
E-mail: knowledge@eatright.org

Center for Food Safety and Applied Nutrition
Food and Drug Administration
U.S. Department of Health and Human Services
Toll-Free: 888-463-6332
Website: http://
www.cfsan.fda.gov

International Food Information Council Foundation
1100 Connecticut Avenue, NW
Suite 430
Washington, DC 20036
Phone: 202-296-6540
Fax: 202-296-6547
Website: http://www.ific.org
E-mail: foodinfo@ific.org

Hearing

Alexander Graham Bell Association for the Deaf and Hard of Hearing (AG Bell)
3417 Volta Place, NW
Washington, DC 20007
Toll-Free: 866-337-5220
Phone: 202-337-5220
Fax: 202-337-8314
TTY: 202-337-5221
Website: http://www.agbell.org
E-mail: info@agbell.org

American Academy of Audiology (AAA)
11730 Plaza America Drive
Suite 300
Reston, VA 20190
Toll-Free: 800-222-2336
Phone: 703-790-8466
Fax: 703-790-8631
TTY: 703-790-8466
Website: http://
www.audiology.org
E-mail: info@audiology.org

American Academy of Otolaryngology-Head and Neck Surgery (AAO-HNS)
One Prince Street
Alexandria, VA 22314-3357
Phone: 703-836-4444
Fax: 703-683-5100
TTY: 703-519-1585
Website: http://www.entnet.org
E-mail: webmaster@entnet.org

American Hearing Research Foundation (AHRF)
8 South Michigan Ave., Suite 814
Chicago, IL 60603-4539
Phone: 312-726-9670
Fax: 312-726-9695
Website: http://www.american-hearing.org

American Speech-Language-Hearing Association (ASHA)
10801 Rockville Pike
Rockville, MD 20852
Toll-Free: 800-638-8255
Phone: 301-897-5700
Fax: 301-571-0457
TTY: 301-897-0157
Website: http://www.asha.org
E-mail: actioncenter@asha.org

American Tinnitus Association (ATA)
P.O. Box 5
Portland, OR 97207
Toll-Free: 800-634-8978
Phone: 503-248-9985
Fax: 503-248-0024
Website: http://www.ata.org
E-mail: tinnitus@ata.org

Hearing Loss Association of America
7910 Woodmont Ave., Suite 1200
Bethesda, MD 20814
Phone: 301-657-2248
Fax: 301-913-9413
TTY: 301-657-2249
Website: http://
www.hearingloss.org
E-mail: info@hearingloss.org

League for the Hard of Hearing (LHH)
50 Broadway
New York, NY 10004
Phone: 917-305-7700
Fax: 917-305-7888
TTY: 917-305-7999
Website: http://www.lhh.org

National Institute on Deafness and Other Communication Disorders
National Institutes of Health
U.S. Department of Health and Human Services
1 Communication Avenue
Bethesda, MD 20892-3456
Toll-Free: 800-241-1044
TTY: 800-241-1055
Website: http://www.nidcd.nih.gov
E-mail: nidcdinfo@nidcd.nih.gov

WISE EARS!® A Public Education Campaign to Prevent Noise-Induced Hearing Loss
Office of Health Communication and Public Liaison
NIDCD
31 Center Drive, MSC 2320
Bethesda, MD 20892-2320
Toll-Free: 800-241-1044
Phone: 301-496-7243
Fax: 301-402-0018
TTY: 800-241-1055
Website: http://www.nidcd.nih.gov/health/wise
E-mail: nidcdinfo@nidcd.nih.gov

Immunizations

Centers for Disease Control and Prevention
1600 Clifton Road
Atlanta, GA 30333.
Toll-Free: 800-311-3435
Phone: 404-639-3534
Website: http://www.cdc.gov/vaccines

National Coalition for Adult Immunization
4733 Bethesda Avenue, Suite 750
Bethesda, MD 20814-5228
Phone: 301-656-0003
Fax: 301-907-0878
Website: http://www.nfid.org
E-mail: ncai@nfid.org

National Immunization Program Public Inquiries
Centers for Disease Control and Prevention
1600 Clifton Road, Mailstop E-05
Atlanta, GA 30333
Toll-Free: 800-CDC-INFO (800-232-4636)
Website: http://www.cdc.gov/vaccines
E-mail: NIPINFO@cdc.gov

Infertility

American College of Obstetricians and Gynecologists (ACOG) Resource Center
409 12th Street, SW
Washington, DC 20024
PO Box 96920
Washington, DC 20090
Phone: 202-863-2487
or 202-638-5577
Fax: 202-484-3917
Toll-Free: 800-762-2264
Website: http://www.acog.org
E-mail: adolhlth@acog.org

American Society for Reproductive Medicine
1209 Montgomery Highway
Birmingham, AL 35216-2809
Phone: 205-978-5000
Website: http://www.asrm.org
E-mail: asrm@asrm.org

InterNational Council on Infertility Information Dissemination, Inc.
P.O. Box 6836
Arlington, VA 22206
Phone: 703-379-9178
Fax: 703-379-1593
Website: http://www.inciid.org
E-mail: alert@inciid.org

RESOLVE
7910 Woodmont Ave., Suite 1350
Bethesda, Maryland 20814
Phone: 301-652-8585
Fax: 301-652-9375
Website: http://www.resolve.org

Society for the Study of Male Reproduction
1100 E. Woodfield Rd., Suite 520
Schaumburg, IL 60173
Phone: 847-517-7225
Fax: 847-517-7229
Website: http://www.ssmr.org

Menopause

American College of Obstetricians and Gynecologists
409 12th Street, SW
Washington, DC 20024
PO Box 96920
Washington, DC 20090
Phone: 202-863-2487
or 202-638-5577
Fax: 202-484-3917
Toll-Free: 800-762-2264
Website: http://www.acog.org
E-mail: adolhlth@acog.org

American Menopause Foundation
350 Fifth Avenue, Suite 2822
New York, NY 10118
Website: http://www.americanmenopause.org

Hormone Foundation
8401 Connecticut Ave., Suite 900
Chevy Chase, MD 20815-5817
Toll-Free: 800-HORMONE
Phone: 301-941-0259
Website: http://www.hormone.org
E-mail: hormone@endo-society.org

North American Menopause Society (NAMS)
P.O. Box 94527
Cleveland, OH 44101
Toll-Free: 800-774-5342
Phone: 440-442-7550
Fax: 440-442-2660
Website: http://www.menopause.org
E-mail: info@menopause.org

Osteoporosis

National Institute on Aging
P.O. Box 8057
Gaithersburg, MD 20898
Bethesda, MD 20892
Toll-Free: 800-222-2225
Phone: 301-496-1752
Fax: 301-496-1072
TTY: 800-222-4225
Website: http://www.nih.gov/nia

National Osteoporosis Foundation
1232 22nd Street N.W.
Washington, DC 20037-1292
Toll-Free: 877-868-4520
Phone: 202-223-2226
Website: http://www.nof.org
E-mail: webmaster@nof.org

Osteoporosis and Related Bone Diseases National Resource Center
National Institutes of Health
2 AMS Circle
Bethesda, MD 20892-3676
Toll-Free: 800-624-BONE (2663)
Phone: 202-223-0344
Fax: 202-293-2356
Website: http://www.niams.nih.gov/bone
E-mail: NIAMSBoneInfo@mail.nih.gov

Tone Your Bones
LRC 358, 1530 3rd Avenue S.
Birmingham, AL 35294-1270
Toll-Free: 888-934-BONE (2663)
Website: http://www.toneyourbones.org

Physical Fitness

American College of Sports Medicine (ACSM)
401 West Michigan Street
Indianapolis, IN 46202-3233
P.O. Box 1440
Indianapolis, IN 46206-1440
Phone: 317-637-9200
Website: http://www.acsm.org/index.asp

National Strength and Conditioning Association (NSCA)
1885 Bob Johnson Dr.
Colorado Springs, CO 80906
Toll Free: 800-815-6826
Phone: 719-632-6722
Website: http://www.nsca-lift.org

President's Council on Physical Fitness and Sports
Department W
200 Independence Avenue, SW
Room 738-H
Washington, DC 20201-0004
Phone: 202-690-9000
Website: http://www.fitness.gov

Shape Up America!
Website: http://www.shapeup.org

Prostate Concerns

American Urological Association (AUA)
1000 Corporate Boulevard
Linthicum, MD 21090
Toll-Free: 800-828-7866
Phone: 410-689-3990
Website: http://
www.auafoundation.org
E-mail:
auafoundation@auafoundation.org

National Cancer Institute (NCI)
Cancer Information Service
6116 Executive Boulevard
Room 3036A
Bethesda, MD 20892-8322
Toll-Free: 800–4CANCER
(800–422–6237)
TTY: 800–332–8615
Website: http://www.cancer.gov
or http://cancernet.nci.nih.gov
E-mail:
cancermail@icicc.nci.nih.gov

Prostatitis Foundation
1063 30th Street, Box 8
Smithshire, IL 61478
Toll-Free: 888-891-4200
Fax: 309-325-7184
Website: http://
www.prostatitis.org
E-mail: mcapstone@aol.com

Sexual Concerns

American Association for Marriage and Family Therapy
112 South Alfred Street
Alexandria, VA 22314-3061
Phone: 703-838-9808
Fax: 703-838-9805
Website: http://www.aamft.org/
families/index_nm.asp

American Association of Sex Educators, Counselors, and Therapists
P.O. Box 1960
Ashland, VA 23005
Phone: 804-752-0026
Fax: 804-752-0056
Website: http://www.aasect.org
E-mail: aasect@aasect.org

American Urological Association
1000 Corporate Boulevard
Linthicum, MD 21090
Toll-Free: 800-828-7866
Phone: 410-689-3990
Website: http://
www.urologyhealth.org

National Kidney and Urologic Diseases Information Clearinghouse
3 Information Way
Bethesda, MD 20892–3580
Toll-Free: 800-891-5390
Fax: 703-738-4929
Website: http://
www2.niddk.nih.gov
E-mail:
nkudic@info.niddk.nih.gov

Society for Sex Therapy and Research
409 12th Street, S.W.
P.O. Box 96920
Washington, DC 20090-6920
Phone: 202-863-1644
Website: http://www.sstarnet.org

Stress/Mental Health

American Psychiatric Association
1000 Wilson Blvd., Suite 1825
Arlington, VA 22209-3901
Toll-Free: 888-35-PSYCH
(888-357-7924)
Phone: 703-907-7300
Fax: 703-907-1085
Website: http://www.psych.org
E-mail: apa@psych.org

American Psychological Association
750 First Street, NE
Washington, DC 20002-4242
Toll-Free: 800-374-2721
Phone: 202-336-5500
TDD/TTY: 202-336-6123
Website: http://www.apa.org

National Alliance on Mental Illness
Colonial Place Three
2107 Wilson Blvd., Suite 300
Arlington, VA 22201-3042
Toll-Free: 800-950-NAMI (6264)
Phone: 703-524-7600
Fax: 703-524-9094
TDD: 703-516-7227
Website: http://www.nami.org
E-mail: info@nami.org

National Institute of Mental Health
Public Information and
Communications Branch
6001 Executive Boulevard,
Room 8184, MSC 9663
Bethesda, MD 20892-9663
Toll-Free: 866-615-6464
Phone: 301-443-4513
Fax: 301-443-4279
TTY: 866-415-8051
Website: http://
www.nimh.nih.gov
E-mail: nimhinfo@nih.gov

National Foundation for Depressive Illness
P.O. Box 2257
New York, NY 10116
Toll-Free: 800-239-1265

Stroke

American Stroke Association
7272 Greenville Ave.
Dallas, TX 75231
Toll-Free: 888-4-STROKE
(478-7653)
Website: http://
www.strokeassociation.org

National Institute of Neurological Disorders and Stroke
P.O. Box 5801
Bethesda, MD 20824
Toll-Free: 800-352-9424
Phone: 301-496-5751
TTY: 301-468-5981
Fax: 301-468-5981
Website: http://
www.ninds.nih.gov
E-mail: braininfo@ninds.nih.gov

National Stroke Association
9707 E. Easter Lane
Englewood, CO 80112-3747
Fax: 303-649-1328
Toll-Free: 800-STROKES
(787-6537)
Website: http://www.stroke.org
E-mail: info@stroke.org

Thyroid Concerns

Hormone Foundation
8401 Connecticut Ave., Suite 900
Chevy Chase, MD 20815-5817
Toll-Free: 800-HORMONE
Phone: 301-941-0259
Website: http://www.hormone.org
E-mail:
hormone@endo-society.org

Thyroid Foundation of America
One Longfellow Pl., Suite 1518
Boston, MA 02114
Toll-Free: 800-832-8321
Fax: 617-534-1515
Website: http://www.allthyroid.org
E-mail: info@allthyroid.org

Traveler's Health

Centers for Disease Control and Prevention
1600 Clifton Road
Atlanta, GA 30333
Toll-Free: 800-311-3435
Phone: 404-639-3534
Website: http://www.cdc.gov/
travel

International Society of Travel Medicine
Phone: 770-736-7060
Website: http://www.istm.org

Vision

Association for Macular Diseases
210 East 64th S., 8th Floor
New York, NY 10021-7471
Phone: 212-605-3719
Website: http://www.macula.org

Foundation Fighting Blindness
11435 Cronhill Drive
Owings Mill, MD 21117-2220
Toll-Free: 888-394-3937
Phone: 410-785-1414
Website: www.blindness.org
E-mail: info@FightBlindness.org

Macular Degeneration Partnership
8733 Beverly Blvd., Suite 201
Los Angeles, CA 90048-1844
Toll-Free: 888-430-9898
Phone: 310-423-6455
Fax: 310-623-1837
Website: www.amd.org

National Eye Institute
National Institutes of Health
31 Center Drive MSC 2510
Bethesda, MD 20892-3655
Phone: 301-496-5248
Website: http://www.nei.nih.gov
E-mail: 2020@nei.nih.gov

Weight Loss

Weight-control Information Network (WIN)
1 WIN Way
Bethesda, MD 20892-3665
Toll-Free: 877-946-4627
Phone: 202-828-1025
Fax: 202-828-1028
Website: http://
win.niddk.nih.gov
E-mail: WIN@info.niddk.nih.gov

Index

Index

619

Health Reference Series

COMPLETE CATALOG

List price $87 per volume. **School and library price $78 per volume.**

Adolescent Health Sourcebook, 2nd Edition

Basic Consumer Health Information about the Physical, Mental, and Emotional Growth and Development of Adolescents, Including Medical Care, Nutritional and Physical Activity Requirements, Puberty, Sexual Activity, Acne, Tanning, Body Piercing, Common Physical Illnesses and Disorders, Eating Disorders, Attention Deficit Hyperactivity Disorder, Depression, Bullying, Hazing, and Adolescent Injuries Related to Sports, Driving, and Work

Along with Substance Abuse Information about Nicotine, Alcohol, and Drug Use, a Glossary, and Directory of Additional Resources

Edited by Joyce Brennfleck Shannon. 683 pages. 2006. 978-0-7808-0943-7.

"It is written in clear, nontechnical language aimed at general readers. . . . Recommended for public libraries, community colleges, and other agencies serving health care consumers."
— *American Reference Books Annual, 2003*

"Recommended for school and public libraries. Parents and professionals dealing with teens will appreciate the easy-to-follow format and the clearly written text. This could become a 'must have' for every high school teacher." — *E-Streams, Jan '03*

"A good starting point for information related to common medical, mental, and emotional concerns of adolescents." — *School Library Journal, Nov '02*

"This book provides accurate information in an easy to access format. It addresses topics that parents and caregivers might not be aware of and provides practical, useable information."
— *Doody's Health Sciences Book Review Journal, Sep-Oct '02*

"Recommended reference source."
— *Booklist, American Library Association, Sep '02*

AIDS Sourcebook, 3rd Edition

Basic Consumer Health Information about Acquired Immune Deficiency Syndrome (AIDS) and Human Immunodeficiency Virus (HIV) Infection, Including Facts about Transmission, Prevention, Diagnosis, Treatment, Opportunistic Infections, and Other Complications, with a Section for Women and Children, Including Details about Associated Gynecological Concerns, Pregnancy, and Pediatric Care

Along with Updated Statistical Information, Reports on Current Research Initiatives, a Glossary, and Directories of Internet, Hotline, and Other Resources

Edited by Dawn D. Matthews. 664 pages. 2003. 978-0-7808-0631-3.

"The 3rd edition of the *AIDS Sourcebook*, part of Omnigraphics' *Health Reference Series*, is a welcome update. . . . This resource is highly recommended for academic and public libraries."
— *American Reference Books Annual, 2004*

"Excellent sourcebook. This continues to be a highly recommended book. There is no other book that provides as much information as this book provides."
— *AIDS Book Review Journal, Dec-Jan '00*

"Recommended reference source."
— *Booklist, American Library Association, Dec '99*

Alcoholism Sourcebook, 2nd Edition

Basic Consumer Health Information about Alcohol Use, Abuse, and Dependence, Featuring Facts about the Physical, Mental, and Social Health Effects of Alcohol Addiction, Including Alcoholic Liver Disease, Pancreatic Disease, Cardiovascular Disease, Neurological Disorders, and the Effects of Drinking during Pregnancy

Along with Information about Alcohol Treatment, Medications, and Recovery Programs, in Addition to Tips for Reducing the Prevalence of Underage Drinking, Statistics about Alcohol Use, a Glossary of Related Terms, and Directories of Resources for More Help and Information

Edited by Amy L. Sutton. 653 pages. 2006. 978-0-7808-0942-0.

"This title is one of the few reference works on alcoholism for general readers. For some readers this will be a welcome complement to the many self-help books on the market. Recommended for collections serving general readers and consumer health collections."
— *E-Streams, Mar '01*

"This book is an excellent choice for public and academic libraries."
— *American Reference Books Annual, 2001*

"Recommended reference source."
— *Booklist, American Library Association, Dec '00*

"Presents a wealth of information on alcohol use and abuse and its effects on the body and mind, treatment, and prevention." — *SciTech Book News, Dec '00*

"Important new health guide which packs in the latest consumer information about the problems of alcoholism." — *Reviewer's Bookwatch, Nov '00*

SEE ALSO *Drug Abuse Sourcebook*

Allergies Sourcebook, 3rd Edition

Basic Consumer Health Information about Allergic Disorders, Such as Anaphylaxis, Hives, Eczema, Rhinitis, Sinusitis, and Conjunctivitis, and Their Triggers, Including Pollen, Mold, Dust Mites, Animal Dander, Insects, Chemicals, Food, Food Additives, and Medications;

Along with Advice about the Diagnosis and Treatment of Allergy Symptoms, a Glossary of Related Terms, a Directory of Resources for Help and Information, and Suggestions for Additional Reading

Edited by Amy L. Sutton. 598 pages. 2007. 978-0-7808-0950-5.

"This book brings a great deal of useful material together. . . . This is an excellent addition to public and consumer health library collections."
— *American Reference Books Annual, 2003*

"This second edition would be useful to laypersons with little or advanced knowledge of the subject matter. This book would also serve as a resource for nursing and other health care professions students. It would be useful in public, academic, and hospital libraries with consumer health collections." — *E-Streams, Jul '02*

∎

Alternative Medicine Sourcebook

SEE Complementary & Alternative Medicine Sourcebook

∎

Alzheimer's Disease Sourcebook, 3rd Edition

Basic Consumer Health Information about Alzheimer's Disease, Other Dementias, and Related Disorders, Including Multi-Infarct Dementia, AIDS Dementia Complex, Dementia with Lewy Bodies, Huntington's Disease, Wernicke-Korsakoff Syndrome (Alcohol-Related Dementia), Delirium, and Confusional States

Along with Information for People Newly Diagnosed with Alzheimer's Disease and Caregivers, Reports Detailing Current Research Efforts in Prevention, Diagnosis, and Treatment, Facts about Long-Term Care Issues, and Listings of Sources for Additional Information

Edited by Karen Bellenir. 645 pages. 2003. 978-0-7808-0666-5.

"This very informative and valuable tool will be a great addition to any library serving consumers, students and health care workers."
— *American Reference Books Annual, 2004*

"This is a valuable resource for people affected by dementias such as Alzheimer's. It is easy to navigate and includes important information and resources."
— *Doody's Review Service, Feb '04*

"Recommended reference source."
— *Booklist, American Library Association, Oct '99*

SEE ALSO *Brain Disorders Sourcebook*

Arthritis Sourcebook, 2nd Edition

Basic Consumer Health Information about Osteoarthritis, Rheumatoid Arthritis, Other Rheumatic Disorders, Infectious Forms of Arthritis, and Diseases with Symptoms Linked to Arthritis, Featuring Facts about Diagnosis, Pain Management, and Surgical Therapies

Along with Coping Strategies, Research Updates, a Glossary, and Resources for Additional Help and Information

Edited by Amy L. Sutton. 593 pages. 2004. 978-0-7808-0667-2.

"This easy-to-read volume is recommended for consumer health collections within public or academic libraries." — *E-Streams, May '05*

"As expected, this updated edition continues the excellent reputation of this series in providing sound, usable health information. . . . Highly recommended."
— *American Reference Books Annual, 2005*

"Excellent reference." — *The Bookwatch, Jan '05*

∎

Asthma Sourcebook, 2nd Edition

Basic Consumer Health Information about the Causes, Symptoms, Diagnosis, and Treatment of Asthma in Infants, Children, Teenagers, and Adults, Including Facts about Different Types of Asthma, Common Co-Occurring Conditions, Asthma Management Plans, Triggers, Medications, and Medication Delivery Devices

Along with Asthma Statistics, Research Updates, a Glossary, a Directory of Asthma-Related Resources, and More

Edited by Karen Bellenir. 609 pages. 2006. 978-0-7808-0866-9.

"A worthwhile reference acquisition for public libraries and academic medical libraries whose readers desire a quick introduction to the wide range of asthma information." — *Choice, Association of College & Research Libraries, Jun '01*

"Recommended reference source."
— *Booklist, American Library Association, Feb '01*

"Highly recommended." — *The Bookwatch, Jan '01*

"There is much good information for patients and their families who deal with asthma daily."
— *American Medical Writers Association Journal, Winter '01*

"This informative text is recommended for consumer health collections in public, secondary school, and community college libraries and the libraries of universities with a large undergraduate population."
— *American Reference Books Annual, 2001*

∎

Attention Deficit Disorder Sourcebook

Basic Consumer Health Information about Attention Deficit/Hyperactivity Disorder in Children and Adults,

Including Facts about Causes, Symptoms, Diagnostic Criteria, and Treatment Options Such as Medications, Behavior Therapy, Coaching, and Homeopathy

Along with Reports on Current Research Initiatives, Legal Issues, and Government Regulations, and Featuring a Glossary of Related Terms, Internet Resources, and a List of Additional Reading Material

Edited by Dawn D. Matthews. 470 pages. 2002. 978-0-7808-0624-5.

"Recommended reference source."
— *Booklist, American Library Association, Jan '03*

"This book is recommended for all school libraries and the reference or consumer health sections of public libraries." — *American Reference Books Annual, 2003*

■

Back & Neck Sourcebook, 2nd Edition

Basic Consumer Health Information about Spinal Pain, Spinal Cord Injuries, and Related Disorders, Such as Degenerative Disk Disease, Osteoarthritis, Scoliosis, Sciatica, Spina Bifida, and Spinal Stenosis, and Featuring Facts about Maintaining Spinal Health, Self-Care, Pain Management, Rehabilitative Care, Chiropractic Care, Spinal Surgeries, and Complementary Therapies

Along with Suggestions for Preventing Back and Neck Pain, a Glossary of Related Terms, and a Directory of Resources

Edited by Amy L. Sutton. 633 pages. 2004. 978-0-7808-0738-9.

"Recommended . . . an easy to use, comprehensive medical reference book." — *E-Streams, Sep '05*

"The strength of this work is its basic, easy-to-read format. Recommended." — *Reference and User Services Quarterly, American Library Association, Winter '97*

■

Blood & Circulatory Disorders Sourcebook, 2nd Edition

Basic Consumer Health Information about the Blood and Circulatory System and Related Disorders, Such as Anemia and Other Hemoglobin Diseases, Cancer of the Blood and Associated Bone Marrow Disorders, Clotting and Bleeding Problems, and Conditions That Affect the Veins, Blood Vessels, and Arteries, Including Facts about the Donation and Transplantation of Bone Marrow, Stem Cells, and Blood and Tips for Keeping the Blood and Circulatory System Healthy

Along with a Glossary of Related Terms and Resources for Additional Help and Information

Edited by Amy L. Sutton. 659 pages. 2005. 978-0-7808-0746-4.

"Highly recommended pick for basic consumer health reference holdings at all levels."
— *The Bookwatch, Aug '05*

"Recommended reference source."
— *Booklist, American Library Association, Feb '99*

"An important reference sourcebook written in simple language for everyday, non-technical users. "
— *Reviewer's Bookwatch, Jan '99*

■

Brain Disorders Sourcebook, 2nd Edition

Basic Consumer Health Information about Acquired and Traumatic Brain Injuries, Infections of the Brain, Epilepsy and Seizure Disorders, Cerebral Palsy, and Degenerative Neurological Disorders, Including Amyotrophic Lateral Sclerosis (ALS), Dementias, Multiple Sclerosis, and More

Along with Information on the Brain's Structure and Function, Treatment and Rehabilitation Options, Reports on Current Research Initiatives, a Glossary of Terms Related to Brain Disorders and Injuries, and a Directory of Sources for Further Help and Information

Edited by Sandra J. Judd. 625 pages. 2005. 978-0-7808-0744-0.

"Highly recommended pick for basic consumer health reference holdings at all levels."
— *The Bookwatch, Aug '05*

"Belongs on the shelves of any library with a consumer health collection." — *E-Streams, Mar '00*

"Recommended reference source."
— *Booklist, American Library Association, Oct '99*

SEE ALSO Alzheimer's Disease Sourcebook

■

Breast Cancer Sourcebook, 2nd Edition

Basic Consumer Health Information about Breast Cancer, Including Facts about Risk Factors, Prevention, Screening and Diagnostic Methods, Treatment Options, Complementary and Alternative Therapies, Post-Treatment Concerns, Clinical Trials, Special Risk Populations, and New Developments in Breast Cancer Research

Along with Breast Cancer Statistics, a Glossary of Related Terms, and a Directory of Resources for Additional Help and Information

Edited by Sandra J. Judd. 595 pages. 2004. 978-0-7808-0668-9.

"This book will be an excellent addition to public, community college, medical, and academic libraries."
— *American Reference Books Annual, 2006*

"It would be a useful reference book in a library or on loan to women in a support group."
— *Cancer Forum, Mar '03*

"Recommended reference source."
— *Booklist, American Library Association, Jan '02*

"This reference source is highly recommended. It is quite informative, comprehensive and detailed in nature, and yet it offers practical advice in easy-to-read language. It could be thought of as the 'bible' of breast cancer for the consumer." — *E-Streams, Jan '02*

"From the pros and cons of different screening methods and results to treatment options, *Breast Cancer Sourcebook* provides the latest information on the subject." — *Library Bookwatch, Dec '01*

"This thoroughgoing, very readable reference covers all aspects of breast health and cancer. . . . Readers will find much to consider here. Recommended for all public and patient health collections." — *Library Journal, Sep '01*

SEE ALSO *Cancer Sourcebook for Women, Women's Health Concerns Sourcebook*

Breastfeeding Sourcebook

Basic Consumer Health Information about the Benefits of Breastmilk, Preparing to Breastfeed, Breastfeeding as a Baby Grows, Nutrition, and More, Including Information on Special Situations and Concerns Such as Mastitis, Illness, Medications, Allergies, Multiple Births, Prematurity, Special Needs, and Adoption

Along with a Glossary and Resources for Additional Help and Information

Edited by Jenni Lynn Colson. 388 pages. 2002. 978-0-7808-0332-9.

"Particularly useful is the information about professional lactation services and chapters on breastfeeding when returning to work. . . . *Breastfeeding Sourcebook* will be useful for public libraries, consumer health libraries, and technical schools offering nurse assistant training, especially in areas where Internet access is problematic." — *American Reference Books Annual, 2003*

SEE ALSO *Pregnancy & Birth Sourcebook*

Burns Sourcebook

Basic Consumer Health Information about Various Types of Burns and Scalds, Including Flame, Heat, Cold, Electrical, Chemical, and Sun Burns

Along with Information on Short-Term and Long-Term Treatments, Tissue Reconstruction, Plastic Surgery, Prevention Suggestions, and First Aid

Edited by Allan R. Cook. 604 pages. 1999. 978-0-7808-0204-9.

"This is an exceptional addition to the series and is highly recommended for all consumer health collections, hospital libraries, and academic medical centers." — *E-Streams, Mar '00*

"This key reference guide is an invaluable addition to all health care and public libraries in confronting this ongoing health issue." — *American Reference Books Annual, 2000*

"Recommended reference source." — *Booklist, American Library Association, Dec '99*

SEE ALSO *Dermatological Disorders Sourcebook*

Cancer Sourcebook, 5th Edition

Basic Consumer Health Information about Major Forms and Stages of Cancer, Featuring Facts about Head and Neck Cancers, Lung Cancers, Gastrointestinal Cancers, Genitourinary Cancers, Lymphomas, Blood Cell Cancers, Endocrine Cancers, Skin Cancers, Bone Cancers, Metastatic Cancers, and More

Along with Facts about Cancer Treatments, Cancer Risks and Prevention, a Glossary of Related Terms, Statistical Data, and a Directory of Resources for Additional Information

Edited by Karen Bellenir. 1,133 pages. 2007. 978-0-7808-0947-5.

"With cancer being the second leading cause of death for Americans, a prodigious work such as this one, which locates centrally so much cancer-related information, is clearly an asset to this nation's citizens and others." — *Journal of the National Medical Association, 2004*

"This title is recommended for health sciences and public libraries with consumer health collections." — *E-Streams, Feb '01*

". . . can be effectively used by cancer patients and their families who are looking for answers in a language they can understand. Public and hospital libraries should have it on their shelves." — *American Reference Books Annual, 2001*

"Recommended reference source." — *Booklist, American Library Association, Dec '00*

SEE ALSO *Breast Cancer Sourcebook, Cancer Sourcebook for Women, Pediatric Cancer Sourcebook, Prostate Cancer Sourcebook*

Cancer Sourcebook for Women, 3rd Edition

Basic Consumer Health Information about Leading Causes of Cancer in Women, Featuring Facts about Gynecologic Cancers and Related Concerns, Such as Breast Cancer, Cervical Cancer, Endometrial Cancer, Uterine Sarcoma, Vaginal Cancer, Vulvar Cancer, and Common Non-Cancerous Gynecologic Conditions, in Addition to Facts about Lung Cancer, Colorectal Cancer, and Thyroid Cancer in Women

Along with Information about Cancer Risk Factors, Screening and Prevention, Treatment Options, and Tips on Coping with Life after Cancer Treatment, a Glossary of Cancer Terms, and a Directory of Resources for Additional Help and Information

Edited by Amy L. Sutton. 715 pages. 2006. 978-0-7808-0867-6.

"An excellent addition to collections in public, consumer health, and women's health libraries." — *American Reference Books Annual, 2003*

"Overall, the information is excellent, and complex topics are clearly explained. As a reference book for the consumer it is a valuable resource to assist them to make informed decisions about cancer and its treatments." — *Cancer Forum, Nov '02*

"Highly recommended for academic and medical reference collections." — *Library Bookwatch, Sep '02*

"This is a highly recommended book for any public or consumer library, being reader friendly and containing accurate and helpful information." — *E-Streams, Aug '02*

"Recommended reference source." — *Booklist, American Library Association, Jul '02*

SEE ALSO *Breast Cancer Sourcebook, Women's Health Concerns Sourcebook*

Cancer Survivorship Sourcebook

Basic Consumer Health Information about the Physical, Educational, Emotional, Social, and Financial Needs of Cancer Patients from Diagnosis, through Cancer Treatment, and Beyond, Including Facts about Researching Specific Types of Cancer and Learning about Clinical Trials and Treatment Options, and Featuring Tips for Coping with the Side Effects of Cancer Treatments and Adjusting to Life after Cancer Treatment Concludes

Along with Suggestions for Caregivers, Friends, and Family Members of Cancer Patients, a Glossary of Cancer Care Terms, and Directories of Related Resources

Edited by Karen Bellenir. 6561 pages. 2007. 978-0-7808-0985-7.

Cardiovascular Diseases & Disorders Sourcebook, 3rd Edition

Basic Consumer Health Information about Heart and Vascular Diseases and Disorders, Such as Angina, Heart Attacks, Arrhythmias, Cardiomyopathy, Valve Disease, Atherosclerosis, and Aneurysms, with Information about Managing Cardiovascular Risk Factors and Maintaining Heart Health, Medications and Procedures Used to Treat Cardiovascular Disorders, and Concerns of Special Significance to Women

Along with Reports on Current Research Initiatives, a Glossary of Related Medical Terms, and a Directory of Sources for Further Help and Information

Edited by Sandra J. Judd. 713 pages. 2005. 978-0-7808-0739-6.

"This updated sourcebook is still the best first stop for comprehensive introductory information on cardiovascular diseases." — *American Reference Books Annual, 2006*

"Recommended for public libraries and libraries supporting health care professionals." — *E-Streams, Sep '05*

"This should be a standard health library reference." — *The Bookwatch, Jun '05*

"Recommended reference source." — *Booklist, American Library Association, Dec '00*

"... comprehensive format provides an extensive overview on this subject." — *Choice, Association of College & Research Libraries*

Caregiving Sourcebook

Basic Consumer Health Information for Caregivers, Including a Profile of Caregivers, Caregiving Responsibilities and Concerns, Tips for Specific Conditions, Care Environments, and the Effects of Caregiving

Along with Facts about Legal Issues, Financial Information, and Future Planning, a Glossary, and a Listing of Additional Resources

Edited by Joyce Brennfleck Shannon. 600 pages. 2001. 978-0-7808-0331-2.

"Essential for most collections." — *Library Journal, Apr 1, 2002*

"An ideal addition to the reference collection of any public library. Health sciences information professionals may also want to acquire the *Caregiving Sourcebook* for their hospital or academic library for use as a ready reference tool by health care workers interested in aging and caregiving." — *E-Streams, Jan '02*

"Recommended reference source." — *Booklist, American Library Association, Oct '01*

Child Abuse Sourcebook

Basic Consumer Health Information about the Physical, Sexual, and Emotional Abuse of Children, with Additional Facts about Neglect, Munchausen Syndrome by Proxy (MSBP), Shaken Baby Syndrome, and Controversial Issues Related to Child Abuse, Such as Withholding Medical Care, Corporal Punishment, and Child Maltreatment in Youth Sports, and Featuring Facts about Child Protective Services, Foster Care, Adoption, Parenting Challenges, and Other Abuse Prevention Efforts

Along with a Glossary of Related Terms and Resources for Additional Help and Information

Edited by Dawn D. Matthews. 620 pages. 2004. 978-0-7808-0705-1.

"A valuable and highly recommended resource for school, academic and public libraries whether used on its own or as a starting point for more in-depth research." — *E-Streams, Apr '05*

"Every week the news brings cases of child abuse or neglect, so it is useful to have a source that supplies so much helpful information. . . . Recommended. Public and academic libraries, and child welfare offices." — *Choice, Association of College & Research Libraries, Mar '05*

"Packed with insights on all kinds of issues, from foster care and adoption to parenting and abuse prevention." — *The Bookwatch, Nov '04*

SEE ALSO: *Domestic Violence Sourcebook*

Childhood Diseases & Disorders Sourcebook

Basic Consumer Health Information about Medical Problems Often Encountered in Pre-Adolescent Children, Including Respiratory Tract Ailments, Ear Infections, Sore Throats, Disorders of the Skin and Scalp, Digestive and Genitourinary Diseases, Infectious Diseases, Inflammatory Disorders, Chronic Physical and Developmental Disorders, Allergies, and More

Along with Information about Diagnostic Tests, Common Childhood Surgeries, and Frequently Used Medications, with a Glossary of Important Terms and Resource Directory

Edited by Chad T. Kimball. 662 pages. 2003. 978-0-7808-0458-6.

"This is an excellent book for new parents and should be included in all health care and public libraries."
—*American Reference Books Annual, 2004*

SEE ALSO: Healthy Children Sourcebook

■

Colds, Flu & Other Common Ailments Sourcebook

Basic Consumer Health Information about Common Ailments and Injuries, Including Colds, Coughs, the Flu, Sinus Problems, Headaches, Fever, Nausea and Vomiting, Menstrual Cramps, Diarrhea, Constipation, Hemorrhoids, Back Pain, Dandruff, Dry and Itchy Skin, Cuts, Scrapes, Sprains, Bruises, and More

Along with Information about Prevention, Self-Care, Choosing a Doctor, Over-the-Counter Medications, Folk Remedies, and Alternative Therapies, and Including a Glossary of Important Terms and a Directory of Resources for Further Help and Information

Edited by Chad T. Kimball. 638 pages. 2001. 978-0-7808-0435-7.

"A good starting point for research on common illnesses. It will be a useful addition to public and consumer health library collections."
—*American Reference Books Annual, 2002*

"Will prove valuable to any library seeking to maintain a current, comprehensive reference collection of health resources. . . . Excellent reference."
—*The Bookwatch, Aug '01*

"Recommended reference source."
—*Booklist, American Library Association, Jul '01*

■

Communication Disorders Sourcebook

Basic Information about Deafness and Hearing Loss, Speech and Language Disorders, Voice Disorders, Balance and Vestibular Disorders, and Disorders of Smell, Taste, and Touch

Edited by Linda M. Ross. 533 pages. 1996. 978-0-7808-0077-9.

"This is skillfully edited and is a welcome resource for the layperson. It should be found in every public and medical library." —*Booklist Health Sciences Supplement, American Library Association, Oct '97*

■

Complementary & Alternative Medicine Sourcebook, 3rd Edition

Basic Consumer Health Information about Complementary and Alternative Medical Therapies, Including Acupuncture, Ayurveda, Traditional Chinese Medicine, Herbal Medicine, Homeopathy, Naturopathy, Biofeedback, Hypnotherapy, Yoga, Art Therapy, Aromatherapy, Clinical Nutrition, Vitamin and Mineral Supplements, Chiropractic, Massage, Reflexology, Crystal Therapy, Therapeutic Touch, and More

Along with Facts about Alternative and Complementary Treatments for Specific Conditions Such as Cancer, Diabetes, Osteoarthritis, Chronic Pain, Menopause, Gastrointestinal Disorders, Headaches, and Mental Illness, a Glossary, and a Resource List for Additional Help and Information

Edited by Sandra J. Judd. 657 pages. 2006. 978-0-7808-0864-5.

"Recommended for public, high school, and academic libraries that have consumer health collections. Hospital libraries that also serve the public will find this to be a useful resource." —*E-Streams, Feb '03*

"Recommended reference source."
—*Booklist, American Library Association, Jan '03*

"An important alternate health reference."
—*MBR Bookwatch, Oct '02*

"A great addition to the reference collection of every type of library." —*American Reference Books Annual, 2000*

■

Congenital Disorders Sourcebook, 2nd Edition

Basic Consumer Health Information about Nonhereditary Birth Defects and Disorders Related to Prematurity, Gestational Injuries, Congenital Infections, and Birth Complications, Including Heart Defects, Hydrocephalus, Spina Bifida, Cleft Lip and Palate, Cerebral Palsy, and More

Along with Facts about the Prevention of Birth Defects, Fetal Surgery and Other Treatment Options, Research Initiatives, a Glossary of Related Terms, and Resources for Additional Information and Support

Edited by Sandra J. Judd. 647 pages. 2006. 978-0-7808-0945-1.

"Recommended reference source."
—*Booklist, American Library Association, Oct '97*

SEE ALSO Pregnancy & Birth Sourcebook

■

Contagious Diseases Sourcebook

Basic Consumer Health Information about Infectious Diseases Spread by Person-to-Person Contact through

Direct Touch, Airborne Transmission, Sexual Contact, or Contact with Blood or Other Body Fluids, Including Hepatitis, Herpes, Influenza, Lice, Measles, Mumps, Pinworm, Ringworm, Severe Acute Respiratory Syndrome (SARS), Streptococcal Infections, Tuberculosis, and Others

Along with Facts about Disease Transmission, Antimicrobial Resistance, and Vaccines, with a Glossary and Directories of Resources for More Information

Edited by Karen Bellenir. 643 pages. 2004. 978-0-7808-0736-5.

"This easy-to-read volume is recommended for consumer health collections within public or academic libraries." —E-Streams, May '05

"This informative book is highly recommended for public libraries, consumer health collections, and secondary schools and undergraduate libraries." —American Reference Books Annual, 2005

"Excellent reference." —The Bookwatch, Jan '05

■

Death & Dying Sourcebook, 2nd Edition

Basic Consumer Health Information about End-of-Life Care and Related Perspectives and Ethical Issues, Including End-of-Life Symptoms and Treatments, Pain Management, Quality-of-Life Concerns, the Use of Life Support, Patients' Rights and Privacy Issues, Advance Directives, Physician-Assisted Suicide, Caregiving, Organ and Tissue Donation, Autopsies, Funeral Arrangements, and Grief

Along with Statistical Data, Information about the Leading Causes of Death, a Glossary, and Directories of Support Groups and Other Resources

Edited by Joyce Brennfleck Shannon. 653 pages. 2006. 978-0-7808-0871-3.

"Public libraries, medical libraries, and academic libraries will all find this sourcebook a useful addition to their collections." —American Reference Books Annual, 2001

"An extremely useful resource for those concerned with death and dying in the United States." —Respiratory Care, Nov '00

"Recommended reference source." —Booklist, American Library Association, Aug '00

"This book is a definite must for all those involved in end-of-life care." —Doody's Review Service, 2000

■

Dental Care & Oral Health Sourcebook, 2nd Edition

Basic Consumer Health Information about Dental Care, Including Oral Hygiene, Dental Visits, Pain Management, Cavities, Crowns, Bridges, Dental Implants, and Fillings, and Other Oral Health Concerns, Such as Gum Disease, Bad Breath, Dry Mouth, Genetic and Developmental Abnormalities, Oral Cancers, Orthodontics, and Temporomandibular Disorders

Along with Updates on Current Research in Oral Health, a Glossary, a Directory of Dental and Oral Health Organizations, and Resources for People with Dental and Oral Health Disorders

Edited by Amy L. Sutton. 609 pages. 2003. 978-0-7808-0634-4.

"This book could serve as a turning point in the battle to educate consumers in issues concerning oral health." —American Reference Books Annual, 2004

"Unique source which will fill a gap in dental sources for patients and the lay public. A valuable reference tool even in a library with thousands of books on dentistry. Comprehensive, clear, inexpensive, and easy to read and use. It fills an enormous gap in the health care literature." —Reference & User Services Quarterly, American Library Association, Summer '98

"Recommended reference source." —Booklist, American Library Association, Dec '97

■

Depression Sourcebook

Basic Consumer Health Information about Unipolar Depression, Bipolar Disorder, Postpartum Depression, Seasonal Affective Disorder, and Other Types of Depression in Children, Adolescents, Women, Men, the Elderly, and Other Selected Populations

Along with Facts about Causes, Risk Factors, Diagnostic Criteria, Treatment Options, Coping Strategies, Suicide Prevention, a Glossary, and a Directory of Sources for Additional Help and Information

Edited by Karen Bellenir. 602 pages. 2002. 978-0-7808-0611-5.

"Depression Sourcebook is of a very high standard. Its purpose, which is to serve as a reference source to the lay reader, is very well served." —Journal of the National Medical Association, 2004

"Invaluable reference for public and school library collections alike." —Library Bookwatch, Apr '03

"Recommended for purchase." —American Reference Books Annual, 2003

■

Dermatological Disorders Sourcebook, 2nd Edition

Basic Consumer Health Information about Conditions and Disorders Affecting the Skin, Hair, and Nails, Such as Acne, Rosacea, Rashes, Dermatitis, Pigmentation Disorders, Birthmarks, Skin Cancer, Skin Injuries, Psoriasis, Scleroderma, and Hair Loss, Including Facts about Medications and Treatments for Dermatological Disorders and Tips for Maintaining Healthy Skin, Hair, and Nails

Along with Information about How Aging Affects the Skin, a Glossary of Related Terms, and a Directory of Resources for Additional Help and Information

Edited by Amy L. Sutton. 645 pages. 2005. 978-0-7808-0795-2.

Diabetes Sourcebook, 3rd Edition

Basic Consumer Health Information about Type 1 Diabetes (Insulin-Dependent or Juvenile-Onset Diabetes), Type 2 Diabetes (Noninsulin-Dependent or Adult-Onset Diabetes), Gestational Diabetes, Impaired Glucose Tolerance (IGT), and Related Complications, Such as Amputation, Eye Disease, Gum Disease, Nerve Damage, and End-Stage Renal Disease, Including Facts about Insulin, Oral Diabetes Medications, Blood Sugar Testing, and the Role of Exercise and Nutrition in the Control of Diabetes

Along with a Glossary and Resources for Further Help and Information

Edited by Dawn D. Matthews. 622 pages. 2003. 978-0-7808-0629-0.

"This edition is even more helpful than earlier versions. . . . It is a truly valuable tool for anyone seeking readable and authoritative information on diabetes."
— American Reference Books Annual, 2004

"An invaluable reference." *—Library Journal, May '00*

Selected as one of the 250 "Best Health Sciences Books of 1999." *—Doody's Rating Service, Mar-Apr '00*

"Provides useful information for the general public."
—Healthlines, University of Michigan Health Management Research Center, Sep/Oct '99

". . . provides reliable mainstream medical information . . . belongs on the shelves of any library with a consumer health collection." *—E-Streams, Sep '99*

"Recommended reference source."
—Booklist, American Library Association, Feb '99

Diet & Nutrition Sourcebook, 3rd Edition

Basic Consumer Health Information about Dietary Guidelines and the Food Guidance System, Recommended Daily Nutrient Intakes, Serving Proportions, Weight Control, Vitamins and Supplements, Nutrition Issues for Different Life Stages and Lifestyles, and the Needs of People with Specific Medical Concerns, Including Cancer, Celiac Disease, Diabetes, Eating Disorders, Food Allergies, and Cardiovascular Disease

Along with Facts about Federal Nutrition Support Programs, a Glossary of Nutrition and Dietary Terms, and Directories of Additional Resources for More Information about Nutrition

Edited by Joyce Brennfleck Shannon. 633 pages. 2006. 978-0-7808-0800-3.

"This book is an excellent source of basic diet and nutrition information." *—Booklist Health Sciences Supplement, American Library Association, Dec '00*

"This reference document should be in any public library, but it would be a very good guide for beginning students in the health sciences. If the other books in this publisher's series are as good as this, they should all be in the health sciences collections."
—American Reference Books Annual, 2000

"This book is an excellent general nutrition reference for consumers who desire to take an active role in their health care for prevention. Consumers of all ages who select this book can feel confident they are receiving current and accurate information." *—Journal of Nutrition for the Elderly, Vol. 19, No. 4, 2000*

SEE ALSO Digestive Diseases & Disorders Sourcebook, Eating Disorders Sourcebook, Gastrointestinal Diseases & Disorders Sourcebook, Vegetarian Sourcebook

Digestive Diseases & Disorders Sourcebook

Basic Consumer Health Information about Diseases and Disorders that Impact the Upper and Lower Digestive System, Including Celiac Disease, Constipation, Crohn's Disease, Cyclic Vomiting Syndrome, Diarrhea, Diverticulosis and Diverticulitis, Gallstones, Heartburn, Hemorrhoids, Hernias, Indigestion (Dyspepsia), Irritable Bowel Syndrome, Lactose Intolerance, Ulcers, and More

Along with Information about Medications and Other Treatments, Tips for Maintaining a Healthy Digestive Tract, a Glossary, and Directory of Digestive Diseases Organizations

Edited by Karen Bellenir. 335 pages. 2000. 978-0-7808-0327-5.

"This title would be an excellent addition to all public or patient-research libraries."
—American Reference Books Annual, 2001

"This title is recommended for public, hospital, and health sciences libraries with consumer health collections." *—E-Streams, Jul-Aug '00*

"Recommended reference source."
—Booklist, American Library Association, May '00

SEE ALSO Eating Disorders Sourcebook, Gastrointestinal Diseases & Disorders Sourcebook

Disabilities Sourcebook

Basic Consumer Health Information about Physical and Psychiatric Disabilities, Including Descriptions of Major Causes of Disability, Assistive and Adaptive Aids, Workplace Issues, and Accessibility Concerns

Along with Information about the Americans with Disabilities Act, a Glossary, and Resources for Additional Help and Information

Edited by Dawn D. Matthews. 616 pages. 2000. 978-0-7808-0389-3.

"It is a must for libraries with a consumer health section." *—American Reference Books Annual, 2002*

"A much needed addition to the Omnigraphics *Health Reference Series*. A current reference work to provide people with disabilities, their families, caregivers or those who work with them, a broad range of information in one volume, has not been available until now. . . . It is recommended for all public and academic library reference collections." — *E-Streams, May '01*

"An excellent source book in easy-to-read format covering many current topics; highly recommended for all libraries." — *Choice, Association of College & Research Libraries, Jan '01*

"Recommended reference source."
— *Booklist, American Library Association, Jul '00*

■

Domestic Violence Sourcebook, 2nd Edition

Basic Consumer Health Information about the Causes and Consequences of Abusive Relationships, Including Physical Violence, Sexual Assault, Battery, Stalking, and Emotional Abuse, and Facts about the Effects of Violence on Women, Men, Young Adults, and the Elderly, with Reports about Domestic Violence in Selected Populations, and Featuring Facts about Medical Care, Victim Assistance and Protection, Prevention Strategies, Mental Health Services, and Legal Issues

Along with a Glossary of Related Terms and Resources for Additional Help and Information

Edited by Dawn D. Matthews. 628 pages. 2004. 978-0-7808-0669-6.

"Educators, clergy, medical professionals, police, and victims and their families will benefit from this realistic and easy-to-understand resource."
— *American Reference Books Annual, 2005*

"Recommended for all collections supporting consumer health information. It should also be considered for any collection needing general, readable information on domestic violence." — *E-Streams, Jan '05*

"This sourcebook complements other books in its field, providing a one-stop resource . . . Recommended."
— *Choice, Association of College & Research Libraries, Jan '05*

"Interested lay persons should find the book extremely beneficial. . . . A copy of *Domestic Violence and Child Abuse Sourcebook* should be in every public library in the United States."
— *Social Science & Medicine, No. 56, 2003*

"This is important information. The Web has many resources but this sourcebook fills an important societal need. I am not aware of any other resources of this type." — *Doody's Review Service, Sep '01*

"Recommended reference source."
— *Booklist, American Library Association, Apr '01*

"Important pick for college-level health reference libraries." — *The Bookwatch, Mar '01*

"Because this problem is so widespread and because this book includes a lot of issues within one volume, this work is recommended for all public libraries."
— *American Reference Books Annual, 2001*

SEE ALSO *Child Abuse Sourcebook*

■

Drug Abuse Sourcebook, 2nd Edition

Basic Consumer Health Information about Illicit Substances of Abuse and the Misuse of Prescription and Over-the-Counter Medications, Including Depressants, Hallucinogens, Inhalants, Marijuana, Stimulants, and Anabolic Steroids

Along with Facts about Related Health Risks, Treatment Programs, Prevention Programs, a Glossary of Abuse and Addiction Terms, a Glossary of Drug-Related Street Terms, and a Directory of Resources for More Information

Edited by Catherine Ginther. 607 pages. 2004. 978-0-7808-0740-2.

"Commendable for organizing useful, normally scattered government and association-produced data into a logical sequence."
— *American Reference Books Annual, 2006*

"This easy-to-read volume is recommended for consumer health collections within public or academic libraries." — *E-Streams, Sep '05*

"An excellent library reference."
— *The Bookwatch, May '05*

"Containing a wealth of information, this book will be useful to the college student just beginning to explore the topic of substance abuse. This resource belongs in libraries that serve a lower-division undergraduate or community college clientele as well as the general public." — *Choice, Association of College & Research Libraries, Jun '01*

"Recommended reference source."
— *Booklist, American Library Association, Feb '01*

SEE ALSO *Alcoholism Sourcebook*

■

Ear, Nose & Throat Disorders Sourcebook, 2nd Edition

Basic Consumer Health Information about Disorders of the Ears, Hearing Loss, Vestibular Disorders, Nasal and Sinus Problems, Throat and Vocal Cord Disorders, and Otolaryngologic Cancers, Including Facts about Ear Infections and Injuries, Genetic and Congenital Deafness, Sensorineural Hearing Disorders, Tinnitus, Vertigo, Ménière Disease, Rhinitis, Sinusitis, Snoring, Sore Throats, Hoarseness, and More

Along with Reports on Current Research Initiatives, a Glossary of Related Medical Terms, and a Directory of Sources for Further Help and Information

Edited by Sandra J. Judd. 659 pages. 2006. 978-0-7808-0872-0.

"Overall, this sourcebook is helpful for the consumer seeking information on ENT issues. It is recommended for public libraries."
—*American Reference Books Annual, 1999*

"Recommended reference source."
—*Booklist, American Library Association, Dec '98*

■

Eating Disorders Sourcebook, 2nd Edition

Basic Consumer Health Information about Anorexia Nervosa, Bulimia Nervosa, Binge Eating, Compulsive Exercise, Female Athlete Triad, and Other Eating Disorders, Including Facts about Body Image and Other Cultural and Age-Related Risk Factors, Prevention Efforts, Adverse Health Effects, Treatment Options, and the Recovery Process

Along with Guidelines for Healthy Weight Control, a Glossary, and Directories of Additional Resources

Edited by Joyce Brennfleck Shannon. 585 pages. 2007. 978-0-7808-0948-2.

"Recommended for health science libraries that are open to the public, as well as hospital libraries. This book is a good resource for the consumer who is concerned about eating disorders." —*E-Streams, Mar '02*

"This volume is another convenient collection of excerpted articles. Recommended for school and public library patrons; lower-division undergraduates; and two-year technical program students."
—*Choice, Association of College & Research Libraries, Jan '02*

"Recommended reference source."
—*Booklist, American Library Association, Oct '01*

SEE ALSO *Diet & Nutrition Sourcebook, Digestive Diseases & Disorders Sourcebook, Gastrointestinal Diseases & Disorders Sourcebook*

■

Emergency Medical Services Sourcebook

Basic Consumer Health Information about Preventing, Preparing for, and Managing Emergency Situations, When and Who to Call for Help, What to Expect in the Emergency Room, the Emergency Medical Team, Patient Issues, and Current Topics in Emergency Medicine

Along with Statistical Data, a Glossary, and Sources of Additional Help and Information

Edited by Jenni Lynn Colson. 494 pages. 2002. 978-0-7808-0420-3.

"Handy and convenient for home, public, school, and college libraries. Recommended."
—*Choice, Association of College & Research Libraries, Apr '03*

"This reference can provide the consumer with answers to most questions about emergency care in the United States, or it will direct them to a resource where the answer can be found."
—*American Reference Books Annual, 2003*

"Recommended reference source."
—*Booklist, American Library Association, Feb '03*

■

Endocrine & Metabolic Disorders Sourcebook

Basic Information for the Layperson about Pancreatic and Insulin-Related Disorders Such as Pancreatitis, Diabetes, and Hypoglycemia; Adrenal Gland Disorders Such as Cushing's Syndrome, Addison's Disease, and Congenital Adrenal Hyperplasia; Pituitary Gland Disorders Such as Growth Hormone Deficiency, Acromegaly, and Pituitary Tumors; Thyroid Disorders Such as Hypothyroidism, Graves' Disease, Hashimoto's Disease, and Goiter; Hyperparathyroidism; and Other Diseases and Syndromes of Hormone Imbalance or Metabolic Dysfunction

Along with Reports on Current Research Initiatives

Edited by Linda M. Shin. 574 pages. 1998. 978-0-7808-0207-0.

"Omnigraphics has produced another needed resource for health information consumers."
—*American Reference Books Annual, 2000*

"Recommended reference source."
—*Booklist, American Library Association, Dec '98*

■

Environmental Health Sourcebook, 2nd Edition

Basic Consumer Health Information about the Environment and Its Effect on Human Health, Including the Effects of Air Pollution, Water Pollution, Hazardous Chemicals, Food Hazards, Radiation Hazards, Biological Agents, Household Hazards, Such as Radon, Asbestos, Carbon Monoxide, and Mold, and Information about Associated Diseases and Disorders, Including Cancer, Allergies, Respiratory Problems, and Skin Disorders

Along with Information about Environmental Concerns for Specific Populations, a Glossary of Related Terms, and Resources for Further Help and Information

Edited by Dawn D. Matthews. 673 pages. 2003. 978-0-7808-0632-0.

"This recently updated edition continues the level of quality and the reputation of the numerous other volumes in Omnigraphics' *Health Reference Series*."
—*American Reference Books Annual, 2004*

"An excellent updated edition."
—*The Bookwatch, Oct '03*

"Recommended reference source."
—*Booklist, American Library Association, Sep '98*

"This book will be a useful addition to anyone's library." —*Choice Health Sciences Supplement, Association of College & Research Libraries, May '98*

". . . a good survey of numerous environmentally induced physical disorders . . . a useful addition to anyone's library."
—*Doody's Health Sciences Book Reviews, Jan '98*

Ethnic Diseases Sourcebook

Basic Consumer Health Information for Ethnic and Racial Minority Groups in the United States, Including General Health Indicators and Behaviors, Ethnic Diseases, Genetic Testing, the Impact of Chronic Diseases, Women's Health, Mental Health Issues, and Preventive Health Care Services

Along with a Glossary and a Listing of Additional Resources

Edited by Joyce Brennfleck Shannon. 664 pages. 2001. 978-0-7808-0336-7.

"Recommended for health sciences libraries where public health programs are a priority."
— *E-Streams, Jan '02*

"Not many books have been written on this topic to date, and the *Ethnic Diseases Sourcebook* is a strong addition to the list. It will be an important introductory resource for health consumers, students, health care personnel, and social scientists. It is recommended for public, academic, and large hospital libraries."
— *American Reference Books Annual, 2002*

"Recommended reference source."
— *Booklist, American Library Association, Oct '01*

"Will prove valuable to any library seeking to maintain a current, comprehensive reference collection of health resources. . . . An excellent source of health information about genetic disorders which affect particular ethnic and racial minorities in the U.S."
— *The Bookwatch, Aug '01*

■

Eye Care Sourcebook, 2nd Edition

Basic Consumer Health Information about Eye Care and Eye Disorders, Including Facts about the Diagnosis, Prevention, and Treatment of Common Refractive Problems Such as Myopia, Hyperopia, Astigmatism, and Presbyopia, and Eye Diseases, Including Glaucoma, Cataract, Age-Related Macular Degeneration, and Diabetic Retinopathy

Along with a Section on Vision Correction and Refractive Surgeries, Including LASIK and LASEK, a Glossary, and Directories of Resources for Additional Help and Information

Edited by Amy L. Sutton. 543 pages. 2003. 978-0-7808-0635-1.

". . . a solid reference tool for eye care and a valuable addition to a collection."
— *American Reference Books Annual, 2004*

■

Family Planning Sourcebook

Basic Consumer Health Information about Planning for Pregnancy and Contraception, Including Traditional Methods, Barrier Methods, Hormonal Methods, Permanent Methods, Future Methods, Emergency Contraception, and Birth Control Choices for Women at Each Stage of Life

Along with Statistics, a Glossary, and Sources of Additional Information

Edited by Amy Marcaccio Keyzer. 520 pages. 2001. 978-0-7808-0379-4.

"Recommended for public, health, and undergraduate libraries as part of the circulating collection."
— *E-Streams, Mar '02*

"Information is presented in an unbiased, readable manner, and the sourcebook will certainly be a necessary addition to those public and high school libraries where Internet access is restricted or otherwise problematic." — *American Reference Books Annual, 2002*

"Recommended reference source."
— *Booklist, American Library Association, Oct '01*

"Will prove valuable to any library seeking to maintain a current, comprehensive reference collection of health resources. . . . Excellent reference."
— *The Bookwatch, Aug '01*

SEE ALSO Pregnancy & Birth Sourcebook

■

Fitness & Exercise Sourcebook, 3rd Edition

Basic Consumer Health Information about the Physical and Mental Benefits of Fitness, Including Cardiorespiratory Endurance, Muscular Strength, Muscular Endurance, and Flexibility, with Facts about Sports Nutrition and Exercise-Related Injuries and Tips about Physical Activity and Exercises for People of All Ages and for People with Health Concerns

Along with Advice on Selecting and Using Exercise Equipment, Maintaining Exercise Motivation, a Glossary of Related Terms, and a Directory of Resources for More Help and Information

Edited by Amy L. Sutton. 663 pages. 2007. 978-0-7808-0946-8.

"This work is recommended for all general reference collections."
— *American Reference Books Annual, 2002*

"Highly recommended for public, consumer, and school grades fourth through college." — *E-Streams, Nov '01*

"Recommended reference source."
— *Booklist, American Library Association, Oct '01*

"The information appears quite comprehensive and is considered reliable. . . . This second edition is a welcomed addition to the series."
— *Doody's Review Service, Sep '01*

■

Food Safety Sourcebook

Basic Consumer Health Information about the Safe Handling of Meat, Poultry, Seafood, Eggs, Fruit Juices, and Other Food Items, and Facts about Pesticides, Drinking Water, Food Safety Overseas, and the Onset, Duration, and Symptoms of Foodborne Illnesses, Including Types of Pathogenic Bacteria, Parasitic Protozoa, Worms, Viruses, and Natural Toxins

Along with the Role of the Consumer, the Food Handler, and the Government in Food Safety; a Glossary, and Resources for Additional Help and Information

Edited by Dawn D. Matthews. 339 pages. 1999. 978-0-7808-0326-8.

"This book is recommended for public libraries and universities with home economic and food science programs." — E-Streams, Nov '00

"Recommended reference source."
— Booklist, American Library Association, May '00

"This book takes the complex issues of food safety and foodborne pathogens and presents them in an easily understood manner. [It does] an excellent job of covering a large and often confusing topic."
— American Reference Books Annual, 2000

Forensic Medicine Sourcebook

Basic Consumer Information for the Layperson about Forensic Medicine, Including Crime Scene Investigation, Evidence Collection and Analysis, Expert Testimony, Computer-Aided Criminal Identification, Digital Imaging in the Courtroom, DNA Profiling, Accident Reconstruction, Autopsies, Ballistics, Drugs and Explosives Detection, Latent Fingerprints, Product Tampering, and Questioned Document Examination

Along with Statistical Data, a Glossary of Forensics Terminology, and Listings of Sources for Further Help and Information

Edited by Annemarie S. Muth. 574 pages. 1999. 978-0-7808-0232-2.

"Given the expected widespread interest in its content and its easy to read style, this book is recommended for most public and all college and university libraries."
— E-Streams, Feb '01

"Recommended for public libraries."
— Reference & User Services Quarterly, American Library Association, Spring 2000

"Recommended reference source."
— Booklist, American Library Association, Feb '00

"A wealth of information, useful statistics, references are up-to-date and extremely complete. This wonderful collection of data will help students who are interested in a career in any type of forensic field. It is a great resource for attorneys who need information about types of expert witnesses needed in a particular case. It also offers useful information for fiction and nonfiction writers whose work involves a crime. A fascinating compilation. All levels."
— Choice, Association of College & Research Libraries, Jan '00

"There are several items that make this book attractive to consumers who are seeking certain forensic data. . . . This is a useful current source for those seeking general forensic medical answers."
— American Reference Books Annual, 2000

Gastrointestinal Diseases & Disorders Sourcebook, 2nd Edition

Basic Consumer Health Information about the Upper and Lower Gastrointestinal (GI) Tract, Including the Esophagus, Stomach, Intestines, Rectum, Liver, and Pancreas, with Facts about Gastroesophageal Reflux Disease, Gastritis, Hernias, Ulcers, Celiac Disease, Diverticulitis, Irritable Bowel Syndrome, Hemorrhoids, Gastrointestinal Cancers, and Other Diseases and Disorders Related to the Digestive Process

Along with Information about Commonly Used Diagnostic and Surgical Procedures, Statistics, Reports on Current Research Initiatives and Clinical Trials, a Glossary, and Resources for Additional Help and Information

Edited by Sandra J. Judd. 681 pages. 2006. 978-0-7808-0798-3.

". . . very readable form. The successful editorial work that brought this material together into a useful and understandable reference makes accessible to all readers information that can help them more effectively understand and obtain help for digestive tract problems."
— Choice, Association of College & Research Libraries, Feb '97

SEE ALSO Diet & Nutrition Sourcebook, Digestive Diseases & Disorders Sourcebook, Eating Disorders Sourcebook

---

Genetic Disorders Sourcebook, 3rd Edition

Basic Consumer Health Information about Hereditary Diseases and Disorders, Including Facts about the Human Genome, Genetic Inheritance Patterns, Disorders Associated with Specific Genes, Such as Sickle Cell Disease, Hemophilia, and Cystic Fibrosis, Chromosome Disorders, Such as Down Syndrome, Fragile X Syndrome, and Turner Syndrome, and Complex Diseases and Disorders Resulting from the Interaction of Environmental and Genetic Factors, Such as Allergies, Cancer, and Obesity

Along with Facts about Genetic Testing, Suggestions for Parents of Children with Special Needs, Reports on Current Research Initiatives, a Glossary of Genetic Terminology, and Resources for Additional Help and Information

Edited by Karen Bellenir. 777 pages. 2004. 978-0-7808-0742-6.

"This text is recommended for any library with an interest in providing consumer health resources."
— E-Streams, Aug '05

"This is a valuable resource for anyone wishing to have an understandable description of any of the topics or disorders included. The editor succeeds in making complex genetic issues understandable."
— Doody's Book Review Service, May '05

"A good acquisition for public libraries."
— American Reference Books Annual, 2005

Head Trauma Sourcebook

Basic Information for the Layperson about Open-Head and Closed-Head Injuries, Treatment Advances, Recovery, and Rehabilitation

Along with Reports on Current Research Initiatives

Edited by Karen Bellenir. 414 pages. 1997. 978-0-7808-0208-7.

Headache Sourcebook

Basic Consumer Health Information about Migraine, Tension, Cluster, Rebound and Other Types of Headaches, with Facts about the Cause and Prevention of Headaches, the Effects of Stress and the Environment, Headaches during Pregnancy and Menopause, and Childhood Headaches

Along with a Glossary and Other Resources for Additional Help and Information

Edited by Dawn D. Matthews. 362 pages. 2002. 978-0-7808-0337-4.

"Highly recommended for academic and medical reference collections." — *Library Bookwatch, Sep '02*

Healthy Aging Sourcebook

Basic Consumer Health Information about Maintaining Health through the Aging Process, Including Advice on Nutrition, Exercise, and Sleep, Help in Making Decisions about Midlife Issues and Retirement, and Guidance Concerning Practical and Informed Choices in Health Consumerism

Along with Data Concerning the Theories of Aging, Different Experiences in Aging by Minority Groups, and Facts about Aging Now and Aging in the Future; and Featuring a Glossary, a Guide to Consumer Help, Additional Suggested Reading, and Practical Resource Directory

Edited by Jenifer Swanson. 536 pages. 1999. 978-0-7808-0390-9.

"Recommended reference source."
— *Booklist, American Library Association, Feb '00*

SEE ALSO *Physical & Mental Issues in Aging Sourcebook*

Healthy Children Sourcebook

Basic Consumer Health Information about the Physical and Mental Development of Children between the Ages of 3 and 12, Including Routine Health Care, Preventative Health Services, Safety and First Aid,

Healthy Sleep, Dental Care, Nutrition, and Fitness, and Featuring Parenting Tips on Such Topics as Bedwetting, Choosing Day Care, Monitoring TV and Other Media, and Establishing a Foundation for Substance Abuse Prevention

Along with a Glossary of Commonly Used Pediatric Terms and Resources for Additional Help and Information.

Edited by Chad T. Kimball. 647 pages. 2003. 978-0-7808-0247-6.

"It is hard to imagine that any other single resource exists that would provide such a comprehensive guide of timely information on health promotion and disease prevention for children aged 3 to 12." —*American Reference Books Annual, 2004*

"The strengths of this book are many. It is clearly written, presented and structured."
— *Journal of the National Medical Association, 2004*

SEE ALSO *Childhood Diseases & Disorders Sourcebook*

Healthy Heart Sourcebook for Women

Basic Consumer Health Information about Cardiac Issues Specific to Women, Including Facts about Major Risk Factors and Prevention, Treatment and Control Strategies, and Important Dietary Issues

Along with a Special Section Regarding the Pros and Cons of Hormone Replacement Therapy and Its Impact on Heart Health, and Additional Help, Including Recipes, a Glossary, and a Directory of Resources

Edited by Dawn D. Matthews. 336 pages. 2000. 978-0-7808-0329-9.

"A good reference source and recommended for all public, academic, medical, and hospital libraries."
— *Medical Reference Services Quarterly, Summer '01*

"Because of the lack of information specific to women on this topic, this book is recommended for public libraries and consumer libraries."
—*American Reference Books Annual, 2001*

"Contains very important information about coronary artery disease that all women should know. The information is current and presented in an easy-to-read format. The book will make a good addition to any library." — *American Medical Writers Association Journal, Summer '00*

"Important, basic reference."
— *Reviewer's Bookwatch, Jul '00*

SEE ALSO *Cardiovascular Diseases & Disorders Sourcebook, Women's Health Concerns Sourcebook*

Hepatitis Sourcebook

Basic Consumer Health Information about Hepatitis A, Hepatitis B, Hepatitis C, and Other Forms of Hepatitis, Including Autoimmune Hepatitis, Alcoholic Hepatitis, Nonalcoholic Steatohepatitis, and Toxic Hepatitis, with

Facts about Risk Factors, Screening Methods, Diagnostic Tests, and Treatment Options

Along with Information on Liver Health, Tips for People Living with Chronic Hepatitis, Reports on Current Research Initiatives, a Glossary of Terms Related to Hepatitis, and a Directory of Sources for Further Help and Information

Edited by Sandra J. Judd. 597 pages. 2005. 978-0-7808-0749-5.

"Highly recommended."
— American Reference Books Annual, 2006

Household Safety Sourcebook

Basic Consumer Health Information about Household Safety, Including Information about Poisons, Chemicals, Fire, and Water Hazards in the Home

Along with Advice about the Safe Use of Home Maintenance Equipment, Choosing Toys and Nursery Furniture, Holiday and Recreation Safety, a Glossary, and Resources for Further Help and Information

Edited by Dawn D. Matthews. 606 pages. 2002. 978-0-7808-0338-1.

"This work will be useful in public libraries with large consumer health and wellness departments."
— American Reference Books Annual, 2003

"As a sourcebook on household safety this book meets its mark. It is encyclopedic in scope and covers a wide range of safety issues that are commonly seen in the home." — E-Streams, Jul '02

Hypertension Sourcebook

Basic Consumer Health Information about the Causes, Diagnosis, and Treatment of High Blood Pressure, with Facts about Consequences, Complications, and Co-Occurring Disorders, Such as Coronary Heart Disease, Diabetes, Stroke, Kidney Disease, and Hypertensive Retinopathy, and Issues in Blood Pressure Control, Including Dietary Choices, Stress Management, and Medications

Along with Reports on Current Research Initiatives and Clinical Trials, a Glossary, and Resources for Additional Help and Information

Edited by Dawn D. Matthews and Karen Bellenir. 613 pages. 2004. 978-0-7808-0674-0.

"Academic, public, and medical libraries will want to add the Hypertension Sourcebook to their collections."
— E-Streams, Aug '05

"The strength of this source is the wide range of information given about hypertension."
— American Reference Books Annual, 2005

Immune System Disorders Sourcebook, 2nd Edition

Basic Consumer Health Information about Disorders of the Immune System, Including Immune System Function and Response, Diagnosis of Immune Disorders, Information about Inherited Immune Disease, Acquired Immune Disease, and Autoimmune Diseases, Including Primary Immune Deficiency, Acquired Immunodeficiency Syndrome (AIDS), Lupus, Multiple Sclerosis, Type 1 Diabetes, Rheumatoid Arthritis, and Graves' Disease

Along with Treatments, Tips for Coping with Immune Disorders, a Glossary, and a Directory of Additional Resources.

Edited by Joyce Brennfleck Shannon. 671 pages. 2005. 978-0-7808-0748-8.

"Highly recommended for academic and public libraries." — American Reference Books Annual, 2006

"The updated second edition is a 'must' for any consumer health library seeking a solid resource covering the treatments, symptoms, and options for immune disorder sufferers. . . . An excellent guide."
— MBR Bookwatch, Jan '06

Infant & Toddler Health Sourcebook

Basic Consumer Health Information about the Physical and Mental Development of Newborns, Infants, and Toddlers, Including Neonatal Concerns, Nutrition Recommendations, Immunization Schedules, Common Pediatric Disorders, Assessments and Milestones, Safety Tips, and Advice for Parents and Other Caregivers

Along with a Glossary of Terms and Resource Listings for Additional Help

Edited by Jenifer Swanson. 585 pages. 2000. 978-0-7808-0246-9.

"As a reference for the general public, this would be useful in any library." — E-Streams, May '01

"Recommended reference source."
— Booklist, American Library Association, Feb '01

"This is a good source for general use."
— American Reference Books Annual, 2001

Infectious Diseases Sourcebook

Basic Consumer Health Information about Non-Contagious Bacterial, Viral, Prion, Fungal, and Parasitic Diseases Spread by Food and Water, Insects and Animals, or Environmental Contact, Including Botulism, E. Coli, Encephalitis, Legionnaires' Disease, Lyme Disease, Malaria, Plague, Rabies, Salmonella, Tetanus, and Others, and Facts about Newly Emerging Diseases, Such as Hantavirus, Mad Cow Disease, Monkeypox, and West Nile Virus

Along with Information about Preventing Disease Transmission, the Threat of Bioterrorism, and Current Research Initiatives, with a Glossary and Directory of Resources for More Information

Edited by Karen Bellenir. 634 pages. 2004. 978-0-7808-0675-7.

"This reference continues the excellent tradition of the *Health Reference Series* in consolidating a wealth of information on a selected topic into a format that is easy to use and accessible to the general public."
— *American Reference Books Annual, 2005*

"Recommended for public and academic libraries."
— *E-Streams, Jan '05*

■

Injury & Trauma Sourcebook

Basic Consumer Health Information about the Impact of Injury, the Diagnosis and Treatment of Common and Traumatic Injuries, Emergency Care, and Specific Injuries Related to Home, Community, Workplace, Transportation, and Recreation

Along with Guidelines for Injury Prevention, a Glossary, and a Directory of Additional Resources

Edited by Joyce Brennfleck Shannon. 696 pages. 2002. 978-0-7808-0421-0.

"This publication is the most comprehensive work of its kind about injury and trauma."
— *American Reference Books Annual, 2003*

"This sourcebook provides concise, easily readable, basic health information about injuries. . . . This book is well organized and an easy to use reference resource suitable for hospital, health sciences and public libraries with consumer health collections."
— *E-Streams, Nov '02*

"Practitioners should be aware of guides such as this in order to facilitate their use by patients and their families."
— *Doody's Health Sciences Book Review Journal, Sep-Oct '02*

"Recommended reference source."
— *Booklist, American Library Association, Sep '02*

"Highly recommended for academic and medical reference collections."
— *Library Bookwatch, Sep '02*

■

Kidney & Urinary Tract Diseases & Disorders Sourcebook

SEE *Urinary Tract & Kidney Diseases & Disorders Sourcebook*

■

Learning Disabilities Sourcebook, 2nd Edition

Basic Consumer Health Information about Learning Disabilities, Including Dyslexia, Developmental Speech and Language Disabilities, Non-Verbal Learning Disorders, Developmental Arithmetic Disorder, Developmental Writing Disorder, and Other Conditions That Impede Learning Such as Attention Deficit/Hyperactivity Disorder, Brain Injury, Hearing Impairment, Klinefelter Syndrome, Dyspraxia, and Tourette's Syndrome

Along with Facts about Educational Issues and Assistive Technology, Coping Strategies, a Glossary of Related Terms, and Resources for Further Help and Information

Edited by Dawn D. Matthews. 621 pages. 2003. 978-0-7808-0626-9.

"The second edition of Learning Disabilities Sourcebook far surpasses the earlier edition in that it is more focused on information that will be useful as a consumer health resource."
— *American Reference Books Annual, 2004*

"Teachers as well as consumers will find this an essential guide to understanding various syndromes and their latest treatments. [An] invaluable reference for public and school library collections alike."
— *Library Bookwatch, Apr '03*

Named "Outstanding Reference Book of 1999."
— *New York Public Library, Feb '00*

"An excellent candidate for inclusion in a public library reference section. It's a great source of information. Teachers will also find the book useful. Definitely worth reading."
— *Journal of Adolescent & Adult Literacy, Feb 2000*

"Readable . . . provides a solid base of information regarding successful techniques used with individuals who have learning disabilities, as well as practical suggestions for educators and family members. Clear language, concise descriptions, and pertinent information for contacting multiple resources add to the strength of this book as a useful tool."
— *Choice, Association of College & Research Libraries, Feb '99*

"Recommended reference source."
— *Booklist, American Library Association, Sep '98*

"A useful resource for libraries and for those who don't have the time to identify and locate the individual publications."
— *Disability Resources Monthly, Sep '98*

■

Leukemia Sourcebook

Basic Consumer Health Information about Adult and Childhood Leukemias, Including Acute Lymphocytic Leukemia (ALL), Chronic Lymphocytic Leukemia (CLL), Acute Myelogenous Leukemia (AML), Chronic Myelogenous Leukemia (CML), and Hairy Cell Leukemia, and Treatments Such as Chemotherapy, Radiation Therapy, Peripheral Blood Stem Cell and Marrow Transplantation, and Immunotherapy

Along with Tips for Life During and After Treatment, a Glossary, and Directories of Additional Resources

Edited by Joyce Brennfleck Shannon. 587 pages. 2003. 978-0-7808-0627-6.

"Unlike other medical books for the layperson, . . . the language does not talk down to the reader. . . . This volume is highly recommended for all libraries."
— *American Reference Books Annual, 2004*

". . . a fine title which ranges from diagnosis to alternative treatments, staging, and tips for life during and after diagnosis."
— *The Bookwatch, Dec '03*

Liver Disorders Sourcebook

Basic Consumer Health Information about the Liver and How It Works; Liver Diseases, Including Cancer, Cirrhosis, Hepatitis, and Toxic and Drug Related Diseases; Tips for Maintaining a Healthy Liver; Laboratory Tests, Radiology Tests, and Facts about Liver Transplantation

Along with a Section on Support Groups, a Glossary, and Resource Listings

Edited by Joyce Brennfleck Shannon. 591 pages. 2000. 978-0-7808-0383-1.

"A valuable resource."
— *American Reference Books Annual, 2001*

"This title is recommended for health sciences and public libraries with consumer health collections."
— *E-Streams, Oct '00*

"Recommended reference source."
— *Booklist, American Library Association, Jun '00*

■

Lung Disorders Sourcebook

Basic Consumer Health Information about Emphysema, Pneumonia, Tuberculosis, Asthma, Cystic Fibrosis, and Other Lung Disorders, Including Facts about Diagnostic Procedures, Treatment Strategies, Disease Prevention Efforts, and Such Risk Factors as Smoking, Air Pollution, and Exposure to Asbestos, Radon, and Other Agents

Along with a Glossary and Resources for Additional Help and Information

Edited by Dawn D. Matthews. 678 pages. 2002. 978-0-7808-0339-8.

"This title is a great addition for public and school libraries because it provides concise health information on the lungs."
— *American Reference Books Annual, 2003*

"Highly recommended for academic and medical reference collections." — *Library Bookwatch, Sep '02*

SEE ALSO *Respiratory Diseases & Disorders Sourcebook*

■

Medical Tests Sourcebook, 2nd Edition

Basic Consumer Health Information about Medical Tests, Including Age-Specific Health Tests, Important Health Screenings and Exams, Home-Use Tests, Blood and Specimen Tests, Electrical Tests, Scope Tests, Genetic Testing, and Imaging Tests, Such as X-Rays, Ultrasound, Computed Tomography, Magnetic Resonance Imaging, Angiography, and Nuclear Medicine

Along with a Glossary and Directory of Additional Resources

Edited by Joyce Brennfleck Shannon. 654 pages. 2004. 978-0-7808-0670-2.

"Recommended for hospital and health sciences libraries with consumer health collections."
— *E-Streams, Mar '00*

"This is an overall excellent reference with a wealth of general knowledge that may aid those who are reluctant to get vital tests performed."
— *Today's Librarian, Jan '00*

"A valuable reference guide."
— *American Reference Books Annual, 2000*

■

Men's Health Concerns Sourcebook, 2nd Edition

Basic Consumer Health Information about the Medical and Mental Concerns of Men, Including Theories about the Shorter Male Lifespan, the Leading Causes of Death and Disability, Physical Concerns of Special Significance to Men, Reproductive and Sexual Concerns, Sexually Transmitted Diseases, Men's Mental and Emotional Health, and Lifestyle Choices That Affect Wellness, Such as Nutrition, Fitness, and Substance Use

Along with a Glossary of Related Terms and a Directory of Organizational Resources in Men's Health

Edited by Robert Aquinas McNally. 644 pages. 2004. 978-0-7808-0671-9.

"A very accessible reference for non-specialist general readers and consumers." — *The Bookwatch, Jun '04*

"This comprehensive resource and the series are highly recommended."
— *American Reference Books Annual, 2000*

"Recommended reference source."
— *Booklist, American Library Association, Dec '98*

■

Mental Health Disorders Sourcebook, 3rd Edition

Basic Consumer Health Information about Mental and Emotional Health and Mental Illness, Including Facts about Depression, Bipolar Disorder, and Other Mood Disorders, Phobias, Post-Traumatic Stress Disorder (PTSD), Obsessive-Compulsive Disorder, and Other Anxiety Disorders, Impulse Control Disorders, Eating Disorders, Personality Disorders, and Psychotic Disorders, Including Schizophrenia and Dissociative Disorders

Along with Statistical Information, a Special Section Concerning Mental Health Issues in Children and Adolescents, a Glossary, and Directories of Resources for Additional Help and Information

Edited by Karen Bellenir. 661 pages. 2005. 978-0-7808-0747-1.

"Recommended for public libraries and academic libraries with an undergraduate program in psychology."
— *American Reference Books Annual, 2006*

"Recommended reference source."
— *Booklist, American Library Association, Jun '00*

Mental Retardation Sourcebook

Basic Consumer Health Information about Mental Retardation and Its Causes, Including Down Syndrome, Fetal Alcohol Syndrome, Fragile X Syndrome, Genetic Conditions, Injury, and Environmental Sources

Along with Preventive Strategies, Parenting Issues, Educational Implications, Health Care Needs, Employment and Economic Matters, Legal Issues, a Glossary, and a Resource Listing for Additional Help and Information

Edited by Joyce Brennfleck Shannon. 642 pages. 2000. 978-0-7808-0377-0.

"Public libraries will find the book useful for reference and as a beginning research point for students, parents, and caregivers."
— American Reference Books Annual, 2001

"The strength of this work is that it compiles many basic fact sheets and addresses for further information in one volume. It is intended and suitable for the general public. This sourcebook is relevant to any collection providing health information to the general public."
— E-Streams, Nov '00

"From preventing retardation to parenting and family challenges, this covers health, social and legal issues and will prove an invaluable overview."
— Reviewer's Bookwatch, Jul '00

Movement Disorders Sourcebook

Basic Consumer Health Information about Neurological Movement Disorders, Including Essential Tremor, Parkinson's Disease, Dystonia, Cerebral Palsy, Huntington's Disease, Myasthenia Gravis, Multiple Sclerosis, and Other Early-Onset and Adult-Onset Movement Disorders, Their Symptoms and Causes, Diagnostic Tests, and Treatments

Along with Mobility and Assistive Technology Information, a Glossary, and a Directory of Additional Resources

Edited by Joyce Brennfleck Shannon. 655 pages. 2003. 978-0-7808-0628-3.

". . . a good resource for consumers and recommended for public, community college and undergraduate libraries." *— American Reference Books Annual, 2004*

Muscular Dystrophy Sourcebook

Basic Consumer Health Information about Congenital, Childhood-Onset, and Adult-Onset Forms of Muscular Dystrophy, Such as Duchenne, Becker, Emery-Dreifuss, Distal, Limb-Girdle, Facioscapulohumeral (FSHD), Myotonic, and Ophthalmoplegic Muscular Dystrophies, Including Facts about Diagnostic Tests, Medical and Physical Therapies, Management of Co-Occurring Conditions, and Parenting Guidelines

Along with Practical Tips for Home Care, a Glossary, and Directories of Additional Resources

Edited by Joyce Brennfleck Shannon. 577 pages. 2004. 978-0-7808-0676-4.

"This book is highly recommended for public and academic libraries as well as health care offices that support the information needs of patients and their families."
— E-Streams, Apr '05

"Excellent reference." *— The Bookwatch, Jan '05*

Obesity Sourcebook

Basic Consumer Health Information about Diseases and Other Problems Associated with Obesity, and Including Facts about Risk Factors, Prevention Issues, and Management Approaches

Along with Statistical and Demographic Data, Information about Special Populations, Research Updates, a Glossary, and Source Listings for Further Help and Information

Edited by Wilma Caldwell and Chad T. Kimball. 376 pages. 2001. 978-0-7808-0333-6.

"The book synthesizes the reliable medical literature on obesity into one easy-to-read and useful resource for the general public."
— American Reference Books Annual, 2002

"This is a very useful resource book for the lay public."
— Doody's Review Service, Nov '01

"Well suited for the health reference collection of a public library or an academic health science library that serves the general population." *— E-Streams, Sep '01*

"Recommended reference source."
— Booklist, American Library Association, Apr '01

"Recommended pick both for specialty health library collections and any general consumer health reference collection." *— The Bookwatch, Apr '01*

Oral Health Sourcebook

SEE Dental Care & Oral Health Sourcebook

Osteoporosis Sourcebook

Basic Consumer Health Information about Primary and Secondary Osteoporosis and Juvenile Osteoporosis and Related Conditions, Including Fibrous Dysplasia, Gaucher Disease, Hyperthyroidism, Hypophosphatasia, Myeloma, Osteopetrosis, Osteogenesis Imperfecta, and Paget's Disease

Along with Information about Risk Factors, Treatments, Traditional and Non-Traditional Pain Management, a Glossary of Related Terms, and a Directory of Resources

Edited by Allan R. Cook. 584 pages. 2001. 978-0-7808-0239-1.

"This would be a book to be kept in a staff or patient library. The targeted audience is the layperson, but the therapist who needs a quick bit of information on a particular topic will also find the book useful."
— Physical Therapy, Jan '02

"This resource is recommended as a great reference source for public, health, and academic libraries, and is another triumph for the editors of Omnigraphics."
— *American Reference Books Annual, 2002*

"Recommended for all public libraries and general health collections, especially those supporting patient education or consumer health programs."
— *E-Streams, Nov '01*

"Will prove valuable to any library seeking to maintain a current, comprehensive reference collection of health resources. . . . From prevention to treatment and associated conditions, this provides an excellent survey."
— *The Bookwatch, Aug '01*

"Recommended reference source."
— *Booklist, American Library Association, Jul '01*

SEE ALSO *Healthy Aging Sourcebook, Physical & Mental Issues in Aging Sourcebook, Women's Health Concerns Sourcebook*

Pain Sourcebook, 2nd Edition

Basic Consumer Health Information about Specific Forms of Acute and Chronic Pain, Including Muscle and Skeletal Pain, Nerve Pain, Cancer Pain, and Disorders Characterized by Pain, Such as Fibromyalgia, Shingles, Angina, Arthritis, and Headaches

Along with Information about Pain Medications and Management Techniques, Complementary and Alternative Pain Relief Options, Tips for People Living with Chronic Pain, a Glossary, and a Directory of Sources for Further Information

Edited by Karen Bellenir. 670 pages. 2002. 978-0-7808-0612-2.

"A source of valuable information. . . . This book offers help to nonmedical people who need information about pain and pain management. It is also an excellent reference for those who participate in patient education."
— *Doody's Review Service, Sep '02*

"Highly recommended for academic and medical reference collections."
— *Library Bookwatch, Sep '02*

"The text is readable, easily understood, and well indexed. This excellent volume belongs in all patient education libraries, consumer health sections of public libraries, and many personal collections."
— *American Reference Books Annual, 1999*

"The information is basic in terms of scholarship and is appropriate for general readers. Written in journalistic style . . . intended for non-professionals. Quite thorough in its coverage of different pain conditions and summarizes the latest clinical information regarding pain treatment."
— *Choice, Association of College and Research Libraries, Jun '98*

"Recommended reference source."
— *Booklist, American Library Association, Mar '98*

Pediatric Cancer Sourcebook

Basic Consumer Health Information about Leukemias, Brain Tumors, Sarcomas, Lymphomas, and Other Cancers in Infants, Children, and Adolescents, Including Descriptions of Cancers, Treatments, and Coping Strategies

Along with Suggestions for Parents, Caregivers, and Concerned Relatives, a Glossary of Cancer Terms, and Resource Listings

Edited by Edward J. Prucha. 587 pages. 1999. 978-0-7808-0245-2.

"An excellent source of information. Recommended for public, hospital, and health science libraries with consumer health collections."
— *E-Streams, Jun '00*

"Recommended reference source."
— *Booklist, American Library Association, Feb '00*

"A valuable addition to all libraries specializing in health services and many public libraries."
— *American Reference Books Annual, 2000*

SEE ALSO *Childhood Diseases & Disorders Sourcebook, Healthy Children Sourcebook*

Physical & Mental Issues in Aging Sourcebook

Basic Consumer Health Information on Physical and Mental Disorders Associated with the Aging Process, Including Concerns about Cardiovascular Disease, Pulmonary Disease, Oral Health, Digestive Disorders, Musculoskeletal and Skin Disorders, Metabolic Changes, Sexual and Reproductive Issues, and Changes in Vision, Hearing, and Other Senses

Along with Data about Longevity and Causes of Death, Information on Acute and Chronic Pain, Descriptions of Mental Concerns, a Glossary of Terms, and Resource Listings for Additional Help

Edited by Jenifer Swanson. 660 pages. 1999. 978-0-7808-0233-9.

"This is a treasure of health information for the layperson."
— *Choice Health Sciences Supplement, Association of College & Research Libraries, May '00*

"Recommended for public libraries."
— *American Reference Books Annual, 2000*

"Recommended reference source."
— *Booklist, American Library Association, Oct '99*

SEE ALSO *Healthy Aging Sourcebook*

Podiatry Sourcebook, 2nd Edition

Basic Consumer Health Information about Disorders, Diseases, Deformities, and Injuries that Affect the Foot and Ankle, Including Sprains, Corns, Calluses, Bunions, Plantar Warts, Plantar Fasciitis, Neuromas, Clubfoot, Flat Feet, Achilles Tendonitis, and Much More

Along with Information about Selecting a Foot Care Specialist, Foot Fitness, Shoes and Socks, Diagnostic Tests and Corrective Procedures, Financial Assistance for Corrective Devices, a Glossary of Related Terms, and a Directory of Resources for Additional Help and Information

Edited by Ivy L. Alexander. 543 pages. 2007. 978-0-7808-0944-4.

"Recommended reference source."
— *Booklist, American Library Association, Feb '02*

"There is a lot of information presented here on a topic that is usually only covered sparingly in most larger comprehensive medical encyclopedias."
— *American Reference Books Annual, 2002*

■

Pregnancy & Birth Sourcebook, 2nd Edition

Basic Consumer Health Information about Conception and Pregnancy, Including Facts about Fertility, Infertility, Pregnancy Symptoms and Complications, Fetal Growth and Development, Labor, Delivery, and the Postpartum Period, as Well as Information about Maintaining Health and Wellness during Pregnancy and Caring for a Newborn

Along with Information about Public Health Assistance for Low-Income Pregnant Women, a Glossary, and Directories of Agencies and Organizations Providing Help and Support

Edited by Amy L. Sutton. 626 pages. 2004. 978-0-7808-0672-6.

"Will appeal to public and school reference collections strong in medicine and women's health. . . . Deserves a spot on any medical reference shelf."
— *The Bookwatch, Jul '04*

"A well-organized handbook. Recommended."
— *Choice, Association of College & Research Libraries, Apr '98*

"Recommended reference source."
— *Booklist, American Library Association, Mar '98*

"Recommended for public libraries."
— *American Reference Books Annual, 1998*

SEE ALSO Breastfeeding Sourcebook, Congenital Disorders Sourcebook, Family Planning Sourcebook

■

Prostate & Urological Disorders Sourcebook

Basic Consumer Health Information about Urogenital and Sexual Disorders in Men, Including Prostate and Other Andrological Cancers, Prostatitis, Benign Prostatic Hyperplasia, Testicular and Penile Trauma, Cryptorchidism, Peyronie Disease, Erectile Dysfunction, and Male Factor Infertility, and Facts about Commonly Used Tests and Procedures, Such as Prostatectomy, Vasectomy, Vasectomy Reversal, Penile Implants, and Semen Analysis

Along with a Glossary of Andrological Terms and a Directory of Resources for Additional Information

Edited by Karen Bellenir. 631 pages. 2005. 978-0-7808-0797-6.

Prostate Cancer Sourcebook

Basic Consumer Health Information about Prostate Cancer, Including Information about the Associated Risk Factors, Detection, Diagnosis, and Treatment of Prostate Cancer

Along with Information on Non-Malignant Prostate Conditions, and Featuring a Section Listing Support and Treatment Centers and a Glossary of Related Terms

Edited by Dawn D. Matthews. 358 pages. 2001. 978-0-7808-0324-4.

"Recommended reference source."
— *Booklist, American Library Association, Jan '02*

"A valuable resource for health care consumers seeking information on the subject. . . . All text is written in a clear, easy-to-understand language that avoids technical jargon. Any library that collects consumer health resources would strengthen their collection with the addition of the *Prostate Cancer Sourcebook*."
— *American Reference Books Annual, 2002*

SEE ALSO Men's Health Concerns Sourcebook

■

Reconstructive & Cosmetic Surgery Sourcebook

Basic Consumer Health Information on Cosmetic and Reconstructive Plastic Surgery, Including Statistical Information about Different Surgical Procedures, Things to Consider Prior to Surgery, Plastic Surgery Techniques and Tools, Emotional and Psychological Considerations, and Procedure-Specific Information

Along with a Glossary of Terms and a Listing of Resources for Additional Help and Information

Edited by M. Lisa Weatherford. 374 pages. 2001. 978-0-7808-0214-8.

"An excellent reference that addresses cosmetic and medically necessary reconstructive surgeries. . . . The style of the prose is calm and reassuring, discussing the many positive outcomes now available due to advances in surgical techniques."
— *American Reference Books Annual, 2002*

"Recommended for health science libraries that are open to the public, as well as hospital libraries that are open to the patients. This book is a good resource for the consumer interested in plastic surgery."
— *E-Streams, Dec '01*

"Recommended reference source."
— *Booklist, American Library Association, Jul '01*

■

Rehabilitation Sourcebook

Basic Consumer Health Information about Rehabilitation for People Recovering from Heart Surgery, Spinal Cord Injury, Stroke, Orthopedic Impairments, Amputation, Pulmonary Impairments, Traumatic Injury, and More, Including Physical Therapy, Occupational Therapy, Speech/Language Therapy, Massage Therapy, Dance Therapy, Art Therapy, and Recreational Therapy

Along with Information on Assistive and Adaptive Devices, a Glossary, and Resources for Additional Help and Information

Edited by Dawn D. Matthews. 531 pages. 1999. 978-0-7808-0236-0.

"This is an excellent resource for public library reference and health collections."
— American Reference Books Annual, 2001

"Recommended reference source."
— Booklist, American Library Association, May '00

■

Respiratory Diseases & Disorders Sourcebook

Basic Information about Respiratory Diseases and Disorders, Including Asthma, Cystic Fibrosis, Pneumonia, the Common Cold, Influenza, and Others, Featuring Facts about the Respiratory System, Statistical and Demographic Data, Treatments, Self-Help Management Suggestions, and Current Research Initiatives

Edited by Allan R. Cook and Peter D. Dresser. 771 pages. 1995. 978-0-7808-0037-3.

"Designed for the layperson and for patients and their families coping with respiratory illness. . . . an extensive array of information on diagnosis, treatment, management, and prevention of respiratory illnesses for the general reader."   — Choice, Association of College & Research Libraries, Jun '96

"A highly recommended text for all collections. It is a comforting reminder of the power of knowledge that good books carry between their covers."
— Academic Library Book Review, Spring '96

"A comprehensive collection of authoritative information presented in a nontechnical, humanitarian style for patients, families, and caregivers."
— Association of Operating Room Nurses, Sep/Oct '95

SEE ALSO Lung Disorders Sourcebook

■

Sexually Transmitted Diseases Sourcebook, 3rd Edition

Basic Consumer Health Information about Chlamydial Infections, Gonorrhea, Hepatitis, Herpes, HIV/AIDS, Human Papillomavirus, Pubic Lice, Scabies, Syphilis, Trichomoniasis, Vaginal Infections, and Other Sexually Transmitted Diseases, Including Facts about Risk Factors, Symptoms, Diagnosis, Treatment, and the Prevention of Sexually Transmitted Infections

Along with Updates on Current Research Initiatives, a Glossary of Related Terms, and Resources for Additional Help and Information

Edited by Amy L. Sutton. 629 pages. 2006. 978-0-7808-0824-9.

"Recommended for consumer health collections in public libraries, and secondary school and community college libraries."
— American Reference Books Annual, 2002

"Every school and public library should have a copy of this comprehensive and user-friendly reference book."
— Choice, Association of College & Research Libraries, Sep '01

"This is a highly recommended book. This is an especially important book for all school and public libraries."
— AIDS Book Review Journal, Jul-Aug '01

"Recommended reference source."
— Booklist, American Library Association, Apr '01

■

Sleep Disorders Sourcebook, 2nd Edition

Basic Consumer Health Information about Sleep and Sleep Disorders, Including Insomnia, Sleep Apnea, Restless Legs Syndrome, Narcolepsy, Parasomnias, and Other Health Problems That Affect Sleep, Plus Facts about Diagnostic Procedures, Treatment Strategies, Sleep Medications, and Tips for Improving Sleep Quality

Along with a Glossary of Related Terms and Resources for Additional Help and Information

Edited by Amy L. Sutton. 567 pages. 2005. 978-0-7808-0743-3.

"This book will be useful for just about everybody, especially the 40 million Americans with sleep disorders."
— American Reference Books Annual, 2006

"Recommended for public libraries and libraries supporting health care professionals." — E-Streams, Sep '05

". . . key medical library acquisition."
— The Bookwatch, Jun '05

■

Smoking Concerns Sourcebook

Basic Consumer Health Information about Nicotine Addiction and Smoking Cessation, Featuring Facts about the Health Effects of Tobacco Use, Including Lung and Other Cancers, Heart Disease, Stroke, and Respiratory Disorders, Such as Emphysema and Chronic Bronchitis

Along with Information about Smoking Prevention Programs, Suggestions for Achieving and Maintaining a Smoke-Free Lifestyle, Statistics about Tobacco Use, Reports on Current Research Initiatives, a Glossary of Related Terms, and Directories of Resources for Additional Help and Information

Edited by Karen Bellenir. 621 pages. 2004. 978-0-7808-0323-7.

"Provides everything needed for the student or general reader seeking practical details on the effects of tobacco use."   — The Bookwatch, Mar '05

"Public libraries and consumer health care libraries will find this work useful."
— American Reference Books Annual, 2005

Sports Injuries Sourcebook, 3rd Edition

Basic Consumer Health Information about Sprains and Strains, Fractures, Growth Plate Injuries, Overtraining Injuries, and Injuries to the Head, Face, Shoulders, Elbows, Hands, Spinal Column, Knees, Ankles, and Feet, and with Facts about Heat-Related Illness, Steroids and Sport Supplements, Protective Equipment, Diagnostic Procedures, Treatment Options, and Rehabilitation

Along with a Glossary of Related Terms and a Directory of Resources for Additional Help and Information

Edited by Sandra J. Judd. 651 pages. 2007. 978-0-7808-0949-9.

"This is an excellent reference for consumers and it is recommended for public, community college, and undergraduate libraries."
— *American Reference Books Annual, 2003*

"Recommended reference source."
— *Booklist, American Library Association, Feb '03*

Stress-Related Disorders Sourcebook

Basic Consumer Health Information about Stress and Stress-Related Disorders, Including Stress Origins and Signals, Environmental Stress at Work and Home, Mental and Emotional Stress Associated with Depression, Post-Traumatic Stress Disorder, Panic Disorder, Suicide, and the Physical Effects of Stress on the Cardiovascular, Immune, and Nervous Systems

Along with Stress Management Techniques, a Glossary, and a Listing of Additional Resources

Edited by Joyce Brennfleck Shannon. 610 pages. 2002. 978-0-7808-0560-6.

"Well written for a general readership, the *Stress-Related Disorders Sourcebook* is a useful addition to the health reference literature."
— *American Reference Books Annual, 2003*

"I am impressed by the amount of information. It offers a thorough overview of the causes and consequences of stress for the layperson. . . . A well-done and thorough reference guide for professionals and nonprofessionals alike." — *Doody's Review Service, Dec '02*

Stroke Sourcebook

Basic Consumer Health Information about Stroke, Including Ischemic, Hemorrhagic, Transient Ischemic Attack (TIA), and Pediatric Stroke, Stroke Triggers and Risks, Diagnostic Tests, Treatments, and Rehabilitation Information

Along with Stroke Prevention Guidelines, Legal and Financial Information, a Glossary, and a Directory of Additional Resources

Edited by Joyce Brennfleck Shannon. 606 pages. 2003. 978-0-7808-0630-6.

"This volume is highly recommended and should be in every medical, hospital, and public library."
— *American Reference Books Annual, 2004*

"Highly recommended for the amount and variety of topics and information covered." — *Choice, Nov '03*

Surgery Sourcebook

Basic Consumer Health Information about Inpatient and Outpatient Surgeries, Including Cardiac, Vascular, Orthopedic, Ocular, Reconstructive, Cosmetic, Gynecologic, and Ear, Nose, and Throat Procedures and More

Along with Information about Operating Room Policies and Instruments, Laser Surgery Techniques, Hospital Errors, Statistical Data, a Glossary, and Listings of Sources for Further Help and Information

Edited by Annemarie S. Muth and Karen Bellenir. 596 pages. 2002. 978-0-7808-0380-0.

"Large public libraries and medical libraries would benefit from this material in their reference collections."
— *American Reference Books Annual, 2004*

"Invaluable reference for public and school library collections alike." — *Library Bookwatch, Apr '03*

Thyroid Disorders Sourcebook

Basic Consumer Health Information about Disorders of the Thyroid and Parathyroid Glands, Including Hypothyroidism, Hyperthyroidism, Graves Disease, Hashimoto Thyroiditis, Thyroid Cancer, and Parathyroid Disorders, Featuring Facts about Symptoms, Risk Factors, Tests, and Treatments

Along with Information about the Effects of Thyroid Imbalance on Other Body Systems, Environmental Factors That Affect the Thyroid Gland, a Glossary, and a Directory of Additional Resources

Edited by Joyce Brennfleck Shannon. 599 pages. 2005. 978-0-7808-0745-7.

"Recommended for consumer health collections."
— *American Reference Books Annual, 2006*

"Highly recommended pick for basic consumer health reference holdings at all levels."
— *The Bookwatch, Aug '05*

Transplantation Sourcebook

Basic Consumer Health Information about Organ and Tissue Transplantation, Including Physical and Financial Preparations, Procedures and Issues Relating to Specific Solid Organ and Tissue Transplants, Rehabilitation, Pediatric Transplant Information, the Future of Transplantation, and Organ and Tissue Donation

Along with a Glossary and Listings of Additional Resources

Edited by Joyce Brennfleck Shannon. 628 pages. 2002. 978-0-7808-0322-0.

"Along with these advances [in transplantation technology] have come a number of daunting questions for potential transplant patients, their families, and their health care providers. This reference text is the best single tool to address many of these questions. . . . It will be a much-needed addition to the reference collections in health care, academic, and large public libraries."
— *American Reference Books Annual, 2003*

"Recommended for libraries with an interest in offering consumer health information." — *E-Streams, Jul '02*

"This is a unique and valuable resource for patients facing transplantation and their families."
— *Doody's Review Service, Jun '02*

■

Traveler's Health Sourcebook

Basic Consumer Health Information for Travelers, Including Physical and Medical Preparations, Transportation Health and Safety, Essential Information about Food and Water, Sun Exposure, Insect and Snake Bites, Camping and Wilderness Medicine, and Travel with Physical or Medical Disabilities

Along with International Travel Tips, Vaccination Recommendations, Geographical Health Issues, Disease Risks, a Glossary, and a Listing of Additional Resources

Edited by Joyce Brennfleck Shannon. 613 pages. 2000. 978-0-7808-0384-8.

"Recommended reference source."
— *Booklist, American Library Association, Feb '01*

"This book is recommended for any public library, any travel collection, and especially any collection for the physically disabled."
— *American Reference Books Annual, 2001*

SEE ALSO *Worldwide Health Sourcebook*

■

Urinary Tract & Kidney Diseases & Disorders Sourcebook, 2nd Edition

Basic Consumer Health Information about the Urinary System, Including the Bladder, Urethra, Ureters, and Kidneys, with Facts about Urinary Tract Infections, Incontinence, Congenital Disorders, Kidney Stones, Cancers of the Urinary Tract and Kidneys, Kidney Failure, Dialysis, and Kidney Transplantation

Along with Statistical and Demographic Information, Reports on Current Research in Kidney and Urologic Health, a Summary of Commonly Used Diagnostic Tests, a Glossary of Related Terms, and a Directory of Resources for Additional Help and Information

Edited by Ivy L. Alexander. 649 pages. 2005. 978-0-7808-0750-1.

"A good choice for a consumer health information library or for a medical library needing information to refer to their patients."
— *American Reference Books Annual, 2006*

Vegetarian Sourcebook

Basic Consumer Health Information about Vegetarian Diets, Lifestyle, and Philosophy, Including Definitions of Vegetarianism and Veganism, Tips about Adopting Vegetarianism, Creating a Vegetarian Pantry, and Meeting Nutritional Needs of Vegetarians, with Facts Regarding Vegetarianism's Effect on Pregnant and Lactating Women, Children, Athletes, and Senior Citizens

Along with a Glossary of Commonly Used Vegetarian Terms and Resources for Additional Help and Information

Edited by Chad T. Kimball. 360 pages. 2002. 978-0-7808-0439-5.

"Organizes into one concise volume the answers to the most common questions concerning vegetarian diets and lifestyles. This title is recommended for public and secondary school libraries." — *E-Streams, Apr '03*

"Invaluable reference for public and school library collections alike." — *Library Bookwatch, Apr '03*

"The articles in this volume are easy to read and come from authoritative sources. The book does not necessarily support the vegetarian diet but instead provides the pros and cons of this important decision. The Vegetarian Sourcebook is recommended for public libraries and consumer health libraries."
— *American Reference Books Annual, 2003*

SEE ALSO *Diet & Nutrition Sourcebook*

■

Women's Health Concerns Sourcebook, 2nd Edition

Basic Consumer Health Information about the Medical and Mental Concerns of Women, Including Maintaining Health and Wellness, Gynecological Concerns, Breast Health, Sexuality and Reproductive Issues, Menopause, Cancer in Women, Leading Causes of Death and Disability among Women, Physical Concerns of Special Significance to Women, and Women's Mental and Emotional Health

Along with a Glossary of Related Terms and Directories of Resources for Additional Help and Information

Edited by Amy L. Sutton. 746 pages. 2004. 978-0-7808-0673-3.

"This is a useful reference book, which makes the reader knowledgeable about several issues that concern women's health. It is recommended for public libraries and home library collections." — *E-Streams, May '05*

"A useful addition to public and consumer health library collections."
— *American Reference Books Annual, 2005*

"A highly recommended title."
— *The Bookwatch, May '04*

"Handy compilation. There is an impressive range of diseases, devices, disorders, procedures, and other physical and emotional issues covered . . . well organized, illustrated, and indexed." — *Choice, Association of College & Research Libraries, Jan '98*

SEE ALSO *Breast Cancer Sourcebook, Cancer Sourcebook for Women, Healthy Heart Sourcebook for Women, Osteoporosis Sourcebook*

Workplace Health & Safety Sourcebook

Basic Consumer Health Information about Workplace Health and Safety, Including the Effect of Workplace Hazards on the Lungs, Skin, Heart, Ears, Eyes, Brain, Reproductive Organs, Musculoskeletal System, and Other Organs and Body Parts

Along with Information about Occupational Cancer, Personal Protective Equipment, Toxic and Hazardous Chemicals, Child Labor, Stress, and Workplace Violence

Edited by Chad T. Kimball. 626 pages. 2000. 978-0-7808-0231-5.

"As a reference for the general public, this would be useful in any library." —*E-Streams, Jun '01*

"Provides helpful information for primary care physicians and other caregivers interested in occupational medicine. . . . General readers; professionals." —*Choice, Association of College & Research Libraries, May '01*

"Recommended reference source." —*Booklist, American Library Association, Feb '01*

"Highly recommended." —*The Bookwatch, Jan '01*

Worldwide Health Sourcebook

Basic Information about Global Health Issues, Including Malnutrition, Reproductive Health, Disease Dispersion and Prevention, Emerging Diseases, Risky Health Behaviors, and the Leading Causes of Death

Along with Global Health Concerns for Children, Women, and the Elderly, Mental Health Issues, Research and Technology Advancements, and Economic, Environmental, and Political Health Implications, a Glossary, and a Resource Listing for Additional Help and Information

Edited by Joyce Brennfleck Shannon. 614 pages. 2001. 978-0-7808-0330-5.

"Named an Outstanding Academic Title." —*Choice, Association of College & Research Libraries, Jan '02*

"Yet another handy but also unique compilation in the extensive *Health Reference Series*, this is a useful work because many of the international publications reprinted or excerpted are not readily available. Highly recommended." —*Choice, Association of College & Research Libraries, Nov '01*

"Recommended reference source." —*Booklist, American Library Association, Oct '01*

SEE ALSO *Traveler's Health Sourcebook*

671

Teen Health Series

Helping Young Adults Understand, Manage, and Avoid Serious Illness

List price $65 per volume. **School and library price $58 per volume.**

Alcohol Information for Teens

Health Tips about Alcohol and Alcoholism

Including Facts about Underage Drinking, Preventing Teen Alcohol Use, Alcohol's Effects on the Brain and the Body, Alcohol Abuse Treatment, Help for Children of Alcoholics, and More

Edited by Joyce Brennfleck Shannon. 370 pages. 2005. 978-0-7808-0741-9.

"Boxed facts and tips add visual interest to the well-researched and clearly written text."
— *Curriculum Connection, Apr '06*

Allergy Information for Teens

Health Tips about Allergic Reactions Such as Anaphylaxis, Respiratory Problems, and Rashes

Including Facts about Identifying and Managing Allergies to Food, Pollen, Mold, Animals, Chemicals, Drugs, and Other Substances

Edited by Karen Bellenir. 410 pages. 2006. 978-0-7808-0799-0.

Asthma Information for Teens

Health Tips about Managing Asthma and Related Concerns

Including Facts about Asthma Causes, Triggers, Symptoms, Diagnosis, and Treatment

Edited by Karen Bellenir. 386 pages. 2005. 978-0-7808-0770-9.

"Highly recommended for medical libraries, public school libraries, and public libraries."
— *American Reference Books Annual, 2006*

"It is so clearly written and well organized that even hesitant readers will be able to find the facts they need, whether for reports or personal information. . . . A succinct but complete resource."
— *School Library Journal, Sep '05*

Body Information for Teens

Health Tips about Maintaining Well-Being for a Lifetime

Including Facts about the Development and Functioning of the Body's Systems, Organs, and Structures and the Health Impact of Lifestyle Choices

Edited by Sandra Augustyn Lawton. 458 pages. 2007. 978-0-7808-0443-2.

Cancer Information for Teens

Health Tips about Cancer Awareness, Prevention, Diagnosis, and Treatment

Including Facts about Frequently Occurring Cancers, Cancer Risk Factors, and Coping Strategies for Teens Fighting Cancer or Dealing with Cancer in Friends or Family Members

Edited by Wilma R. Caldwell. 428 pages. 2004. 978-0-7808-0678-8.

"Recommended for school libraries, or consumer libraries that see a lot of use by teens."
— *E-Streams, May '05*

"A valuable educational tool."
— *American Reference Books Annual, 2005*

"Young adults and their parents alike will find this new addition to the *Teen Health Series* an important reference to cancer in teens."
— *Children's Bookwatch, Feb '05*

Complementary and Alternative Medicine Information for Teens

Health Tips about Non-Traditional and Non-Western Medical Practices

Including Information about Acupuncture, Chiropractic Medicine, Dietary and Herbal Supplements, Hypnosis, Massage Therapy, Prayer and Spirituality, Reflexology, Yoga, and More

Edited by Sandra Augustyn Lawton. 405 pages. 2006. 978-0-7808-0966-6.

Diabetes Information for Teens

Health Tips about Managing Diabetes and Preventing Related Complications

Including Information about Insulin, Glucose Control, Healthy Eating, Physical Activity, and Learning to Live with Diabetes

Edited by Sandra Augustyn Lawton. 410 pages. 2006. 978-0-7808-0811-9.

Diet Information for Teens, 2nd Edition

Health Tips about Diet and Nutrition

Including Facts about Dietary Guidelines, Food Groups, Nutrients, Healthy Meals, Snacks, Weight Control, Medical Concerns Related to Diet, and More

Edited by Karen Bellenir. 432 pages. 2006. 978-0-7808-0820-1.

"Full of helpful insights and facts throughout the book. ... An excellent resource to be placed in public libraries or even in personal collections."
— *American Reference Books Annual, 2002*

"Recommended for middle and high school libraries and media centers as well as academic libraries that educate future teachers of teenagers. It is also a suitable addition to health science libraries that serve patrons who are interested in teen health promotion and education."
— *E-Streams, Oct '01*

"This comprehensive book would be beneficial to collections that need information about nutrition, dietary guidelines, meal planning, and weight control. ... This reference is so easy to use that its purchase is recommended."
— *The Book Report, Sep-Oct '01*

"This book is written in an easy to understand format describing issues that many teens face every day, and then provides thoughtful explanations so that teens can make informed decisions. This is an interesting book that provides important facts and information for today's teens."
— *Doody's Health Sciences Book Review Journal, Jul-Aug '01*

"A comprehensive compendium of diet and nutrition. The information is presented in a straightforward, plain-spoken manner. This title will be useful to those working on reports on a variety of topics, as well as to general readers concerned about their dietary health."
— *School Library Journal, Jun '01*

Drug Information for Teens, 2nd Edition

Health Tips about the Physical and Mental Effects of Substance Abuse

Including Information about Marijuana, Inhalants, Club Drugs, Stimulants, Hallucinogens, Opiates, Prescription and Over-the-Counter Drugs, Herbal Products, Tobacco, Alcohol, and More

Edited by Sandra Augustyn Lawton. 468 pages. 2006. 978-0-7808-0862-1.

"A clearly written resource for general readers and researchers alike."
— *School Library Journal*

"This book is well-balanced. ... a must for public and school libraries."
— *VOYA: Voice of Youth Advocates, Dec '03*

"The chapters are quick to make a connection to their teenage reading audience. The prose is straightforward and the book lends itself to spot reading. It should be useful both for practical information and for research, and it is suitable for public and school libraries."
— *American Reference Books Annual, 2003*

"Recommended reference source."
— *Booklist, American Library Association, Feb '03*

"This is an excellent resource for teens and their parents. Education about drugs and substances is key to discouraging teen drug abuse and this book provides this much needed information in a way that is interesting and factual."
— *Doody's Review Service, Dec '02*

Eating Disorders Information for Teens

Health Tips about Anorexia, Bulimia, Binge Eating, and Other Eating Disorders

Including Information on the Causes, Prevention, and Treatment of Eating Disorders, and Such Other Issues as Maintaining Healthy Eating and Exercise Habits

Edited by Sandra Augustyn Lawton. 337 pages. 2005. 978-0-7808-0783-9.

"An excellent resource for teens and those who work with them."
— *VOYA: Voice of Youth Advocates, Apr '06*

"A welcome addition to high school and undergraduate libraries." — *American Reference Books Annual, 2006*

"This book covers the topic in a lucid manner but delves deeper into every aspect of an eating disorder. A solid addition for any nonfiction or reference collection."
— *School Library Journal, Dec '05*

Fitness Information for Teens

Health Tips about Exercise, Physical Well-Being, and Health Maintenance

Including Facts about Aerobic and Anaerobic Conditioning, Stretching, Body Shape and Body Image, Sports Training, Nutrition, and Activities for Non-Athletes

Edited by Karen Bellenir. 425 pages. 2004. 978-0-7808-0679-5.

"Another excellent offering from Omnigraphics in their *Teen Health Series.* ... This book will be a great addition to any public, junior high, senior high, or secondary school library."
— *American Reference Books Annual, 2005*

Learning Disabilities Information for Teens

Health Tips about Academic Skills Disorders and Other Disabilities That Affect Learning

Including Information about Common Signs of Learning Disabilities, School Issues, Learning to Live with a Learning Disability, and Other Related Issues

Edited by Sandra Augustyn Lawton. 337 pages. 2005. 978-0-7808-0796-9.

"This book provides a wealth of information for any reader interested in the signs, causes, and consequences of learning disabilities, as well as related legal rights and educational interventions. . . . Public and academic libraries should want this title for both students and general readers."

— American Reference Books Annual, 2006

■

Mental Health Information for Teens, 2nd Edition

Health Tips about Mental Wellness and Mental Illness

Including Facts about Mental and Emotional Health, Depression and Other Mood Disorders, Anxiety Disorders, Behavior Disorders, Self-Injury, Psychosis, Schizophrenia, and More

Edited by Karen Bellenir. 400 pages. 2006. 978-0-7808-0863-8.

"In both language and approach, this user-friendly entry in the *Teen Health Series* is on target for teens needing information on mental health concerns."
— Booklist, American Library Association, Jan '02

"Readers will find the material accessible and informative, with the shaded notes, facts, and embedded glossary insets adding appropriately to the already interesting and succinct presentation."
— School Library Journal, Jan '02

"This title is highly recommended for any library that serves adolescents and parents/caregivers of adolescents."
— E-Streams, Jan '02

"Recommended for high school libraries and young adult collections in public libraries. Both health professionals and teenagers will find this book useful."
— American Reference Books Annual, 2002

"This is a nice book written to enlighten the society, primarily teenagers, about common teen mental health issues. It is highly recommended to teachers and parents as well as adolescents."
— Doody's Review Service, Dec '01

■

Sexual Health Information for Teens

Health Tips about Sexual Development, Human Reproduction, and Sexually Transmitted Diseases

Including Facts about Puberty, Reproductive Health, Chlamydia, Human Papillomavirus, Pelvic Inflammatory Disease, Herpes, AIDS, Contraception, Pregnancy, and More

Edited by Deborah A. Stanley. 391 pages. 2003. 978-0-7808-0445-6.

"This work should be included in all high school libraries and many larger public libraries. . . . highly recommended."
— American Reference Books Annual, 2004

"*Sexual Health* approaches its subject with appropriate seriousness and offers easily accessible advice and information."
— School Library Journal, Feb '04

Skin Health Information for Teens

Health Tips about Dermatological Concerns and Skin Cancer Risks

Including Facts about Acne, Warts, Hives, and Other Conditions and Lifestyle Choices, Such as Tanning, Tattooing, and Piercing, That Affect the Skin, Nails, Scalp, and Hair

Edited by Robert Aquinas McNally. 429 pages. 2003. 978-0-7808-0446-3.

"This volume, as with others in the series, will be a useful addition to school and public library collections."
— American Reference Books Annual, 2004

"There is no doubt that this reference tool is valuable."
— VOYA: Voice of Youth Advocates, Feb '04

"This volume serves as a one-stop source and should be a necessity for any health collection."
— Library Media Connection

■

Sports Injuries Information for Teens

Health Tips about Sports Injuries and Injury Protection

Including Facts about Specific Injuries, Emergency Treatment, Rehabilitation, Sports Safety, Competition Stress, Fitness, Sports Nutrition, Steroid Risks, and More

Edited by Joyce Brennfleck Shannon. 405 pages. 2003. 978-0-7808-0447-0.

"This work will be useful in the young adult collections of public libraries as well as high school libraries."
— American Reference Books Annual, 2004

■

Suicide Information for Teens

Health Tips about Suicide Causes and Prevention

Including Facts about Depression, Risk Factors, Getting Help, Survivor Support, and More

Edited by Joyce Brennfleck Shannon. 368 pages. 2005. 978-0-7808-0737-2.

■

Tobacco Information for Teens

Health Tips about the Hazards of Using Cigarettes, Smokeless Tobacco, and Other Nicotine Products

Including Facts about Nicotine Addiction, Immediate and Long-Term Health Effects of Tobacco Use, Related Cancers, Smoking Cessation, Tobacco Use Prevention, and Tobacco Use Statistics

Edited by Karen Bellenir. 440 pages. 2007. 978-0-7808-0976-5.

DATE DUE

SEP 2 0 2011		
NOV 2 9 2011		
GAYLORD		PRINTED IN U.S.A.

Health Reference Series